Transforming Voice and Communication with Transgender and Gender-Diverse People

AN EVIDENCE-BASED PROCESS

Transforming Voice and Communication with Transgender and Gender-Diverse People

AN EVIDENCE-BASED PROCESS

Adrienne B. Hancock, PhD, CCC-SLP
Linda L. Siegfriedt, MEd, CCC-SLP

PLURAL PUBLISHING INC.

PLURAL PUBLISHING
INC.

5521 Ruffin Road
San Diego, CA 92123

Email: information@pluralpublishing.com
Website: https://www.pluralpublishing.com

Typeset in 11/13 Garamond by Flanagan's Publishing Services, Inc.
Printed in the United States of America by Integrated Books International

Library of Congress Cataloging-in-Publication Data:
Names: Hancock, Adrienne B., author. | Siegfriedt, Linda, author.
Title: Transforming voice and communication with transgender and gender-diverse people : an evidence-based process / Adrienne B. Hancock, Linda Siegfriedt.
Description: San Diego : Plural Publishing, [2020] | Includes bibliographical references and index.
Identifiers: LCCN 2019017792| ISBN 9781635500899 (alk. paper) | ISBN 1635500893 (alk. paper)
Subjects: | MESH: Speech Therapy | Voice Training | Voice Quality | Communication | Transgender Persons | Case Reports
Classification: LCC RC423 | NLM WM 475.3 | DDC 616.85/500867--dc23
LC record available at https://lccn.loc.gov/2019017792

CONTENTS

PREFACE

This book is not about the larynx. It is about people in a transformation process. Clients who wish to transform their voice and communication navigate physical, mental, and emotional work. As a guide for this process, whether you are a speech-language pathologist or voice teacher, your role is to inform and facilitate transformation. We designed this book to help you do just that.

We share our knowledge and experience with the hope that you will understand our approach well enough to develop your own. Our evidence-based guidance for the practitioner is presented here in chronological progression, from personal and practical preparations through rationale and instructions for techniques and ending with troubleshooting and maintenance strategies.

The first section, "Start Smart," begins with a chapter about developing and monitoring the provider's self-awareness because we believe a mindful provider is crucial for the safety and success of the process. Information about the populations is provided next to develop the provider's cultural humility and sensitivity. This section closes with practical considerations for working with marginalized populations and ways to mitigate barriers to their accessing care. Real examples of inspirational colleagues demonstrate how this work can be done well with thoughtful planning.

When you are ready to "Press On" through the collaborative stage of this process with the client, the second section of the book will guide you through the best practice standards for gender-related voice and communication services. Assessment is tailored to the client's circumstances and needs, and extends beyond basic vocal function assessment. Intervention is presented in stages of "Ready, Set, Go" to highlight the importance of taking time to establish a collaborative, informed, and evidence-based plan ("Get Ready") and prepare the client's body and mind ("Get Set") before launching into direct voice work ("Go").

Endurance in this process must continue through the end to "Finish Strong." This final section acknowledges that the process involves unique challenges. Several real case examples illustrate how application of evidence-based strategies fosters completion of the client's program. Intentional planning for generalization and independence leads to an affirming send-off—although there are valuable ways to stay connected, too. Finally, the last chapter features personal reflections from people who have experienced transformations already.

This text is intended for an audience with basic knowledge of voice and communication mechanisms and clinical and/or instructional methods. However, because we routinely receive requests for information from providers at all levels of voice experience for more information and guidance about how to go about working with these populations, we have provided some fundamental information within each training area to be more inclusive to all providers called to do this work. We encourage students and new providers to refer to voice textbooks and references as needed to further develop more comfort and confidence in working with voice in general.

In our experience journeying alongside clients, we have found a world of possibilities we could not otherwise imagine. We are cisgender women and were surprised as anyone when we found ourselves together with a caseload of clients about which we knew very little. Since then, we have felt great satisfaction and sensed the importance of serving these populations, each within our own unique skill set and inspired desires. As gender-diverse people gain greater access to healthcare, information, and the right to choose their own path, all of us will be privileged to receive their talents and gifts.

ACKNOWLEDGMENTS

We are grateful to transgender and gender-diverse clients and research participants over the years; they are our best teachers and our motivation to educate and advocate for their benefit. We would especially like to thank Aeva, Ali, Dena, Grace, Lizzy, Morgan, Reana, and SJ for their trust and for sharing their deepest experiences with us. There are also many clinicians who forged a space for this practice in the field of speech-language pathology and the international community of transgender healthcare professionals, and we are particularly in awe of Richard Adler and Joan Regnell. We are grateful for the encouragement, support, and patience from our colleagues and students in the Department of Speech, Language, and Hearing Sciences at The George Washington University in Washington, D.C. We thank Julia Donovan and Stephanie Ferreira for their assistance preparing this book. Over a decade ago, students started us on this journey with gender-diverse people; today, students are still our hope for progress.

From Adrienne:
It is my privilege to contribute through teaching, research, and writing. I appreciate my mentors in this, including Dr. Leonard "Chick" LaPointe, who first taught me what a person-centered philosophy felt like, and Dr. Shelley Brundage, who has a talent for elevating both skill and spirit of others. I am grateful for Linda Siegfriedt, my collaborator in aims of work and life, whose attention to wholeness enriched this book as well as my experience. My deepest gratitude goes to the people who have allowed me to listen to or be a part of their transformation stories.

With love, I acknowledge and thank my husband Jeremy for his steadying support and grace, and precious Elizabeth for her focus on family fun. I appreciate my parents, Bob and Sue Blanchard, and family for making loving others be such a standard part of life. Finally, in all things, I acknowledge Jesus as my Lord and ultimate model for serving marginalized people.

From Linda:
I am grateful for the opportunity and privilege to contribute as a clinical provider, instructor, and coauthor. With appreciation, I acknowledge my clients whose strength and purpose have inspired me to listen with my soul and give with my heart. I am thankful for my coauthor and friend Adrienne Hancock who has been a joy and has shown me how to be a force in the expression of inner passion and dedication.

I would like to thank my parents Leo and Lucille Abdelahad and my siblings Sandy and Michael for their love and support, and my friends and relatives for their incredible enthusiasm, all of which gave momentum to the evolution of this book. In acknowledgment of her gracious presence and insight, I thank my dear friend Cathy Burgess. And most significantly, in recognition of his amazing light I thank my husband Klyde whose love and inspiring words supported me to express my truest self.

REVIEWERS

Plural Publishing, Inc. and the authors would like to thank the following reviewers for taking the time to provide their valuable feedback during the development process:

Eric R. Bronner, MM, MS, CMVT-MT, CSVW-III
Voice Faculty, Roger Williams University
Master Teacher, McClosky Institute of Voice
Voice Practitioner, Private Studio

Matthew L. Garrett, PhD
Associate Professor, Choral Music Education
Interim Director, University Center for Innovation in Teaching and Education
Case Western Reserve University

Tracy R. Grady, MM, BM
Voice Faculty, Baldwin Wallace University Conservatory of Music
Cofounder and Director, Cleveland Transgender Choir

Amy J. Hadley, EdD, CCC-SLP
Associate Professor
Communication Disorders
Stockton University

Grace Hao, PhD, CCC-SLP
Professor
Communication Disorders
North Carolina Central University

Wanda A. Kapaun, MS, CCC-SLP
Founder/Provider
Home Speech Therapy, PLLC

Ciara Leydon, PhD
Sacred Heart University
Blair Menn, MA, CCC-SLP
Kaiser Permanente Medical Center

Gwen L. Nolan, MS, CCC-SLP
Assistant Clinical Professor
Department of Communication Sciences and Disorders
University of Missouri

Loraine Sims, DMA
Associate Professor
Edith Killgore Kirkpatrick Professor of Voice
Louisiana State University

Wendy Vastine, BFA-Theatre, MA-SLP
Transformative Voice

Josie Zanfordino, MA, CCC-SLP
Say It Proud Speech Therapy

TERMINOLOGY USED IN THIS BOOK

Words matter. As more of society recognizes that, appropriateness of terminology changes frequently. This evolution of language is normal and healthy, but the current pace requires vigilance! We accept the responsibility to use words carefully so more people are made visible and protected. Consensus regarding terminology is increasingly difficult due to the variety of voices included in the space. People who use the same term may use it with slightly different meaning, particularly across cultures.

When choosing words for this book, we sought advice from members of the gender-diverse community, experts in gender production, and professional organizations. Yet, terms in this book may fall short of our intent to be both sensitive and clear. They will inevitably become outdated. Even our own recent research articles and presentations use terms that we would not choose today. You will notice some terms in this book, particularly those describing participants in research studies, are within quotation marks. This is intended to acknowledge that the term would perhaps not be the current choice, but nonetheless was used at that time to describe a particular group. Quotations marks maintain reporting accuracy in perpetuity. We did not feel comfortable, for instance, assuming that 14 people described in an article as "male-to-female transsexuals" would all be described as "trans feminine" today, or whenever our words will be read.

Words matter because people matter. Words can lift people up or tear people down. We trust that open dialogue—truly listening and responding with compassion—can alleviate division and fear seeded in words.

To the future, may it bring peace and unity.

PART I

Start Smart

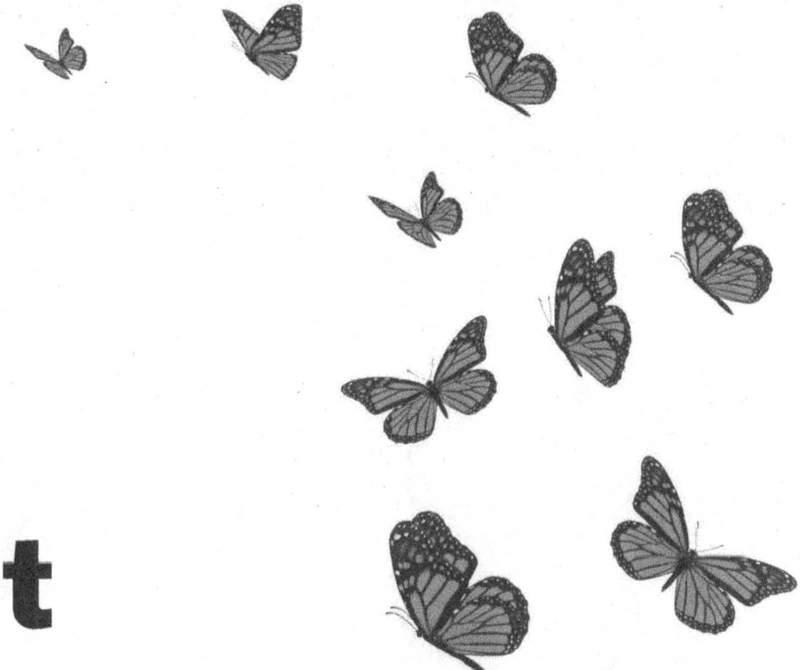

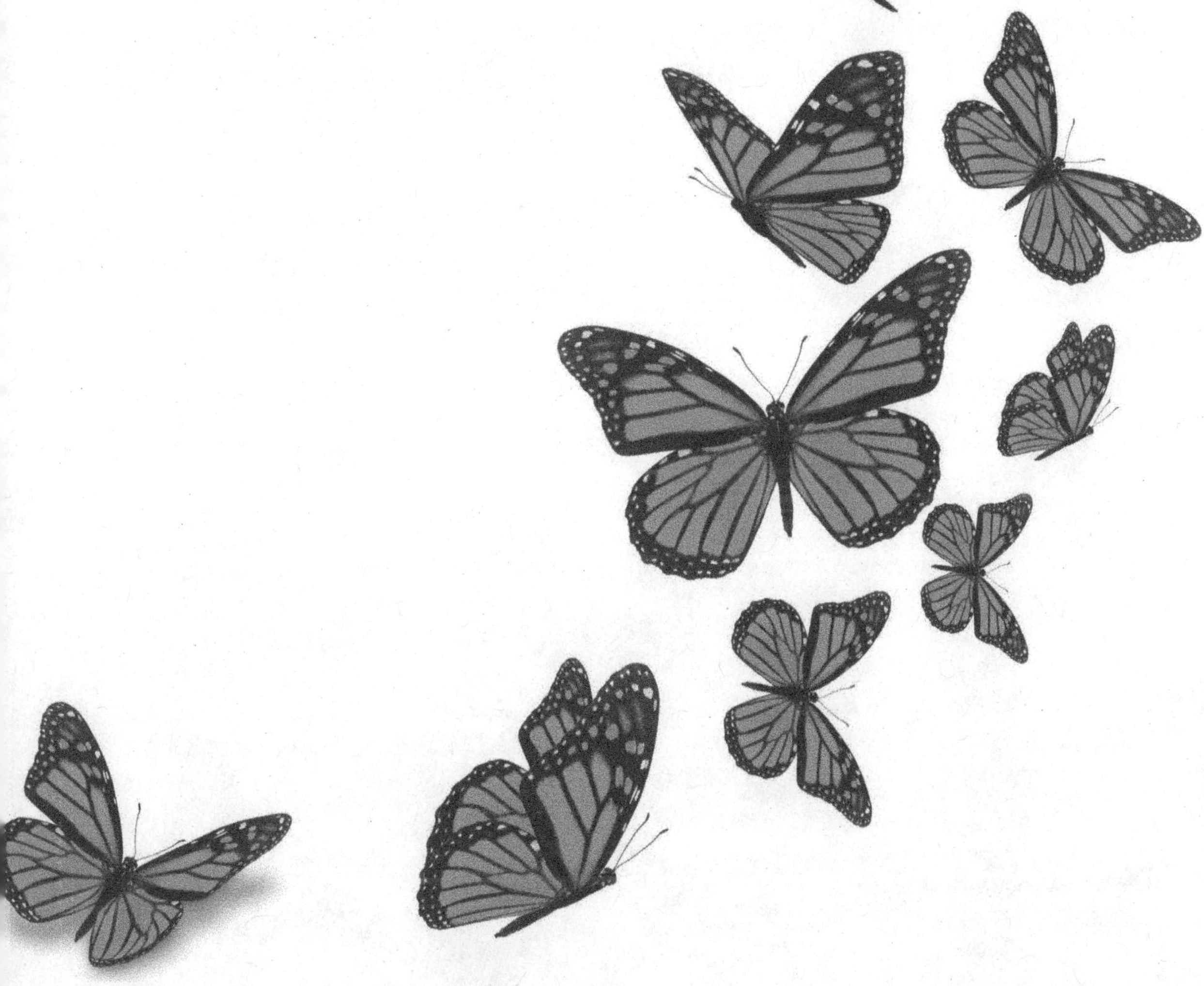

CHAPTER 1

The Mindful Provider

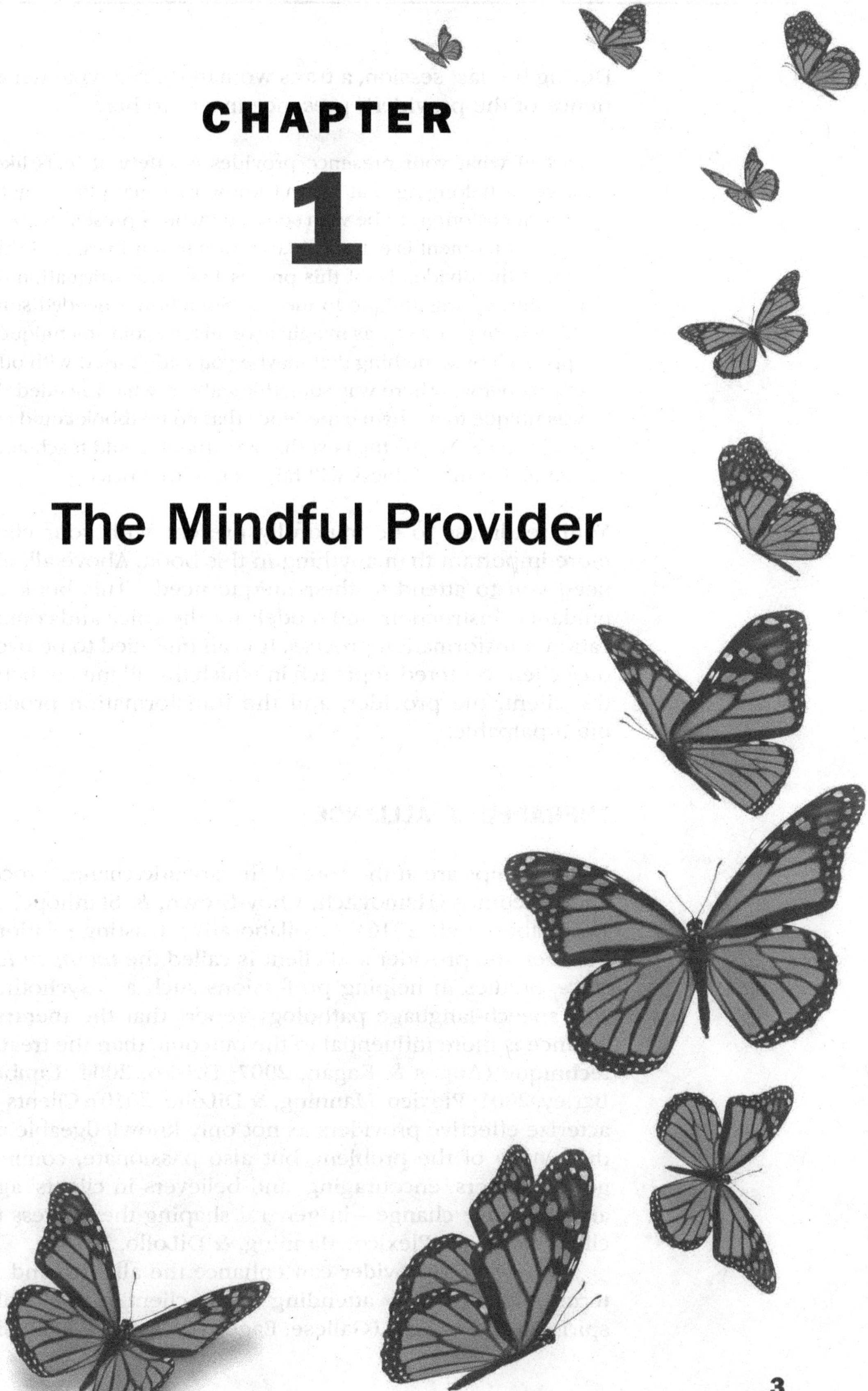

During her last session, a trans woman shared what her experience of the provider's presence meant to her:

> Part of what your presence provides is safety. It feels like a place of belonging that I don't know that many of us get to experience often. To be with someone who is present with you at every moment is extraordinarily rare in our lives. . . . I think one of the dividends [of this process] was the affirmation that my journey was unique to me. . . . Somehow I needed something from you that was imaginative, maybe some technique or approach or something that maybe you hadn't used with other clients before. There was something about what I needed that was unique to my own experience that no textbook could ever really teach. Maybe the best that a textbook could teach about that is that mindfulness will take you to that place.

Your readiness to be mindfully present with your client is more important than anything in this book. Above all, clients need you to attend to their unique needs. This book offers guidance, instruction, and models for the voice and communication transformation process. It is all intended to be overlaid on a client-centered approach in which the alignment between the client, the provider, and the transformation process is often palpable.

THERAPEUTIC ALLIANCE

Relationships are at the core of therapeutic change processes and outcomes (Hamovitch, Choy-Brown, & Stanhope, 2018; Kornhaber et al., 2016). A collaborative, trusting relationship between the provider and client is called the *therapeutic alliance.* Studies in helping professions such as psychotherapy and speech-language pathology report that the therapeutic alliance is more influential to the outcome than the treatment technique (Angus & Kagan, 2007; Drisko, 2004; Lambert & Barley, 2001; Plexico, Manning, & DiLollo, 2010). Clients characterize effective providers as not only knowledgeable about the nature of the problem, but also passionate, committed, good listeners, encouraging, and believers in clients' agency and cognitive change—in general shaping the process to be client centered (Plexico, Manning, & DiLollo, 2010).

One way a provider can enhance the alliance and long-term outcomes is by attending to the client's emotional and spiritual experiences (Gallese, Eagel, & Migrone, 2007; Siegal,

2010; Spillers, 2007). Understanding another's mind, specifically their intentions, expressions, emotions, and somatic sensations, can be challenging and complicated. Current models of interpersonal relationships indicate this is not simply taking another's perspective. Rather, it is a "mandatory, nonconscious, and prereflexive mechanism that is not the result of a deliberate and conscious cognitive effort aimed at interpreting the intentions hidden in the overt behavior of others" (Gallese, Eagel, & Migone, 2007). For example, a parent's empathy for their crying baby's distress elicits a response to comfort the baby, not to start crying like the baby (see Gallese, Eagel, & Migone, 2007 for discussion of the neuronal underpinning of interpersonal relations). *Therapeutic empathy* does not mean you feel exactly how the client feels or know exactly what they are thinking; it means your behavioral response to the client is appropriate because of your accurate perception of them in that moment (Angus & Kagan, 2007).

At the heart of therapeutic alliance and empathy is *attunement*: the provider's awareness of and responsiveness to the client's thought processes, emotions, behaviors, and experiences (Erskine, Moursund, & Trautmann, 1999). The unconscious perception and response to subtle cues is brought to the conscious level (Gallese et al., 2007). Providers can lean into the session to facilitate the next step in the clinical plan or lean back and allow the moment to direct the process. There are times to lean in and act, and there are times to lean back and allow. In this sense, there is an ebb and flow in each session (Marks-Tarlow, 2012). Attunement requires the practioner be:

- Fully present, focusing on what is happening in the moment,
- aware of their own internal process,
- aware of and sensitive to the client's process,
- involved in the relationship, and
- open to being moved and affected by the relationship.

All the knowledge and science in the world will not be applied effectively if we are not attuned to what is unfolding in each session. Attunement provides the art complement to our science, the music to the clinical dance (Marks-Tarlow, 2014; Risser, 2015). When we are attuned, we are receptive to what is happening in the moment. It is in this state that intuition is allowed to play a role and insights show themselves. When this happens, there is an impulse toward what needs to be said or done.

Clinical Intuition

A gut feeling. A heart wrench for someone else's emotional pain. An intangible knowing. A sensation of direction from a greater source. Have you experienced any of these? Intuition can manifest in a variety of ways, but it is fundamentally a source of knowledge (Vaughan, 1979; Marks-Tarlow, 2014). Many consider it a recognition (Simon, 1992; Kahneman & Klein, 2009). In a review of neurobiological underpinnings of intuition, Marks-Tarlow (2014) concludes that "the mind is embodied in the brain, though the brain is embedded in the body; and the embodied nature of clinical intuition is precisely how clinicians tune into nuance, variability, and the full complexity of relationship, as expressed moment to moment."

For the practioner, clinical intuition about the client or the process provides an additional source of information and clinical guidance (Bove & Rizzi, 2009). It is not common sense, but it may be considered one's clinical sense. Providers attuned to their clinical intuition realize that the effectiveness of evidence-based practice (EBP) models lies not just in the components of empirical evidence, clinical expertise, and patient needs, but also in the synergy among them. The ingredient of clinical intuition is what transforms good EBP into great EBP. The sections below will guide you to include intuition in client-centered care in a way that is effective and ethical.

If you have hesitations, you are not alone. We invite you to explore those hesitations as you keep reading. Decision-making literature in the helping professions acknowledges clinical intuition but debates its role and value in a professional capacity (Kahneman & Klein, 2009; Rogerson, Gottlieb, Handelsman, Knapp, & Younggren, 2011). Some scholars posit intuitive judgments arise from experience and subconscious attention to cues; people have been able to raise those cues to consciousness and develop some very effective interventions (e.g., Newborn Intensive Care Unit [NICU] nurses able to identify sepsis in babies before the medical tests can). In contrast, skeptical scholars have demonstrated that intuitive judgments are prone to systematic biases and are therefore made at the cognitive level. It is worthwhile to wonder when intuition can be trusted and explore the conditions that hone intuition as a skill.

In a paper comparing views of expert intuition, Kahneman and Klein (2009) describe points of agreement in the field of decision-making science. First, knowledge and experience are necessary for valid intuition, but not always enough. While a NICU nurse's intuition about a baby's health is better than that of someone who is not a NICU nurse, long-term forecasts of political events by experts are not more accurate than those made by untrained readers of newspapers (refer to Kahneman & Klein, 2009 for several examples from the research literature). Key differences in these scenarios are the predictability of the task and the opportunity for feedback (i.e., sick babies are more consistent than political events and their outcomes are known more quickly). Skilled intuitions will develop best for talented individuals in "an environment with sufficient regularity, which provides valid cues to the situation" (Kahneman & Klein, 2009, p. 520). An important corollary is that one's intuition is not inherent and static; rather, it is developed and improves.

Second, many people follow intuitions without checking them, either because it is difficult or because they simply do not bother. Experts are better at knowing when they don't know; nonexperts don't know what they don't know, and their overconfidence is potentially disastrous. Occasional accuracy reinforces an illusion of skill in these individuals. However, it is widely accepted that people use nonrational thinking and bias. We must be mindful of those processes to prevent them from clouding our interpretation of the intuitive moment; otherwise, we may be in a bias blind spot (Pronin & Kugler, 2007; Rogerson et al., 2011).

Third, one's intuition about some things may be better than their intuition about other things. This point may be particularly relevant for providers who have experience with patients who have voice disorders, but not with gender-diverse people electing voice modification. Do not overgeneralize your confidence in your clinical intuition to situations in which you have less expertise.

Challenges to understanding or using intuition in EBP will occur even in optimal circumstances. Balancing the potential benefits of intuition with clients' care and needs is an ethical responsibility, and practitioners should err on the side of safety (Rogerson et al., 2011). Concerns can be mitigated by developing skills to decide when and how to act on an intuition. Thus, ethical integration of intuition in our sessions includes not only noticing the nudge, but also intentional filtering and action. Several models of moral and ethical decisions include both an automatic intuitive level and a controlled critical evaluation level (Jeffrey, 2012; Kitchener, 1984).

The following sections are based on the six areas of the Clinical Intuition Exploration Guide, listed in Box 1–1 (Jeffrey, 2012). Due to the broad and individual nature of intuitive experiences, the areas are not intended to be prescriptive or

Box 1–1. Clinical Intuition Exploration Guide

1. Attunement: invite clinical intuition by being open and ready
2. Experience: heighten awareness of your clinical intuition
3. Interpretation: wonder what it could mean
4. Decision Making: consider what to do with it
5. Action: share your intuition with the client, or not
6. Evaluation: reflect and learn

(Jeffrey, 2012)

linear, but rather to provide a useful scaffold for responsibly incorporating clinical intuition during the client's transformation process. With experience, you will find some of these areas may become effortless or take less time for you. The first three relate to facilitating intuition and the last three to a meaningful analysis of it.

Step 1: Attunement

Attunement requires two levels of awareness (Jeffrey, 2012). First, a general clarity and understanding of one's self and role in the process. It is difficult to attend to others and correctly attribute intuitions when our own issues are unsettled. As intuitions may be experienced in a variety of ways, it is good to ready your mind, body, emotions, or any other part of yourself that may distract or detract from attunement. This preparation should not be considered an emptying, but rather an intentional tidying, calming, or slowing of one's self so that attention is available to clearly focus on another. The client-centered approach in this text cannot be facilitated by a clinician unable to attune to the client because of their own flustered state.

A popular and effective self-regulation strategy is meditation (Walsh & Shapiro, 2006). Active mind–body practices—those with multiple foci of attention such as meditation or yoga—can improve one's ability to regulate thoughts and emotions, enabling adaptive responses to stress both during the meditation that, when practiced regularly, carry over into daily life. Brain areas related to self-control, social cognition, language, and judgment (e.g., superior temporal lobe, medial prefrontal cortex) are uniquely related to active meditation styles (Acevedo, Pospos, & Lavretsky, 2016).

The second level of awareness required for attunement is a more focused sort of attention in day-to-day life, specifically focusing on the here and now. This is sometimes referred to as present-moment awareness, or mindfulness. Jon Kabat-Zinn (2016) says of mindfulness: "Mindfulness is awareness and means paying attention in a particular way; on purpose, in the present moment, and non-judgmentally." It is distinct from concentration-based approaches to meditation, such as transcendental meditation or mantras, which aim to sustain focus of attention on a single stimulus (Baer, 2003). Neural underpinnings of mindfulness practice, as opposed to active meditation styles such as yoga, include areas associated with sensory and emotional integration, self-control, body awareness, and movement (Acevedo, Pospos, & Lavretsky, 2016). Mindfulness helps us to shift from the automatic to the intentional, from problem solving to problem observing in-the-moment.

Below are a few simple approaches to these levels of attunement (i.e., general well-being through meditation and in-the-moment mindfulness) that we have successfully used with clients and students over many years. They can increase a generalized sense of well-being and satisfaction when integrated into a healthy lifestyle on a regular basis. Rituals and habits such as a good night sleep, eating well, regular exercise, implementing self-responsibility, and practicing kindness and gratitude also serve the process. The two approaches introduced below are fully described and expanded in Chapter 6 with scripts and instructions for incorporation into intervention. Box 1–2 lists apps that our clients have found to be helpful. Feel free to search the internet for a variety of approaches that suits your needs.

Box 1–2. Apps for Meditation and Mindfulness

- The Mindfulness App
- Headspace
- Calm
- Mindbody
- Buddhify
- Insight Timer
- Smiling Mind
- Meditation Timer Pro

Providers with their own meditation and mindfulness practice not only increase their ability to attune with others, but also can offer their personal experience to support clients through their own process (Siegal, 2010). If there is an approach below that appeals to you, try it for a few minutes each day for 6 to 8 weeks and re-evaluate your ability to become aware of yourself, the present moment, and your clients. Whichever approach resonates with you, remember that starting anything new requires time, patience, and compassion. It will not be long before greater awareness and more frequent experiences of attunement become a part of your life.

General Awareness and Meditation. Authenticity, the process of being genuine or real, is the result of our outer actions aligning with our inner selves instead of our past conditioning. If we, as providers, expect our clients to be able to observe and assess their authenticity in our training sessions, then we should be willing to do the same. Over time, daily meditation helps us identify our authentic selves and increase congruence between who we are and how we present ourselves to the world—a goal with parallels to our clients' journeys.

Meditation appears to have existed in the Hindu tradition since approximately 1500 years BCE (Before Common Era). Its major focus is to become observant of the workings of the mind. Sometimes, we allow the mind to run free and sort of drag us along, even if we do not like where it is going. Our thoughts have a big impact on how we see the world and on what we say and do. Many thoughts are created out of habituated patterns and memories from significant experiences and people in our lives, versus of our own choosing on a conscious level. Focusing our mind through meditation helps us become aware of these thoughts in a disciplined way. Walsh and Shapiro (2006) define meditation as "a family of self-regulation practices that focus on training attention and awareness in order to bring mental processes under greater voluntary control and thereby foster general mental well-being and development and/or specific capacities such as calm, clarity, and concentration" (p. 229).

The root word of meditation, *meditari*, is Latin, meaning "to reflect on, to study, and to practice." Importantly, meditation is a verb. Meditation is best approached as a process. Trying too hard or telling ourselves, for example, "I will stop my mind now," will pull us out of the present moment. Being suspended, if you will, in a process is what allows one to be receptive and attuned to the dynamics of each moment.

Before you start:

1. Sit in a comfortable position in a quiet space where you will not be disturbed or distracted.
2. Set a timer for few minutes the first time (5 minutes is fine) and gradually increase your time as it feels right to you.
3. Close your eyes and begin gently as you follow the instructions below.

You may notice your thoughts as they come and go. If thoughts come in, observe them as if they are clouds passing gently above on a clear day. It is not considered bad or good that thoughts come into your experience. You don't have to get rid of thoughts; you don't have to hold on to thoughts. Simply cultivate awareness without judgment as you follow the meditation process. It is helpful to acknowledge and accept all that comes to you as you practice meditation. Relax and just observe what you may sense during your experience.

Following the Breath. The basic process in this exercise is to allow your breathing to be natural as you pay attention to it. Here are the steps in detail:

1. Sit in a relaxed position and allow the breath to flow naturally through the nose.
2. Allow your attention follow all the little shifts that the breath makes along the journey of the breathing cycle in and out.
3. Notice how the body breathes for you without any effort or conscious thought on your part. Can you allow the body to take over?
4. Observe the airflow itself as it passes through the throat then back again. Note that the air passing through the nostrils may vary from left to right and cycle to cycle.
5. Can you sense the motion of the abdomen and the chest as the breath flows in and out?
6. Feel what is happening and how this feeling shifts.
7. If in the process you observe thoughts, simply notice that they are there and watch them pass. Then return to your breath.

Deep Breathing. The basic process in this exercise is to breathe through the nose slowly, taking the deepest breath in and letting it out slowly. Here are the steps:

1. Take in a breath as slowly and as deeply as you can until you reach the top of your breath cycle.
2. Pause at the top of the breath briefly, noticing the pause.
3. Then just as slowly release the breath all the way out.
4. Pause at the bottom of the breath briefly, observing the pause.
5. Repeat.
6. Notice everything about your body as it shifts from inhalation to exhalation:
   - ☐ The movement of the body.
   - ☐ The airflow itself as it passes through the body.
   - ☐ The air tracking through the nostrils may vary in motion and intensity.
   - ☐ Observe and investigate. Feel what is happening and how this feeling shifts.
7. Any thoughts that arise are simply there to be observed; when they pass, return to the breath once again.

Body Scan. With a light, gentle approach, slowly scan the body with curiosity (e.g., "I wonder how this is going to feel?").[1]

Starting at your feet: Feel the sensation of the bottoms and tops of your feet, your toes, and your heels. Then slowly move upward to your ankles, lower legs, and knees, feeling each part by part. Take your time. Feel slowly and deeply. You may feel a subtle sensation of tingling or a coolness or warmth. It may even change from part to part. Notice it all. At your own pace, move all the way up your body part by part to the top of your head.

Focus on feeling the body versus thinking about the body. If thoughts or judgments arise, which are automatic and habitual patterns, simply become aware and then move back to feeling the body. It is the act of returning to the sensations, paying attention with friendly curiosity, that is important. Feel each part for whatever the sensation is. There will be some parts that you may not feel, or they may be different each time you approach them; that is perfectly fine. Simply note, "How interesting, I cannot really feel my left arm right now," and continue through the rest of the body without any judgment that there is something wrong with your experience. It is in

---

[1]Scripts for guiding the Deep Breathing Meditation and the Body Scan Meditation are in Appendix 6–A.

the returning to the observation, watching, and the awareness that allows it to be an experience.

Yoga. Yoga is a mind–body practice with origins in ancient India. It has become a popular form of exercise for flexibility, strengthening, and coping with stress and tension. There are many practices available today in boutiques, health clubs, church basements, and outdoor spaces. It is accessible to many, though perhaps some bodies will require modifications to standard practices. Some clubs have a variety of levels ranging from students who are inactive to those used to more rigorous physical activity.

There are many benefits to yoga beyond physical strength and flexibility (Walsh & Shapiro, 2006). Yoga instructors guide participants to enhance the mind–body connection and to improve body awareness in the poses and the active flow of the breath. Their guidance through the class often includes the opportunity to become more alert and attentive to mental, emotional, and physical experiences that may otherwise be unnoticeable due to day-to-day distractions.

Present-Moment Awareness and Mindfulness. To explore how to bring the focused attention and present-moment awareness (i.e., mindfulness) experienced in your meditation practices into your clinical sessions, we will describe a few examples of how we can be mindful even in everyday moments. Some of the resources below are modified from Linda's mindfulness-based stress reduction (MBSR) training at the University of Massachusetts in Worcester, MA, and Vipassana meditation practice training at the Vipassana Meditation Center in Shelburne, MA, as well as personal experience in developing this process over many years working with a variety of people. In an empirical review, MBSR's effectiveness was superior to control groups in several studies (Baer, 2003).

Awareness of Breath. As you go through your day, follow your breath's motion. Notice how your body breathes for you. There is nothing to do. Feel your breath in your abdomen or chest, notice how it flows in and out of the nose and mouth. At various points throughout the day, become mindful of the breath.

- Every time you change an activity in daily rituals is an opportunity to check in and take a mindful breath. For instance, think, "I rise from sleep and breathe, take a shower and breathe, get dressed and breathe, have breakfast and breathe, get in my car and breathe."

- When driving, become aware of conscious breathing at stop signs and red lights, in traffic jams, and in parking lots.
- During hourly sessions at work, take a conscious breath at the start of each session, feeling the body's natural motion of the breath each time. Keep expanding the time that you are aware of your breath as your session progresses.
- When you teach your clients to breathe, refresh your own breathing too.
- If you feel distressed or distracted, simply use this as a cue to focus of the flow of your breath, and watch relaxation expand in your experience.

Awareness of Thought. Observe thoughts throughout the day. The purpose is not to crave no thought, but rather to be aware of whatever your experience is. Thoughts may be benign, such as "Oh, there I was just thinking about what happened yesterday with my daughter" or "I just noticed that I am thinking about how it will go when I meet my colleague today at lunch." Other thoughts may tempt you down a path of distracting self-analysis, daydreaming, or judgment, such as "I can't believe I ate that . . . it will show tomorrow . . . I wonder if anyone notices my stomach . . . I'll never be able to fit into . . ." Notice and let the thought pass without judging it. Some people imagine putting it on a shelf for later. In that moment you don't have to decide what, if anything, the thought means. This frees you to become more familiar with the experience of presence, which is what happens between your thoughts. With practice, mental distraction diminishes and we become more present and calm.

Awareness of the Emotions. The emotions that exist in all of us can range from fear, anger, and grief on one end of the spectrum to joy, compassion, and love on the other. We experience emotions in our bodies. These sensations are the basis of expressions such as "butterflies in my stomach" or "love in my heart." When positive emotions such as love or compassion arise, we can become more aware of them as we savor them in appreciation. However, when more unpleasant emotions arise, it can be quite disconcerting. It is not uncommon to find oneself eating, talking, or otherwise being distracted by the mental, emotional, or physical uneasiness of negative emotions. Noticing these behaviors is another way to become aware (e.g., "Am I eating because I am hungry, or because am I upset about something?").

When we quiet ourselves and stay aware of the arising emotions, letting ourselves feel them consciously, we may notice the sensations slowly release—similar to releasing the air of an inflated balloon. It takes about 90 seconds to experience the release of unpleasant emotions. Once the discomfort subsides, we often feel clearer, freer, and lighter.

Awareness of Your Body. During daily activities, notice where your body is in time and space and how its feeling can make you more aware of the moment. For example, during each stage of your day, stop and become aware and feel your body as you remind yourself that "I am here," "this is me," "I am connected to the earth," "I feel the water on my skin," "I feel the sunshine on my face," "I feel the air against my skin," "I feel my weight in the chair," "I feel my feet against the floor," and so on.

Using a body awareness approach redirects one's attention away from distracting thoughts to what is real in the moment. Here are a few exercises that can be done during simple daily activities:

- Walking: When walking, feel the connection of your feet to the floor or the ground if walking outside. Feel the way your arms swing, the way you shift your weight, and the way you alternate moving your legs. Notice the way your feet feel within the boundary of your shoes or how your gait changes when you come back to awareness. Everything subtly changes: our alignment, the evenness of pressure on the bottoms of our feet, the flow of our movements, and so on. During one of Linda's conscious walks, she discovered that the persistent pain in her hip suddenly stopped after a couple of minutes into the walk. When she went back to her work day, walking down the hallway, it came back. This seemed impossible, and she thought, "What could I be doing consciously that I was not doing the rest of the time?" She explored this on her next walk and found that when she was aware, there was greater comfort in her body. There seemed to be a connection between her mental activity (related to worry) and physical unease. When she walked consciously, she slowed down and found that she simply was more aligned and relaxed. Because her attention was on the experience of walking, there was less mental activity and stress. This appeared to leave her with greater sense of confidence and well-being.

- Sitting: When sitting at the computer or with a client, feel the weight of your body in the chair, resting against the back of the chair, with your feet against the floor. Note when you change position, cross your ankles or legs, shift your arms or hands, and take a breath. Feel the fabric of your clothing against your skin. Notice if your body is tired and wants to lean to one side or another. Observe the experience when you sit at work, versus sitting in your home, versus when you sit in the coffee shop. All of this can make you more aware and sensitive to what is going on in and around you.
- Eating: When Linda and her husband go to their special restaurant on their anniversary, they take their time. It is a total sensory experience for them, taking in the artistry of the chef's creation: the colors and designs of the foods dancing across the plate, the blending of aromas, the contrasting of textures, and the complementing of delicate flavors. They savor the experience and are highly aware. You do not have to go to a restaurant to have the same experience. When eating, really slow down and give yourself time to taste all the flavors, explore all the textures and temperatures, feel the fork in your hand as you pick up your food, and take in all the colors and aromas.

Over time with regular practice, we gain greater awareness in daily life of our emotions, our body, and our thoughts. The more open and ready we are in the present moment, the better able we are to attune to the client and experience intuition.

Step 2: Experience

If we have acknowledged and prepared ourselves for intuition to have a role in this process, we still need to heighten our sensitivity to our intuition, whatever form it may take for us. This may take time and experience. It could be easy to miss the intuition, or the opportunity to act on the intuition. Below is a recent example of when Linda noticed and used intuition in a treatment session at her university's clinic:

> Over the course of several sessions, the client showed up on time, did her homework, and appeared very grateful and motivated. It was clear that on a physical level, my student and I could elicit higher pitch, oral resonance, and a lowering of volume, yet there was no generalization from session to session. We shared these observations with her, adding that we felt that she had the physical potential to achieve her vocal goals but appeared uncomfortable about participating fully in certain aspects of the process. She had no comment and presented a blank expression. The potential benefit for psychological counseling was discussed.
>
> The student provider and I agreed that I would sit in on the next session. She would guide the client through the general relaxation, massage, and breathing components of the session (essentially what is described in Chapter 6) and I would then do the direct voice training portion (described in Chapter 7).
>
> I remember preparing to go into that session and had a few clinical, technically oriented ideas in my back pocket that I was going to try if it felt right. As I approached the room, I intentionally cleared my mind to focus my attention on the present moment. I was taking off the protective armor of having to be the one with the answers. Instead, I wanted to be attuned to the client and set myself up to be a receiver to be completely aware of and receptive to the process. I had no idea what to expect. There was only trust that being attuned would lead me in the best direction. I wanted to just let it happen. It has served me well. When you trust in this process, you will find yourself doing it more and more.
>
> I began by asking the client how she felt things were going. She paused and then said, "I found something I did with my voice over the weekend that seemed to help." I could feel the air in the room suddenly get very still. After listening to her additional comments, I stopped her and casually asked, "Could you show me what you did over the weekend with your voice that helped?" She nodded.
>
> Over the next 20 minutes, what unfolded was the shaping and generalization of a good target voice from her personally developed approach. It was the most productive that we had been with her the entire semester. There was nothing particularly

special about her approach, other than it was hers. This client was telling us that she was ready to change, and this was a way she could feel it was authentic.

I found out later that that the client had made the same statement to the graduate provider earlier in the same session, but as a new clinician she had been so focused on trying to do the training that she either missed or dismissed the cue. The student clinician learned, as we all continue to learn, that sometimes even our best plan and preparation may be insufficient.

Linda's experience was marked by a feeling of stillness in the air. She had prepared herself, in the moment and through years of practice doing so, to be open and willing to experience any intuition in the process. The moment came, and she was able to sense and respond quickly in this session. There may have been several ways to interpret and act—or not—on her awareness of that stillness in the air. In this case, asking the client to expand on an offhanded comment propelled the process out of a rut and back into an authentic experience for all. The other aspects of responsible use of intuition described below often happen quickly for her now after years of mindful clinical practice, but the effect depends on attunement to the client, the moment, and intuition.

Step 3: Interpretation

In the brief suspension between sensing the intuition and conscious response to it, explore the possible meanings and how they might relate to your or the client's life. As you are only a part of this process, you likely will not be able to know exactly what your intuitive feeling means, but this is a time to filter for the influence of your values, beliefs, and biases. The intuition may be for you rather than the client, or for later rather than now. Preparations to be attuned, such as through meditation or mindfulness practices presented above, pay off here. "Assessing the intersection of the self and one's professional role," as Jeffrey (2012) describes it, is critical in ethical practice and can—should—be done before, during, and after time with a client.

A strong therapeutic alliance is also helpful here, as the client may provide the insight as to why an otherwise meaningless act had an enormous impact on the transformation process. The following client provides such an insight about a simple touch given during a breathing exercise:

> "I would never have imagined in a million years how much emotion was involved in voice training. It is far more than I ever thought it would be. Far more. The lesson I learned is that you cannot disentangle being connected to yourself physically and emotionally. There was one important session where I learned this. We were working with my posture and my breath. I have this really distinct memory . . . you [the provider] just sort of put your hand on my back and my hand on my stomach and I just completely fell apart. That's when I started bawling."
>
> She continues, "I've had time to reflect on what was going on for me. Your touch triggered so much of that. I think part of it is that I have been deprived of it for so long, but part of it was the sense that my voice and my breath and my spirit all came from this common tender place that I couldn't find before. It was always there, right? I just had not ever been able to let those feelings come out before that day. How you knew what to do or say to make that happen, I do not know, I just sense that it was a part of the presence, the awareness of that moment in time. That moment changed me. It was there that my feelings were born."

The more mindful we are, the more we can sense what is going on for another person and intuit our next move in a session. Our intuition can show itself as an impulse to pause, touch a shoulder, or say something unexpected without knowing exactly why. They are often subtle enough to be of no risk to express to the client. It is not uncommon for these experiences to provide the exact perception the client needs to break through a barrier or issue within the session.

Step 4: Decision Making

Throughout the relationship, as real intuitions come to you, you will make decisions about the potential impact of the intuition. This is not just what the intuition means, but what it could mean for the process. Jeffrey (2012) recommends reflecting on the possible harm or benefit of sharing the intuition as a second ethics check (the first being whether one's self has colored the intuition or meaning ascribed to it). The sharing of the intuition should never be self-serving, but rather benefit the client. Ask yourself, "Who would this serve?" This is essentially the weighing of the "what ifs." Some examples:

- What if I told them about my discomfort with that word they keep using?

- What if I told them I think they should not do that?
- What if I urged them to feel this way about it?
- What if I suggested we go try it at this place?

Several sessions may pass as you toggle between interpreting meaning, considering impact, and weighing how to act. It may be helpful to discuss with a colleague or supervisor/mentor. Alternatively, some intuitions to say or do something can be acted upon instantly—either because of their benign nature or because a quick response is required (e.g., you suspect self-harming behavior). Even in these cases, subsequent evaluation of the decision can inform future intuitive experiences.

Step 5: Action

While the decision-making step is largely considering the "what ifs," the action step is about considering the "how to." Jeffrey (2012) points out that the intuitive moment can be honored whether it is shared with the client immediately, eventually, or not at all. If you decide to act, consider when the client would be most receptive to it, as well as how you would respond if it is not received well.

Keep in mind that dwelling in the critical-evaluative level of intuition can interfere with the power derived from a strong therapeutic alliance and attunement. Just as we don't recommend a purely gut-driven approach, we caution against a rigid program void of interpersonal connection and courage to be vulnerable with each other. Again, therapeutic alliance and attunement will steer this stage well. Here is an example of when Linda practiced attunement in a session:

> During one of my client's generalization sessions at a restaurant, the client expressed the concern that people were looking at her as she walked from the table to the restroom and back again. She shared that concern with me as she returned to our table saying, "I feel that everyone is looking at me and judging me. Like they know I'm transgender." An insight that she needed a new framework for how she saw herself came into my awareness as I looked at her, and I responded, "I wonder if you ever considered that they were looking at how beautiful you are with your striking dress, gorgeous long blond hair, and the way you carry yourself? Not a lot of people can do that!"

While my clinical agenda was to support the generalization of her voice in social and public communication contexts, my awareness told me that this was an important moment for her. I was attuned to the need for this client to see herself in a new way. It was not actually a thought in my mind at that time, but an impulse to respond with the words that I did. I did not know what I was going to say in advance. The client and I heard the words come out together. At the same time there was a "knowing" that the words were especially poignant for that client, at that specific time. They provided a mirror for her—showed her to herself through my eyes.

We have kept in touch since she completed her communication training and at almost a year later, she still tells me that comment changed her life. It reframed the experience for her and allowed her to alter the repetitive dialogue in her thinking and expand into a new possibility. She can feel good about the way she looks and sounds. She can feel proud of all that she has accomplished and gone through in her life now that she is free from the self-consciousness of her voice and of her physical self.

Step 6: Evaluation

Reflection on whether, how, and why an action stemming from an intuition was effective is a useful exercise. Recognize when it happens, appreciate it, and encourage yourself to continue responsible and effective use of intuition. Likewise, consideration of the times you or the client are not progressing can strengthen your skills and improve use of intuition in the future. Be assured there will be plenty of these learning opportunities! Below is Linda's reflection regarding one such experience:

I once had a client who was really struggling with voice training. She would tell me how hard it was every week. I kept thinking that I needed to do a better job so it wasn't so hard for her, so I would work harder at making it easier for her. It became stressful for me to see her.

I now wonder what could have happened if I had relaxed and was able to be more attuned to her in those moments. She was simply telling me about her struggle and how shockingly difficult she finds this work, particularly compared to the rest of her life, which always seemed to come easily to her. She just really needed me to get that. It had nothing at all to do with my work.

If I was more mindful at the time, perhaps I could have asked myself, "Am I really missing something here? Or is this client really struggling and just sharing her experience?" It could have changed the whole dynamic.

SUMMARY

Much of this book will inform the science aspect of our journey, but we have intentionally started by acknowledging the value of the therapeutic alliance as the complementary art. Development of skilled intuition expands our potential to provide client-centered care. When we practice the processes presented above, we can become more attuned—that is, aware and responsive—to our clients' needs.

Not surprisingly, it is also helpful if clients are aware and responsive in the present moment. We feel it is critical for our clients to begin intervention sessions by "getting set" themselves (as described in Chapter 6). Preconceived ideas, habits, and judgments about themselves and the clinical situation may need to be set aside so more of the natural transformation process can unfold. Yet clients cannot set aside what they do not know is there. Your awareness practice will help you guide your client in their own practice. This is yet another way that learning to incorporate both the art and science of this process leads to powerful voice and communication transformation.

REFERENCES

Acevedo, B. P., Pospos, S., & Lavretsky, H. (2016). The neural mechanisms of meditative practices: Novel approaches for healthy aging. *Current Behavioral Neuroscience Report*, *3*, 328–339.

Angus, L., & Kagan, F. (2007). Empathetic relational bonds and personal agency in psychotherapy: Implications for psychotherapy supervision, practice, and research. *Psychotherapy: Theory, Research, Practice, Training*, *44*(4), 371–377.

Baer, R. A. (2003) Mindfulness training as a clinical intervention: A conceptual and empirical review. *Clinical Psychology: Science and Practice*, *10*(2), 125–143.

Bove, S., & Rizzi, M. (2009). Listening to intuition: Reflections on unconscious processes in the therapeutic relationship. *Transactional Analysis Journal*, *39*, 39–45.

Erskine, R. G., Moursund, J. P., & Trautmann, R. L. (1999). *Beyond empathy: A therapy of contact-in-relationship*. London, UK: Taylor & Francis.

Gallese, V., Eagle, M. N., & Migone, P. (2007). Intentional attunement: Mirror neurons and the neural underpinnings of interpersonal relations. *Journal of American Psychoanalytic Association*, *55*(1), 131–176.

Hamovitch, E. K., Choy-Brown, M., & Stanhope, V. (2018). Person-centered care and the therapeutic alliance. *Community Mental Health Journal*, *54*, 951–958.

Jeffrey, A. (2012). The clinical intuition exploration guide: A decision-making tool for counsellors and supervisors. *Family Journal*, *20*(1), 37–44.

Kabat-Zinn, J. (2016). *Mindfulness for beginners: Reclaiming the present moment and your life*. Boulder, CO: Sounds True.

Kahneman, D., & Klein, G. (2009). Conditions for intuitive expertise. *American Psychologist*, *64*(6), 515–526.

Kitchener, K. (1984). Intuition, critical evaluation and ethical principles: The foundation for ethical decisions in counselling psychology. *Counselling Psychologist*, *12*(3), 43–55.

Marks-Tarlow, T. (2012). *Clinical intuition in psychotherapy: The neurobiology of embodied response*. New York, NY: W. W. Norton.

Marks-Tarlow, T. (2014). The interpersonal neurobiology of clinical intuition. *Smith College Studies in Social Work*, *84*(2-3), 219–236.

Price, A., Zulkosky, K., White, K., & Pretz, J. (2017). Accuracy of intuition in clinical decision-making among novice clinicians. *Journal of Advanced Nursing*, *73*(5), 1147–1157.

Pronin, E., & Kugler, M. B. (2007). Valuing thoughts, ignoring behavior: The introspection illusion as a source of the bias blind spot. *Journal of Experimental Social Psychology*, *43*, 565–578.

Risser, R. (2015). Balancing the art and science of the singing voice. *Perspectives on Voice and Voice Disorders*, *25*, 110–115.

Rogerson, M. D., Gottlieb, M. C., Handelsman, M. M., Knapp, S., & Younggren, J. (2011). Nonrational processes in ethical decision making. *American Psychologist*, *66*(7), 614–623.

Siegel, D. J. (2010). *The mindful therapist: A clinician's guide to mindsight and neural integration*. New York, NY: W. W. Norton.

Spillers, C. (2007). An existential framework for understanding the counseling needs of clients. *American Journal of Speech-Language Pathology*, *16*, 191–197.

Walsh, R., & Shapiro, S. L. (2006). The meeting of meditative disciplines and western psychology: A mutually enriching dialogue. *American Psychologist*, *61*(3), 227–239.

CHAPTER 2

Cultural Considerations

"The rainbow is a division of white light into many beautiful colors."

Speech-language pathologists (SLPs) will recognize this definition of a rainbow from a standard reading passage used in assessment of speech (Fairbanks, 1960). The rainbow provides a convenient illustration for considering the cultural aspects of gender identity, presentation, and attribution. From this technical definition of the rainbow, we learn that a source's majesty can be realized by observing its many beautiful parts. So it is with humanity. Variation in gender expression affords a view of humanity's majesty. Just as with understanding sexual attraction as only gay or straight, to view gender as only male or female is to be color-blind when looking at a rainbow.

We must seek to recognize and include all variations of humanity. Some racial equity initiatives promote a "color-blind" approach, intending to remove the barriers of bias against people of color. This likely is well-intended, but it homogenizes and dismisses rich cultural variations in humanity. Similarly, when we call for a transgender person to be treated "like a cisgender person," we implicitly suggest that whatever is different about a trans person should be ignored, reduced, or even eliminated, as though the difference is either invalid or unbearable. Instead, we can call for practices that include all, regardless of gender identity. A simple example is the use of forms that provide a fill-in line for gender rather than a male or female checkbox. The difference may seem subtle, unless you are in a minority group and know how it is to always be measured and treated by standards designed for the majority. More of these inclusive practices will be presented in Chapter 3.

When Adrienne was in preschool, she learned the ROYGBIV acronym for the colors of the rainbow, including indigo between blue and violet. When she went to a new school and started kindergarten, she was surprised there was no mention of indigo when we were given construction paper to make rainbow mobiles. She knew about indigo. She knew there was nothing wrong with indigo and that, in fact, her rainbow would be inaccurate without it. She asked for indigo paper. Even though her accuracy was acknowledged by science and the teachers themselves, she was only given reasons to make do with the colors presently available. Then paper rainbows were hung from the ceiling and indigo was represented nowhere.

Learning about and including indigo in the rainbow art project would have improved the accuracy as well as aesthetic of the classroom. Imagine what learning about and including LGBTQ communities can do for our society. Crucial to the premise of this chapter is the following principle learned in kindergarten: The rainbow is a division of white light into many beautiful colors, even more than are typically represented.

CULTURAL HUMILITY

Merriam-Webster's 2014 word of the year was *culture*. The word with the biggest spike in lookups during 2014, culture is increasingly used to encompass many elements of a particular group and may be applied in a broad (e.g., American culture) or narrow (e.g., corporate cultures) sense. One might expect to find the definition of culture to include the knowledge, beliefs, values, customs, and arts of a particular society, group, place, or time. Merriam-Webster includes those in the definition, but the first four definitions are of a slightly different nature:

1. Cultivation, tillage.
2. The act of developing the intellectual and moral faculties, especially by education.
3. Expert care and training.
4. (a) enlightenment and excellence of taste acquired by intellectual and aesthetic training; (b) acquaintance with and taste in fine arts, humanities, and broad aspects of science as distinguished from vocational and technical skills; a person of culture.

Using every sense of the word, then, we invite you to culture yourself in the culture of others. Your personal cultivation might begin with an honest self-assessment of your knowledge and attitudes about a population's cultures and subcultures, but should continue by considering your skill for applying that information to shape your behavior and cultivate a practice of inclusive care for your clients. Chapters 2 and 3 are designed to help you do just that.

Although cultural competency was initially conceptualized as a measurable milestone and end product of education, most recent models of cultural competency present it as a process continually developing with education, training, and experience. See National Center for Cultural Competence at Georgetown University (2019) for a variety of definitions, and note the evolution of the term's usage since 1989. *Cultural competency* is typically thought of as a skill set that allows a clinician to learn and integrate a client's cultural aspects in a particular setting. In other words, one does not become competent with a culture; one becomes competent in learning about a culture and using it to enhance interactions. Cultures and their influence are dynamic. In this sense, a professional's level of cultural competency is unique to each client interaction. This is clear in the definition of cultural competency offered by the Centers for Disease Control and Prevention, which focuses on the capacity to function effectively within the context of a culture (National Prevention Information Network, 2015). Professional cultural competence is described by the American Speech-Language-Hearing Association (ASHA, 2019) as "understanding and appropriately responding to the unique combination of cultural variables that the professional and client/patient bring to interactions."

Some experts extend the goal beyond tolerant, nondiscriminatory attitudes and behaviors and insist a culturally competent professional should recognize and dismantle systematic privilege and marginalization (Kumas-Tan, Beagan, Loppie, MacLeod, & Frank, 2007). *Cultural humility* is proposed as a term preferable to cultural competency because it implies adoption of an attitude that acknowledges and encourages a lifelong process of learning how one's own self affects the care they provide (Tervalon & Murray-Garcia, 1998). Viewing culture as a fluid and dynamic construct of several aspects coming together uniquely in an individual, cultural humility is consistent with a person-centered approach to care. Whereas cultural competence models can be seen as reinforcing stereotypes and "othering" minorities by highlighting their differences from the majority cultures, a posture of cultural humility promotes respect for all, recognition and minimization of power differences through explicit recognition of biases, and ongoing self-reflection (Yeager & Bauer-Wu, 2014).

Culturally-appropriate, inclusive care is deserved and increasingly required in professional standards. The American Speech-Language-Hearing Association (2016) Principles of Ethics IC states, "Individuals shall not discriminate in the delivery of professional services or in the conduct of research and scholarly activities on the basis of race, ethnicity, sex, gender identity/gender expression, sexual orientation, age, religion, national origin, disability, culture, language, or dialect."

This chapter is designed to equip and prime providers to consider gender-related cultural issues as a component of excellent care. As do most models of cultural competency in health fields, we begin with information about these marginalized populations to influence clinician's attitudes and motivate skill building. We acknowledge that though some terms, practices, and understandings about gender are widely adopted, there are people for which those terms are inadequate at best and hurtful at worst. The terms used throughout this book were carefully considered and selected for clarity and sensitivity and based on best practice at the time of publication. The book was also reviewed by people of minority gender identities for their guidance.

The following information is offered as a foundational starting point for the professional dedicated to providing culturally appropriate services. Readers are encouraged to explore additional resources now and periodically through the future, particularly resources written by members of the communities we aim to serve (see Appendix 2–A). Make a plan to keep yourself updated, such as by subscribing to Google alerts for relevant topics or following LGBTQ health organizations on social media (Margolies, Joo, & McDavid, n.d.).

CORE CONCEPTS

Populations

Most babies are assigned female at birth (AFAB) or assigned male at birth (AMAB), according to the doctor's judgment of physical characteristics observable at birth. Disorders of sex development (DSD), commonly known as intersex conditions, occur when reproductive or sexual anatomy "doesn't seem to fit the typical definitions of female or male" (Intersex Society of North America, 2019); these conditions may not be identified until puberty, fertility assessments, autopsy, or ever. Estimates for number of people whose bodies differ from standard male or female are as high as 1 in 100 births, with 1 or 2 in 1,000 babies receiving surgery to "normalize" genital appearance (Blackless et al., 2000). Prevalence can vary according to attributed cause; approximately 1 in 3,000 people are born with only one X chromosome (i.e., Turner syndrome), while 1 in 600 are born with XXY chromosome (i.e., Klinefelter syndrome) and 1 in 1,000 with XYY (Hook & Warburton, 1983; Nielsen & Wohlert, 1990; World Health Organization [WHO], 2018).

Although traditionally any presence of a Y chromosome indicates male sex, biological scientists are increasingly recognizing the inaccuracy of that definition. A 2015 feature in *Nature* explains why the biological boundary between binary sexes is quite blurry, even in utero. Sex determination involves more than 20 genes. For example, gene mutations can result in a person with XY chromosomes having a typical cisgender female body or atypical or rudimentary gonads; people with XX chromosomes can develop physical features thought of as male if certain hormones are present, or if they also carry the SRY gene (Ainsworth, 2015). Conditions such as Complete Androgen Insensitivity Syndrome (CAIS), when people have Y chromosomes and internal testes but female external genitalia, or Congenital Adrenal Hyperplasia (CAH), which causes XX individuals to have high amounts of male sex hormones and therefore ambiguous genitalia at birth, are increasingly studied and further examples of the complexity of sex even from the biological perspective. The WHO (2015) sums it up this way: "there are not only females who are XX and males who are XY, but rather, there is a range of chromosome complements, hormone balances, and phenotypic variations that determine sex." Science, like the prism in the opening quote of this chapter, is helping to reveal the many beautiful colors of biological sex and challenge the binary conception of gender.

Increased recognition of variation in sex is valuable for destabilizing structural biases of a binary system that lead to discrimination of those outside the binary. Still, sex is distinct from gender. It should not be assumed that trans or nonbinary people have a DSD, or that cisgender people do not. For example, in a study of 14 women with CAIS, all expressed satisfaction with psychosexual development and having been raised as female; none desired gender reassignment (Wisniewski, 2000). As such, "Gender dissatisfaction occurs more frequently in individuals with DSD than in the general population but is difficult to predict from karyotype, prenatal androgen exposure, degree of genital virilization, or assigned gender" (Lee, Houk, Ahmed, & Hughes, 2006, p. e489). For more information on DSD diagnostic practice standards and statistics on gender identity outcome, see the statement from the International Consensus Conference on Intersex by Lee et al. (2006).

Terminology

Social organization and adoption of customs based on biological sex creates conceptions of gender. Debate over whether gender is based in nature or nurture is ongoing, but it seems to be a bit of both (for more information on this topic see Ainsworth, 2015; Lee et al., 2006; Roughgarden, 2009; WHO, 2018). Comparison studies of brain anatomy, genetics, and hormone exposure pre- and postnatally support some degree of organic, biologic basis for gender identity, but a causal mechanism—or more likely mechanisms—of gender identity remain unclear (see summaries by Saraswat, Weinand, & Safer, 2015; Winter et al., 2016). What is clear, though, is that at a young age, perhaps three or four years, children are aware of their own gender (i.e., *gender identity, subjective gender position*) and begin to understand it in context of the culture of gender around them. Children quickly become aware of gender norms in their culture, including associations between gender and appearance, social and familial roles, occupations, and interests. *Gender role* refers to behaviors that the population considers characteristic of one gender. A girl who is a "tomboy," for example, is said to have a male gender role because she has interests culturally atypical for her gender identity group, but she does not have a self-representation of a gender inconsistent with her sex assigned at birth.

The position that gender is not exclusively biologically determined, but rather interactive and constructed by the conversation partners and influenced by their cultures, is increasingly supported by science and accepted in some societies (Bucholtz & Hall, 2005; Butler, 1993, 1999; Lee, et al., 2006; West & Zimmerman, 1987). Two concepts related to this constructionist perspective are relevant for a profession about communication: gender presentation and gender attribution. *Gender presentation* is related to how one communicates their gender identity through physical appearance, voice, or other behaviors. *Gender attribution* is how a person is perceived and classified as belonging to a gender group. Self-attribution and attribution by others are typically observed through forms of address and referral (i.e., pronouns). Misgendering occurs when there is incongruence between any of these gender constructs (i.e., one's gender identity, desired gender presentation, desired self-attribution, or desired gender attribution by others).

One's *sexual orientation* is less about their own sex and gender than whom they are sexually attracted toward. At least three constructs can be used to indicate sexual orientation: behavior, attraction, and identity (Mayer et al., 2008). *Gay* and *straight* are considered to be more colloquial synonyms of *homosexual* and *heterosexual*, respectively, but terminology can be influential. An experiment embedded in the 2012 American National Election Survey found that ballots using the term *homosexual* in place of *gay* were associated with lower levels of support for LGBT rights, particularly in some social groups and personality styles (Smith, Murib, Motta, Callaghan, & Theys, 2018). Regardless, the common adjectives *gay* or *homosexual* (attraction toward a person of the same gender), *straight* or *heterosexual* (attraction toward a person of the opposite gender), and *bisexual* (attraction toward a person of the same or opposite gender) are problematic, especially for transgender and gender nonconforming people, for two reasons. First, they describe the correspondence of gender between two people, so when one person's gender is hidden, fluid, or changing, the accuracy of the term is in question. It is misleading to suggest a trans man who has always been attracted to females changed his sexual orientation when he transitioned his gender presentation to male. Second, the terms assume a binary gender organization and thus exclude people with a nonbinary gender positioning. The current solution is to simply state the nature of attraction. One is "sexually attracted to women," "sexually attracted to all genders," and so on.

The sexual orientation of your client is likely irrelevant to the plan of care, except as it relates to the clinician building rapport and being culturally sensitive enough to avoid assumptions. For example, referring to a client's wife when he has a husband. These *heteronormative assumptions* create barriers to excellent care for members of the larger LGBT community. In a survey of 192 patients with a communication impairment identifying as LGBT, the majority did not disclose their LGBT membership because they feared being "perceived or treated negatively by their clinicians," yet they felt it would be important to disclose so their partners could be included in the process. Most people perceived their audiologist or SLP to have a "bias toward a heterosexual orientation," most often perceived from case history and intake forms (Kelly & Robinson, 2011, p. 89).

Terminology changes and expands, and the speed of change is increasing with the use of social media. *Queer* was once a derogatory term but in the 1990s was reclaimed as a self-description for people opposing heterosexual social norms, whether they were transgender or not (Stryker, 2017). To learn more about current terminology and labels from members of the LGBTQ community, see videos by the Honest Accomplice Theatre Group's (2019) "The Trans Literacy Project," available online (http://honestaccomplice.org/the-trans-literacy-project/). The Human Rights Campaign (HRC) and the American Psychological Association (APA) and other resources in Appendix 2–A are also trustworthy sources for current terminology, though it is important to recognize that:

> Some words referring to practices or identities that are termed "transgender" . . . are culturally or ethnically specific, such as the hijra in India, the Polynesian mahu, South American travesti, or Native American "two-spirit." The seemingly inexhaustible global catalog of specialized terms for gender variety shows how impossible it really is to group such a wide range of phenomena together under the single term "transgender" without keeping that word's definition very flexible and without paying close attention to who is using it to refer to whom, and for what reasons. (Stryker, 2008, p. 23)

Thus, it is important to routinely evaluate the terminology you use and always ask the client their preferences.

Operational Definitions

Complexity and variety of identities creating subgroups within an already small population pose challenges for social and scientific processes that require operational definitions to measure and serve these populations (National Academies Press, 2011). For example, until very recently, trans populations were described using a variation of the typical binary: male-to-female or female-to-male. Yet, there is growing concern that ignoring the variation is inaccurate and problematic. The U.S. Institute of Medicine Committee on LGBT Health Issues and Research Gaps and Opportunities (National Academies Press, 2011) lamented the underreporting and false positives resulting from studies asking participants to simply self-identify as "transgender"; the term may not be uniformly understood and is not used by all gender-diverse people. Beyond the perpetuation of marginalizing minorities, there is also the issue of evidence-based practice. If participants in empirical studies of interventions are not described precisely enough for the reader to determine the internal and external validity of the results, any application to individual clients must be guarded.

Since visibility of variation in gender identity has increased, more research studies have included multiple options for self-identification, or even fillable spaces (Conron, Scout, & Austin, 2008). A common recommendation is the two-step identification process, in which the participant is asked, separately, the sex they were assigned at birth and their current gender identity. Cross-reference of these two variables are used to classify respondents' gender classification. The Gender Identity in U.S. Surveillance Group that published best practices for asking questions on surveys dedicated a chapter to further special considerations for adolescents, race/ethnicity, socioeconomic status, and intersex status (Greytak et al., 2014), yet research on the applicability of standard practices for people who are not "white, young, college-educated, native-born United States [citizens]" is still limited (Bauer, Braimoh, Scheim, & Dharma, 2017, p. 4). One analysis of multiple-step approaches used in two popular American and Canadian surveys concluded with recommendation to alter the answer options for gender identity to four: male, female, indigenous or other cultural gender minority identity (e.g., two-spirit), and something else, and to add a third question about the gender currently lived in day-to-day life (Bauer et al., 2017). Although most of the published recommended practices are developed for research purposes, they are useful for clinical documentation as well. More about this will be covered in Chapter 4 when we present the assessment process.

Diversity

Gender Identity

The position of the World Professional Association of Transgender Health (WPATH) is that "the expression of gender characteristics, including identities, that are not stereotypically associated with one's assigned sex at birth is a common and culturally-diverse human phenomenon [that] should not be judged as inherently pathological or negative" (WPATH Board of Directors, 2010). However, stress of stigma and discrimination resulting from minority gender identities and characteristics can result in mental health concerns and psychological distress. This position was also adopted in the *Diagnostic and Statistical Manual of Mental Disorders* (5th ed., *DSM-5*), which replaced "Gender Identity Disorder" with "Gender Dysphoria." *Gender dysphoria* refers to discomfort or distress caused by a discrepancy between a person's gender identity and that person's sex assigned at birth, whereas *gender nonconformity* refers to a difference from the cultural gender norms and is a matter of diversity (WPATH, 2011, p. 5). As the term *gender nonconforming* has fallen out of favor for highlighting what people are *not* rather than what they *are*, gender-diverse terminology is gaining traction in popular and scientific outlets (APA, 2015).

When a person's gender identity is congruent with the sex assigned at birth, they are considered *cisgender* (Figure 2–1). If their gender identity is incongruent with the sex assigned at birth, they are considered *transgender.*[1] *Cis* is Latin for "same side of"; *trans* is Latin for "other side of." *Transfeminine* people were AMAB but do not identify as male; *transmasculine* people were AFAB but do not identify as female. A shortened term (e.g., trans female or trans woman) is sometimes used to distinguish between cis and trans people, though it should be noted that not all trans people would classify themselves trans because they may be nonbinary or may not like any modifier used with their gender identity.

Some people do not identify or position themselves in one of these binary categories of gender at all and view gender as nonbinary, or more of a continuum with unbound degrees

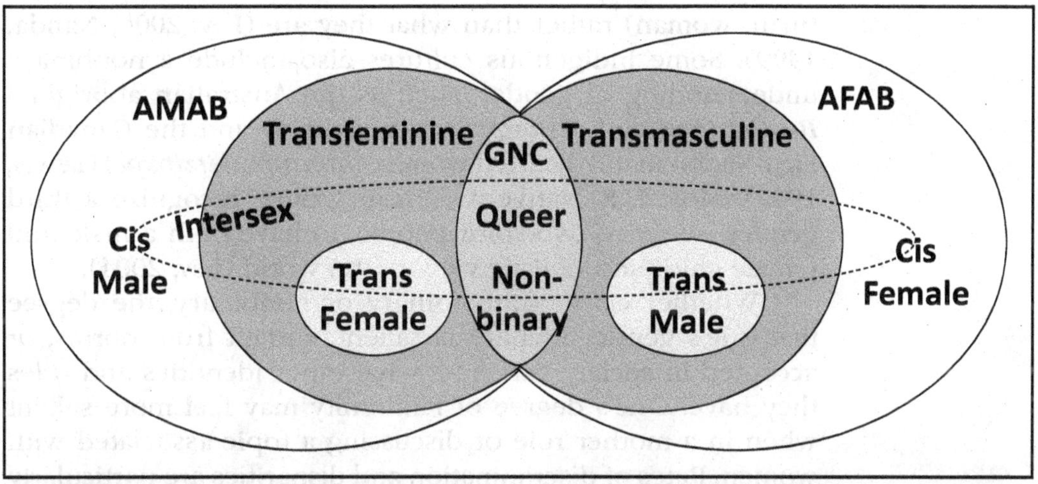

Figure 2–1. Relationships of the terms commonly used to describe gender positioning. AMAB = assigned male at birth, AFAB = assigned female at birth. Source: Hancock, A., and Azul, D. (2017). *Cultural and clinical considerations for EBP with transgender and gender non-conforming people* [ASHA Presentation]. Los Angeles, CA.

[1]Some professional health organizations use a broader definition of the term *transgender* to include any variance from cultural gender norms, such as cross-dressing, regardless of gender identity. The term *transsexual* has been defined more narrowly to specify the person's desire to change their physical body and/or presentation to align with norms for another gender. Perhaps because of mainstream public's confusion of gender and sexuality, the term *transsexual* is less frequently used now.

of variation. Rather than identify as cisgender or transgender, these people may identify as nonbinary, gender nonconforming, gender-variant, gender-fluid, genderqueer, or another term they find fitting. In one study of interviews with 14 German transmasculine people, the diversity of subjective gender positions was apparent when six different terms were used: male, nonbinary, queer male, agender, bigender, ambivalent/changeable (Azul, 2016). Furthermore, in Western culture, *female* and *male* are more often used in a biomedical sense, whereas *woman* and *man* are common in social sciences.

Although gender norms commonly follow sex as either male or female, some cultures acknowledge variations. Evidence that the Hindu Indian culture acknowledges and incorporates the notion of gender diversity are the *hijra* people of India. Typically intersex or castrated people AMAB, hijra do not identify as male nor female so are seen as a separate third gender (Lev, 2004). Although Indian cultures have established roles for hijra—even esteemed roles in the cases of association with deities or figures of Hinduism—self-descriptions of their gender identities are still often about what they are not (man, woman) rather than what they are (Lev, 2004; Nanda, 1999). Some indigenous cultures also include a nonbinary understanding of gender, such as the Australian aboriginal *Brotherboys* and *Sistergirls* (Kerry, 2014) and the Canadian First Nation manly-hearted women (*ninauposkitzipxpe*) (Lewis, 1941). Most U.S. Native American groups recognize a third gender category, two-spirit people, to have both a male and female spirit and holistic view of the world (Lev, 2004).

Whether cis or trans, binary or nonbinary, the degree that one's gender identity is salient, variant from norms, or accepted in society varies by what other identities and roles they have. One's degree of femininity may feel more salient when in a mother role or discussing a topic associated with women. Rates of discrimination and disparities are particularly high for people with identities in the intersection of multiple minority or marginalized groups (Kattari, Walls, Whitfield, & Langenderfer, 2017). Reports of harassment, discrimination, and victimization vary by age, with people less than 35 years of age reporting the highest rates (Kattari & Hasche, 2016). In the National Transgender Discrimination Survey, the average statistic of white trans respondents is almost always better than the corresponding statistic for the trans and nonbinary people who were also American Indian, Asian, Black, Latino/a, or multiracial (Grant et al., 2010).

Understanding a client's gender identity involves understanding how it changes and functions in contexts of all roles the client experiences. Diversity of gender identities exists both across and within individuals. Learning the nature of your client's gender identity and positioning in their cultures will require conversation because, as discussed in the following section, gender identity cannot always be assumed from gender presentation.

Gender Presentation and Attribution

Clothing, jewelry, hairstyles, and cosmetics can visually communicate one's gender instantly. Or can they? In modern Western culture, ear lobe piercing tends to be associated with females. Yet, earrings were worn by male soldiers in ancient Persia by both "sons and daughters" of the Israelites, and by "courtiers and gentlemen of courage" during the English Renaissance ("Earring" n.d.). Today most children's clothing is designed for a culture of binary gender: blue and gray outfits with dinosaurs and trucks for young boys, pink and pastel outfits with flowers and princesses for young girls. However, as recently as the early 20th century, drawing attention to a child's gender was considered precocious sexuality; boys would not begin to be distinguishable by wearing trousers until age 4 or 5, and then only if they indicated interest (Paoletti, 2012).[2] Perhaps the most recent dramatic shift is women wearing trousers. Men wearing dresses has not come to the same level of ubiquity, likely because even the power of marketing has not overcome sexism and homophobia.

Historical evidence demonstrates that means to communicate gender are culturally bound and change over time. Therefore, cultural context must be considered when communicating gender—whether for one's own expression or for attributing gender to someone else, such as with personal pronouns. Much of the research applied to gender presentation goals in this book was conducted in the gender cultures of the North American, European, and Australian regions. Currently, these societies largely hold to a gender binary with little tolerance for natural variation. Gender attributions by others are predominately binary and are pervasive beginning at the 20-week gestation ultrasound, when a doctor presents a pink or blue card to the mother. Distinctions between adult men and women have been the subject of numerous publications

[2]Paoletti (2012) attributes the current gender divergence in children's clothing stores is attributable to marketing genius in the 1950–1970s, when American families were having fewer kids and therefore buying less clothes. Gender-specific clothing mitigated utility of "hand me downs."

and conversations—again, since ancient times and across all disciplines and societal contexts. Some distinctions are grounded in good science; others are not. This has extended to descriptions of how men and women present their gender in verbal and nonverbal communication.

Most approaches to changing the client's gender presentation or influencing gender attribution developed during the height of popularity for gender-linked behavior and language and thus rely heavily on binary gender norms. Yet relatively recent work in sociolinguistics provides evidence against a strictly "female" and "male" language style. According to two meta-analyses of papers published since 1968 and 1977, if variables such as size and gender composition of group or length and topic of conversation are included in the analysis, then the effect of speaker's gender on their language choices is small (Leaper & Ayres, 2007; Leaper & Robnett, 2011). Even factors seemingly external to the research context contribute —in small degrees—to reported outcomes. For example, studies with women (versus men) as first author or published between 1977 and 1991 (versus 1992 to 2008) were more likely to report that women used more tentative language than men used (Leaper & Robnett, 2011).

As with language structure and use, voice and articulation characteristics are thought to distinguish adult cisgender men and women. There is stronger evidence for a gender dichotomy in voice and articulation, though plenty of overlap and complexities exist in these areas as well. Chapter 5 will include more detail about these communication variables for consideration in development of an intervention plan. When behaviors and levels for target outcomes are considered, it is important to remember that the client's desired gender presentation, self-attribution, and attribution by others may not conform to the binary gender norms available and held by most of society, nor to the conceptualization of gender held by the provider. Communication about these concepts is fundamental to the formation of therapeutic alliance and the intervention process. Chapter 4 describes an interview during initial assessment that can inform the clinician about the central and most influential component of service: the client.

Insensitivity

Using the wrong name or pronoun is called *misgendering*, and it should be avoided. It may be challenging to use the client's pronouns, particularly if their gender presentation does not match your conception of the gender presentation typical of that pronoun. Using they/them pronouns—an attribution commonly desired by gender nonbinary people—for a single person may run counter to etiquette and grammar lessons of yesteryear but so did adoption of "Ms." to avoid guessing between "Mrs." or "Miss" when it was introduced in the 1970s. It can be challenging, even for supportive people, to change habits when a friend or family member transitions and chooses a new name and pronouns. The focus and effort spent to use the correct attributions will be well worth it. Being misgendered can make people feel disrespected and invalidated. Intentionally using the wrong pronoun or *dead name* (i.e., the name given at birth that is no longer used by the person) can be hurtful and even considered an act of violence, according to Laverne Cox, a transgender activist and actress (see her speech at https://www.youtube.com/watch?v=6cytc0p4Jwg). Research from the University of Texas confirms that using chosen names at school, work, home, and with friends can have positive effects for transgender adolescents, such as lowering symptoms of severe depression and lessening suicidal ideations and attempts (Russell, Pollitt, Li, & Grossman, 2018).

Questions and comments about the person's gender identity should respect their gender positioning as valid. Terms such as *real woman* instead of *cisgender woman* connote that trans women are "fake women." Some people avoid the adjective *preferred* when discussing gender pronouns because pronoun use is about accuracy more than preference. Well-intentioned compliments on "passing" may only draw attention to the fact that the person is being judged by a societal standard rather than being accepted simply as they are.

In our experience with students and clinicians new to working with gender-diverse clients, using the wrong pronoun or offending the client ranks high on their list of apprehensions. A few resources for learning and practicing respectful attribution are listed in Box 2–1.

When we make a mistake with the pronoun, we immediately apologize and correct ("sorry, I meant *she*.") and move on. Prolonged apology or highlighting the issue may make the person more uncomfortable and involve more emotional labor for them than us, so just take responsibility and do better next time. Whatever effort or time or comfort we sacrifice to create a habit of using the correct attribution will be negligible compared to the burdens LGBT populations have been carrying for centuries.

Box 2–1

Lessons on Misgendering and Respect for Pronouns

- A 55-minute educational resource for classes to learn about the importance of pronouns and how to avoid misgendering.
  https://www.glsen.org/sites/default/files/Misgendering-and-Respect-for-Pronouns.pdf

They/Them Pronouns

- A first-person account by a person who uses they/them pronouns addresses common questions they receive.
  http://www.teenvogue.com/story/they-them-questions-answered

How to React After Accidentally Misgendering Someone

- A resource providing recommendations about how to acknowledge the mistake of misgendering someone. The author provides rationale for why it is important to use the correct gender attribution.
  http://www.pdxqcenter.org/how-to-react-after-accidentally-misgendering-someone/

HISTORICAL CONTEXT

Shaping of a Culture

Learning about the historical baggage carried by many gender-diverse people makes it easier to understand why continued misgendering and discrimination can be so disturbing. Awareness of the variety of gender expressions throughout history and across cultures can shape one's response to gender variance (Lev, 2004). Further, it is important to understand the unique histories of populations so often viewed as one group with growing number of letters: LGBTQQIA+ (Lesbian, Gay, Bisexual, Transgender, Queer, Questioning, Intersex, Allies, and more). Education about this history is typically relegated to LGBT History Month, but an increasing number of organizations and websites are making accessible the stories from distant and recent past that shape a more gender-diverse culture (see Box 2–2 for resources to explore). When history

Box 2–2

Archive

- Search the database by time period, person, place, subject, documents, bibliographies, visual material, oral histories, and timelines. The archive also serves as a place of community participation to make LGBT history easily accessible to a wide audience. http://outhistory.org/

Interactive Timeline

- Prominent dates of political, social, and cultural events in LGBTQ history. http://www.pbs.org/outofthepast/

The Committee on Lesbian, Gay, Bisexual, and Transgender History (CLGBTH)

- An affiliate of the American Historical Association, this committee webpage facilitates communication between scholars whose work in various disciplines focuses on LGBTQ history. Resources include newsletters, recognition for notable work in lesbian, gay, bisexual, transgender, and queer history, and academic resources collected and created by the CLGBTH. http://clgbthistory.org/

Queers in history: The comprehensive encyclopedia of historical gays, lesbians, bisexuals, and transgenders (Stern, 2009)

- A compilation of biographical information on prominent political, religious, academic, and cultural figures who were/are gay, lesbian, bisexual, or transgender. It encompasses aspects of LGBT culture from 2450 BC to present day.

Transgender history: The roots of today's revolution (Stryker, 2017)

- Investigates transgender history in the United States with a focus on political and social change throughout the 20th century. Written by a self-identified transsexual lesbian woman, it includes major movements and historical figures, as well as depictions of transgenderism in popular culture.

is reported by members of the dominant classes, stories of minorities are often lost or told with bias (Lev, 2004). Therefore, learning history from personal records of gender-diverse people in history (i.e., letters) or modern historians with perspectives more similar to their subjects' is always preferable.

In the Beginning

Ancient historical records include people who changed their attire, behavior, and even anatomy to live in gender roles other than what they were assigned at birth. Ancient Jewish texts of the Talmud include terms for a person who has both "male" and "female" sexual characteristics (*androgynos*), a person whose sexual characteristics are indeterminate or obscured (*tumtum*), a person who is AFAB but develops male characteristics and is infertile (*ay'lonit*), and a person AMAB but develops female characteristics (*saris hamah*), each with different legal regulations and implications (Sojourn, 2015). Gender variance in Greco-Roman cultures often involved religious or spiritual practices, such as the Greek worshippers of the goddess Cybele, who castrated themselves and referred to themselves as female. Greek history and mythology also have many stories of cross-dressing. Royal families of Roman courts cross-dressed, and changing genders was acknowledged; even a Roman emperor, Elagabalus, is said to have requested castration to change his sex (Lev, 2004). As Christianity spread and new converts were encouraged to abandon the culture of paganism and idol worship, various cultural practices were established as sins against God. In some Christian cultures, the "effeminate" and "homosexual" are still described as unrighteous, or separated from God, right alongside idolaters, adulterers, thieves, slave traders, and liars (1 Corinthians 6:9-11 NIV; 1 Timothy 1:3-11 NIV).[3]

Medical Investigations and Interventions

Fast forward to the late 1800s, when research emerged suggesting a biological basis for transgender and homosexual

[3]Scholars believe Greek words *arsenokoites* (abuse), translated as *homosexual* and *malakos* (soft), translated as *effeminate* in most of the New Testament references likely refers to the pagan practices of men forcing young boys to have sex with them or males enslaved for prostitution by pagan temples.

feelings (not yet differentiated) and undermining the common notion that sexual or gender variance was sinful behavior. Doctors began describing transgender people as in need of medical, rather than spiritual, intervention. Several medical researchers (e.g., Karl Heinrich Ulrichs, Karl Maria Kertbeny) advocated for inclusion of people who were simply in the tails of a normal distribution curve (Stryker, 2017).

Magnus Hirschfeld, one of the most influential researchers to write about the biological basis of variations in human sexuality and gender, formed several organizations during the early 1900s to advocate social reform and justice for sexual minorities. In 1910 Hirschfeld wrote the first book about treatment for transgender people, including raising children according to their expressed gender rather than sex assigned at birth, and in 1931 arranged for his friend Dora Richter to have the first documented "male-to-female genital transformation surgery" (Stryker, 2017). Hirschfeld's Institute for Sexual Science was destroyed by Nazis in 1933 after Hitler called Hirschfeld "the most dangerous Jew in Germany" (Stryker, 2017). This violent act was not the only nor last attack on the LGBTQ communities around the world, but it demonstrates the persecution that kept, and in many places continues to keep, these minority groups marginalized and at risk.

Research on the "causes and cures" for sexual and gender variants continued, often experimenting with psychiatric hospital patients from convenient and vulnerable populations such as men serving in the military whose sexuality had been discovered. These studies were funded by sources such as the California Sex Deviates Research Act of 1950 (Stryker, 2017).[4]

While American researchers were beginning to recognize a distinction between gay men and people we would now call transgender, barriers to medical services for transgender health were being reinforced (e.g., legal testimony that genital modification would constitute mayhem, the willful destruction of healthy tissue, which exposed surgeons who performed such surgery to criminal prosecution). Body modification services had been available in Europe and Asia, but in 1952 media attention around the world centered on Christine Jorgensen, an American ex-GI who went to Copenhagen, Denmark, and

[4]Under current guidelines and best practices for ethical research, LGBT populations may be considered vulnerable, as gender and sexual variance carry social stigma and disadvantages. Therefore, research with these populations may require additional considerations and protections in research, such as additional measures to protect research participants' rights or privacy (Shivayogi 2013).

had a successful genital transformation surgery. Questions and confusions about sexual orientation, physical sex, and gender expression were thrust into the societal spotlight and continue to be negotiated there today.

Political, social, and economic climates of America in the 1960s bred increasing resistance to discrimination and denied services in the form of protests, demonstrations, and occasionally actual food fights (e.g., Cooper's Donuts in 1959, Dewey's lunch counter in 1965, Compton's Cafeteria in 1966). By June of 1969 a so-called "gay revolution" (which included trans and gender-diversity issues) was inevitable and conditions were primed for perhaps the most infamous demonstration of police resistance in LGBTQ history: the riot at Stonewall Inn. On this occasion, police came to do a routine raid on the gay bar but met resistance. The confrontation went on for days and included thrown beer bottles, fire, and some say even a line of drag queens dancing a can-can to mock police (Stryker, 2017).

In 1966, Dr. Harry Benjamin, ahead of many other medical professionals, argued that a person's gender identity could not be changed, and therefore the best and only remaining solution was to change the person's body. Johns Hopkins University Medical School established the first "sex change" program in the United States, followed by the University of Minnesota, Stanford University, and the University of Texas (Stryker, 2017). However, the objectives of these early programs were more related to maintaining traditional gender expressions and heterosexuality than to alleviate suffering from dysphoria. The Harry Benjamin International Gender Dysphoria Association (HBIGDA)—which later became WPATH—developed the diagnostic criteria for gender identity disorder as well as a set of intervention guidelines for psychotherapy, hormone therapy, and surgery, which became known as the Standards of Care.

Social Politics of Medicine

Gender identity disorder (GID) was added to the *DSM-IV* (1994) —the edition after *homosexualism* was removed from it. This almost simultaneous depathologizing of homosexuality and pathologizing of gender variance was, and still is, perceived as marking a major rift between the LGB and TQ communities. Some attribute the addition of GID to the *DSM* to sociopolitical movements more than medical evidence. In particular, lesbian feminists were speaking against trans women and drag queens, groups they felt mocked what it is to be a woman, were not "real women." and were therefore unwelcome in the feminist movement (Stryker, 2017). For example, in her book *The Transsexual Empire: The Making of a She-Male,* Janice Raymond compares Nazi doctors designing a superior race to the doctors performing gender reassignment surgery to maintain a binary and patriarchal order (original 1979, republished in 1994 with new introduction reiterating her position). More recently, radical feminist theory is critical of gender as a cultural—not biological—tool to repress people of the female sex. Some radical feminists argue that trans women AMAB who demand other people accept their gender and allow them into physical or emotional spaces reserved for people AFAB are just another example of AMAB people disregarding and disrespecting AFAB people (see Barrett, 2016). This position is referred to as *trans-exclusionary radical feminism*, or TERF, although that term has obvious bias itself.

In the 1960s well-known gay-rights activists with queer identities were overlooked and even outright banned from participating in pride parades by the mainstream gay activist organizations. Two examples are Sylvia Rivera and Marsha Johnson: The self-described drag queens founded a shelter for gay and trans teens and championed civil rights for people marginalized for their sexual orientation, gender, race, or socioeconomic status. The queer movement of the 1990s became relatively more trans-inclusive when organizations began adding the "T" to the "LGB" descriptor (Stryker, 2017, p. 170). Yet, some still lament celebrations of marriage-equality laws and other civil rights victories for sexual orientation minorities while trans people are "left behind" and "remain at risk for discrimination and violence" (Boylan, 2011). Transphobic rhetoric continues to divide factions of LGBTQ+ communities.

It is difficult to pinpoint when the "Q" for Queer and "I" for Intersex began to be included in the acronym, but GLAAD officially recommended them in its media reference guide in 2016. GLAAD cited the growing number of people, especially young people, identifying as queer. Those populations are usually included in the meaning, even if not in the LGBT acronym. Cheryl Chase, founder of the Intersex Society of North America, moved to San Francisco to align intersex politics with queer and transgender politics because she saw similarities between how the medical establishment recommended and performed surgeries to normalize bodies of intersex and transgender people to fit into a gender binary and heteronormative culture (Stryker, 2017).

To summarize medical and social history of trans people in recent history: Very shortly after trans people were recognized and able to access gender-specific care, they were marginalized and pathologized by the medical community and even within what is typically portrayed as a unified LGBTQ community. After more than a decade, in a move slightly away from pathologizing gender diversity, gender identity disorder was changed to gender dysphoria (GD) and separated from sexual dysfunctions and paraphilic disorders in the 5th edition of the *DSM* (*DSM-5*, 2013). A key criterion of GD is the patient's distress regarding the incongruence between gender identity and sex assigned at birth. In other words, a trans person does not meet the criteria for a diagnosis of a psychiatric disorder unless they experience gender dysphoria. The eleventh International Classification of Disease (ICD-11) moved the diagnosis of gender incongruence to a new chapter on sexual health rather than mental health (Winter et al., 2016).

Guidelines for voice and communication services were introduced to the WPATH Standards of Care in the 7th edition (2011). Empirical research, provider experience, and client testimonials were instrumental in this recognition of voice and communication as part of health care for some trans and gender-diverse individuals. No requirement of psychological or medical status is necessarily needed for voice and communication work, although some health payor systems are more apt to cover services directly linked to a client's diagnosis. This freedom is somewhat unique to our discipline. For example, guidelines for endocrine treatment published by the *Journal of American Medical Association* in 2017 require a diagnosis of gender dysphoria and counseling regarding potential medical and fertility prior to hormone therapy for adults seeking cross-sex hormones. Adolescents seeking hormones to suppress pubertal hormones also need confirmation from a multidisciplinary team of medical and mental health professionals that their gender dysphoria/incongruence is persistent and they are mentally able to give consent.

Trauma and Tragedy

Despite increase in care standards at regional and international levels, they still need to be "negotiated, approved, and implemented by the public and private health authorities of various countries, in the context of broader socioreligious and sociopolitical issues, within the normative climate of heterosexism" (Wylie et al., 2016). Therefore, it is important to learn the standards of care as well as the nature and underpinnings of the predominant gender culture. A timeline of significant civil liberties and protections provided to gender-diverse populations illustrates the changes in socioreligious and sociopolitical climate in recent history (see Box 2–3).

Box 2–3

1952	The American Psychiatric Association lists homosexuality as a sociopathic personality disturbance in the Diagnostic and Statistical Manual (it is removed in 1973).
1953	U.S. President Eisenhower signs executive order that bans homosexual people from working for the federal government.
1961	Illinois is first U.S. state to decriminalize homosexuality by repealing sodomy laws.
1969	Transgender and gender-diverse people are among those who resisted arrest in a routine bar raid by police on the Stonewall Inn in New York City, igniting the modern LGBT rights movement.
1972	Sweden is the first country to allow transgender people to legally change their sex after meeting specific requirements.
1975	The first U.S. federal gay rights bill is introduced to address discrimination based on sexual orientation.
1975	South Australia is the first Australian state to decriminalize male homosexual activity.
1980	Gender identity disorder first appears in the American Psychiatric Association's *DSM-III*.
1986	The U.S. Supreme Court rules in Bowers v. Hardwick that the Constitution allows states to pass and enforce sodomy laws targeting homosexuals.
1987	The Constitution of Sweden bans discrimination against gay men, lesbians, and bisexual people.

1992	Minnesota state legislature enacts the first statewide law banning discrimination against transgender people.
1996	Hawaii Judge Chang rules that the state does not have a legal right to deprive same-sex couples of the right to marry.
1998	First U.S. Transgender Day of Remembrance.
2003	The U.S. Supreme Court strikes down the "homosexual conduct" law, thereby decriminalizing same-sex sexual conduct.
2004	In South Africa, the Alteration of Sex Description and Sex Status Act allows transsexual and intersex people to change their legally recognized sex.
2006	First openly transgender U.S. official to win statewide office: Kim Coco Iwamoto to Hawaii Board of Education.
2006	First openly transgender person ordained in Reform Judaism.
2008	Sweden alters its constitution to offer protection from discrimination based on transgender identity or expression.
2011	Girl Scouts of the United States of America welcomes transgender girls (Boy Scouts of America follow suit in 2017).
2013	*DSM-5* refers to gender dysphoria rather than gender identity disorder.
2014	Malaysian Putrajaya Court of Appeal ruled a ban on cross-dressing unconstitutional.
2014	Laverne Cox is the first openly transgender person nominated for an Emmy award.
2015	The U.S. Supreme Court rules that states cannot ban same-sex marriage.
2016	U.S. lifts ban on transgender people serving openly in the U.S. military.
2017	California and Oregon are the first U.S. states to legally recognize nonbinary gender as an option on identity documents.

Unfortunately, inequality and intolerance still exist. Even with some protections, trans populations are susceptible to crimes of hate, including violence. Transgender Day of Remembrance in the U.S. started in 1998 in San Francisco and now is nationally recognized and held annually in November to honor and remember people who are killed for being—or perceived as being—transgender or gender-diverse. Days of remembrance like this are now observed around the world. In addition to services and vigils, educational events and exhibits increase awareness of the threats trans and gender nonconforming people face daily. The HRC hosts a website with information about the individuals remembered and current antitransgender violence rates in the United States.

HEALTH DISPARITIES AND BARRIERS TO CARE

Serious psychological distress for people in trans populations contributes to attempted suicide rates nearly 9 times that of the U.S. population (i.e., 40% to 46% compared to 2% to 4.6%, Grant et al., 2010; James et al., 2016; Testa et al., 2017). Transgender people with disabilities are even more likely to experience psychological distress (59%), attempt suicide (54%), and report mistreatment by health care providers (42%) (James et al., 2016). Transgender people of color experience disparities at higher rates than their white peers. For example, the HIV rate in the U.S. population is 0.3%, whereas in transgender populations it is 1.4% overall but 6.7% among Black trans people and 19% among Black trans women (James et al., 2016).

Gender-based victimization, gender-based rejection, gender-based discrimination, and identity nonaffirmation are external stressors that can lead to three types of internal stressors: negative expectations for future events, internalized transphobia, and nondisclosure of one's identity, as proposed in the Gender Minority Stress and Resilience (GMSR) model (Testa, Habarth, Peta, Balsam, & Bockting, 2015). These stressors, particularly when mediated by interpersonal variables of thwarted belongingness (e.g., social disconnection, lack of support) and perceived burdensomeness (e.g., self-hatred, feeling like a liability/burden), are significant predictors of suicidal ideation (Testa et al., 2017). For example, odds of a transgender or gender-diverse person attempting suicide or misuse of drugs or alcohol to cope with discrimination significantly rise with increasing levels of family rejection (Augustus, 2016).

Continued marginalization, inequity in health care, and minority stress explains why one-third of transgender patients have not disclosed their gender identity to their medical providers (James et al., 2016; Mayer et al., 2008), and half have delayed or forgone medical treatment due to fear of mistreatment or affordability (Cruz, 2014; Grant et al., 2010). Hiding one's gender identity takes a toll on health.

Levesque et al. (2013) cited several barriers to health care stemming from both provider and patient. Practical actions to diminish such barriers are presented in Chapter 3; a brief overview of the barriers and resulting disparities will be presented here to illustrate the circumstances of many LGBTQ populations. Fundamental barriers to care relate to the client's ability to perceive their need, learn about their care options, and trust providers to deliver appropriate care. Additionally, barriers related to physical accessibility (i.e., mobility, transportation to skilled and knowledgeable providers, social support) and cost can prevent access to health care. Currently most insurance plans in the U.S. exclude transition-related care from coverage. Even if care is accessed, desired health consequences are dependent upon the patient's ability to engage (e.g., whether they receive empowerment, adherence, support) and the provider's technical and interpersonal competence to provide coordinated care.

A significant barrier to accessing care is fear of mistreatment by health care providers. In a 2016 U.S. survey, 33% of transgender people reported being mistreated by a provider (James et al., 2016). An earlier survey specified that 19% had been refused care due to their gender identity, 28% had been verbally harassed, and 2% physically assaulted while receiving medical care (Grant et al., 2010). Descriptions from more than 150 transgender patients highlighted six themes of mistreatment: gender insensitivity, displays of discomfort, denied services, substandard care, verbal abuse, and forced care (Kosenko, Rintamaki, Raney, & Maness, 2013). Patient perception of a negative experience, regardless of providers' intent, can deter them from seeking care in the future.

Disparities and barriers to access are present in the communication field as well. Only 50% of transgender survey respondents understood that SLPs could provide gender-related services, and only 3% said they would be "interested in seeking services from an SLP in voice and/or communication training" (Sawyer, Perry, & Dobbins-Scaramelli, 2014, p. 159). The reasons for this are still unclear, but may relate to heterosexual bias of SLPs perceived by clients (Kelly & Robinson, 2011). In a survey of SLPs from the U.S., Australia, Canada, and New Zealand, accuracy on questions about LGBTQ culture was near 50% and self-ratings confirmed their knowledge level was lower than their comfort or willingness to serve transgender populations. Fifty-one percent of SLPs were not sure what to address in transgender voice intervention, which is not surprising considering 47% indicated that it was never addressed at all in their professional degree program (Hancock & Haskin, 2015).

Trans care is often excluded from medical training, and patients anticipate that providers will not know how to meet their medical needs (Roberts & Fantz, 2014). A study by Poteat, German, and Kerrigan (2013) demonstrated that provider uncertainty breeds stigmatizing attitudes and even abuse of power, ultimately continuing the systems of inequality that contribute to health consequences. To combat this, providers can self-evaluate and continually improve their own knowledge and attitudes toward trans and gender-diverse people, particularly in context of providing professional services to them.

SELF-EVALUATION

Humans like to categorize. In fact, sometimes we need to categorize. How else would we match our socks, prevent social chaos, even protect ourselves from foe? The need to categorize people is fundamental in the human brain (Amodio, 2014). We don't hesitate to categorize ourselves, either. For a variety of proposed reasons, we are biased to like the category we are in better than any other category. This biased, preferential evaluation is prejudice, and it leads to efforts to clearly distinguish one's own group from the "other" group. In social contexts this creates stereotypes, or "conceptual attributes associated with a group . . . which may refer to trait or circumstantial characteristics," and they are learned early in life, as evidenced by the rhyme, "Snips of snails and puppy dog tails, that's what little boys are made of! . . . Sugar and spice and all things nice, that's what little girls are made of!" (Amodio, 2014, p. 669).

Unfortunately, preferences often manifest in negative opinions, judgments, or attitudes about the "other" group. When those prejudices are communicated—in words or action —discrimination occurs.

Hidden Bias

We are often unaware of our prejudices and resulting discriminatory behavior. Hidden biases—those not apparent and even in contradiction to conscious commitments to equality—are referred to as *implicit biases*. Existence of bias is confirmed by studies of brain imaging. For example, for Caucasian people with hidden racial bias, a part of the brain associated with emotional learning and response to social threat (i.e., amygdala) was more active when shown faces of African Americans than when shown Caucasian faces (Phelps et al., 2000). This may be a function of learned threat response to racial outgroups, apprehension about appearing to others to be prejudiced, or simply a goal-directed response to attend more to members of one's own social group (Amodio, 2014).

Researchers at Harvard University, the University of Virginia, the University of Washington, and Yale proport to identify implicit bias better than measures of self-reporting do through tests of reaction time available online at Project Implicit (https://implicit.harvard.edu/implicit/takeatest.html). Currently there are versions of the Implicit Association Test (IAT) for race (Black-white), religion, sexuality (gay-straight), and a variety of other categories. Georgetown University's National Center for Cultural Competence (n.d.) offers a free online course about conscious and unconscious bias in health care and resulting disparities (https://nccc.georgetown.edu/bias/).

Implicit bias does not have to lead to discrimination. Self-regulation can counter effects of prejudices and stereotypes on behavior (Amodio, 2014). A new body of research suggests that even when individual scores on the IAT do not predict behavior, the average score in a community does predict behavior in that community. In communities with white people who have higher racial bias, as measured by people in those communities taking the IAT online, police kill African Americans at disproportionately high rates (Hehman, Flake, & Calanchini, 2017). As this research is correlational and not causal, violence cannot be attributed to community bias directly; however, this research is evidence that we should consider bias effects at the community level as well as the individual level, because they may be different. According to social psychologists such as Dr. Mahzarin Banaji of Harvard, as a member of a community, you are "both influenced by and influencing the larger social group around [you]" (Vedantam, 2018).[5]

[5]Impacts of bias in the individual and community are further explored in the National Public Radio (NPR) Hidden Brain podcast with Shankar Vedantam's March 9, 2018 show: "Radio Replay: The Mind of the Village" (https://www.npr.org/templates/transcript/transcript.php?storyId=591895426)

Solutions

Though social goals and legislation have improved conditions for some LGBTQ populations, discrimination still exists. Popular studies demonstrating that people with equivalent—or even superior—qualifications are treated differently at job interviews offer, perhaps inadvertently, a method to avoid discrimination. In a study of selection for a symphony orchestra, the use of a curtain to block the judges' view of the musician led to increased hiring of female musicians (Goldin & Rouse, 2000). Note the bias was not eliminated, it was just prevented from affecting the outcome. When attributes produce such discrimination, "it is worth considering when such cues are undesirable and should be moved from perception" (Lai & Banaji, in press, p. 10).

Neuroscience, too, indicates that eliminating the implicit bias may not be possible so discrimination interventions should target cognitive processes that regulate behavior.

Specifically, interventions should increase awareness of the potential for bias, train attention to specific cues, and then prepare specific responses to anticipated cues. For example, if we meet a trans person very different from ourselves, we will likely have bias, so we will remind ourselves to respond more carefully and sensitively. Such in-the-moment reminders have been suggested for improving equity in prescribing pain medication to white and African-American patients (Vedantam, 2018).

Over the past decade, numerous LGBTQ cultural competency trainings appeared; most aim to reduce disparities and discriminatory behaviors by influencing knowledge and attitudes about a culture or subcultures. However, a 2016 review of evidence for cultural competence interventions found no qualifying research on culturally competent services for trans people specifically (Butler et al., 2016). In other words, the effectiveness of trainings for cultural competency working with trans people has not been evaluated because it doesn't exist yet.

The effectiveness of general LGBTQ cultural competency trainings is largely unmeasured, in part due to disagreement about what constitutes cultural competency and how best to measure it (Henderson, Horne, Hills, & Kendall, 2018). There are more than 50 instruments purporting to measure cultural competency, and those most frequently used incorporate several questionable assumptions about what constitutes cultural competency (e.g., culture is only about ethnicity and race,

Caucasian people don't have a culture). Furthermore, several instruments—particularly those used to measure effectiveness of trainings—measured awareness and knowledge but not skill (Kumas-Tan et al., 2008). That said, there is evidence that general cultural sensitivity training can improve health care provider attitudes and patient health outcomes (Majumdar, Browne, Roberts, & Carpio, 2004).

Reflection and Response

The path to extinguish discrimination begins with an honest and thorough self-examination of the bias—explicit or implicit—that we each carry. What are your feelings toward lesbian women? Gay men? Queer and gender-diverse people? Transgender people? When 271 SLPs answered these questions using a 1 to 5 scale (1 = mostly negative, 5 = mostly positive), responses skewed toward positive feelings, but mean ratings were near 4.3 for each population posed (Hancock & Haskin, 2015). Even people with overall positive perceptions or who identify as a member of the LGBTQ community themselves can have bias and unintentionally discriminate. A less standardized way to evaluate one's biases is to evaluate one's actions, particularly when fatigued, stressed, or distracted. Careful self-reflection can search for sources of bias that may be manifesting discrimination. For example:

- How much do you know about the trans populations and how do you know your understanding is accurate? Are you familiar with the books and documentaries in Appendix 2–A?
- Are you more comfortable around one of the populations than another (i.e., trans men, trans women, genderqueer)?
- Do you hesitate to serve these populations professionally due to a stigma that you would face from society, coworkers, or your own family by doing so?
- When you serve individuals, what is the influence of your own notions about gender?

You can compare some of your views to more than 4,500 American adults surveyed by Pew Research Center (http://www.pewresearch.org/fact-tank/2017/12/05/how-do-your-views-on-gender-compare-with-those-of-other-americans/).

For a more in-depth self-assessment and customized educational resources, take the Cultural and Linguistic Competence Health Practitioner Assessment developed by Georgetown University National Center for Cultural Competence (https://www.clchpa.org/).

Influence Others

After increasing awareness of one's own bias and noticing the circumstances in which it might be acted upon, reasonable responses should be developed. Preventing discrimination is possible but requires intentional and longitudinal commitment (Forscher, Lai, Axt, Ebersole, & Herman, under review).

- How will you remind yourself to actively consider whether your post on social media may be insensitive to someone?
- What cue will you use to actively make sure individuals with minority identities are included in conversations and decision making?
- When will you review your workplace and consider the inclusive practices outlined in the next chapter?
- How often will you visit the website of a LGBTQ organization to monitor how news is affecting marginalized populations?

In addition to shaping our own thinking and practices, we can work to eliminate perpetuation of stereotypes and resulting discrimination in our larger communities. People in our own family, social or religious community, school district, and work environment will learn and live in a culture that increasingly recognizes diversity and challenges the status quo. Professionals have an obligation to train students and junior employees to deliver inclusive care and develop their own cultural competence. Lead by example.

Speak out against injustices as well as oversimplified generalizations about a group of people. Encourage a variety of perspectives to be included in discussions and support people who may feel vulnerable because of sharing their minority status or view. Even smaller gestures, such as exposure to authentic role models, can thwart early pressures to adopt negative stereotypes (Gunter, 2013). Appendix 2–A includes educational resources, including formalized curriculum for creating antibias education, such as the online modules offer-ed by Teaching Tolerance (https://www.tolerance.org/professional-development/critical-practices-for-antibias-education).

While some of the available materials (e.g., the Teaching Tolerance website) assume a young audience, these lessons are important to impart to anyone still able to learn, whether child, young adult, or just young at heart. People's own cultural identities (e.g., age, race, gender) will shape their needs and contributions. Those with majority identities can think critically about their privileges or potential influence they have; those with minority identities may need support to feel safe as themselves.

SUMMARY

The tendency to narrowly define and describe gender identities permeates society, but as information collects from studies of biology to behavior we see more and more of the many beautiful shades that exist. There is more work to be done to make the lesser-known variations of gender more visible. The discriminatory effect of prejudice diminishes only when we acknowledge, monitor, and consciously act in opposition to often deeply-rooted bias.

Our job begins with knowing our client. Everything else we do will be centered on that knowledge. Learning about their gender identity and positioning in their culture, their preferences for gender attribution and presentation, as well as the deep roots of marginalization and disparities that still affect every part of their life and being is foundational to delivering culturally appropriate service.

REFERENCES

Ainsworth, C. (2015). Sex redefined. *Nature*, *518*(7539), 288–291.

American Psychological Association (APA). (2015). *Key concepts in understanding gender diversity and sexual orientation among students*. Retrieved from https://www.apa.org/pi/lgbt/programs/safe-supportive/lgbt/key-terms.pdf

American Speech-Language-Hearing Association (ASHA). (2016). *Code of ethics*. Retrieved from https://www.asha.org/Code-of-Ethics/

American Speech-Language-Hearing Association (ASHA). (2019). *Cultural competence*. Retrieved from https://www.asha.org/practice-portal/professional-issues/cultural-competence/

Amodio, D. M. (2014). The neuroscience of prejudice and stereotyping. *Nature Reviews, 15*(10), 670–682.

Augustus, K. (2016). Family rejection as a predictor of suicide attempts and substance misuse among transgender and gender nonconforming adults. *LGBT Health, 3*(3).

Azul, D. (2016). Gender-related aspects of transmasculine people's vocal situations: Insights from a qualitative content analysis of interview transcripts. *International Journal of Language and Communication Disorders, 51*(6), 672–684.

Barrett, R. (2016). *Female erasure: What you need to know about gender politics' war on women, the female sex and human rights.* Pacific Palisades, CA: Tidal Time Publishing.

Bauer, G. R., Braimoh, J., Scheim, A. I., & Dharma, C. (2017). Transgender-inclusive measures of sex/gender for population surveys: Mixed methods evaluation and recommendations. *PLOS ONE, 12*(5), e0178043.

Blackless, M., Charuvastra, A., Derryck, A., Fausto-Sterling, A., Lauzanne, K., & Lee, E. (2000). How sexually dimorphic are we? Review and synthesis. *American Journal of Human Biology, 12*(2), 151–166.

Boylan, J. F. (2011). We want cake, too. *New York Times.* Retrieved from https://www.nytimes.com/2011/08/12/opinion/we-want-cake-too.html

Bucholtz, M., & Hall, K. (2005). Identity and interaction: A sociocultural linguistic approach. *Discourse Studies, 7*(4-5), 585–614.

Butler, J. (1993). *Bodies that matter: On the discursive limits of "sex."* New York, NY: Routledge.

Butler, J. (1999). *Gender trouble: Feminism and the subversion of identity.* New York, NY: Routledge.

Butler, M. (2016). Improving cultural competence to reduce health disparities. *Comparative Effectiveness Review No. 170.* AHRQ Publication No. 16-EHC006-EF. Rockville, MD: Agency for Health Care Research and Quality.

Conron, K. J., Scout, N., & Austin, S. B. (2008). Everyone has a right to, like, check their box: Findings on a measure of gender identity from a cognitive testing study with adolescents. *Journal of LGBT Health Research, 4*(1), 1–9.

Cruz, T. (2014). Assessing access to care for transgender and gender nonconforming people: A consideration of diversity in combating discrimination. *Social Science and Medicine, 110*, 65–73.

Earring. (n.d.). In *Wikipedia*. Retrieved from https://en.wikipedia.org/wiki/Earring

Fairbanks, G. (1960). *Voice and articulation drillbook* (2nd ed., pp. 124–139). New York, NY: Harper & Row.

Forscher, P. S., Lai, C. K., Axt, J. R., Ebersole, C. R., Herman, M., Devine, P. G., & Nosek, B. A. (Under review). *A meta-analysis of procedures to change implicit bias.* Retrieved from https://psyarxiv.com/dv8tu/ Preprint doi:10.31234/osf.io/dv8tu

Goldin, C., & Rouse, C. (2000). Orchestrating impartiality: The impact of "blind" auditions on female musicians. *American Economic Review*, *90*, 715–741.

Grant, J., Mottet, L., Tanis, J., Herman, J., Harrison, J., & Keisling, M. (2010). *National transgender discrimination survey report on health and health care*. National Gay and Lesbian Task Force Foundation.

Greytak, E., Gill, A., Conron, K., Matthews, P. A., Scout, N., Reisner, S., . . . Tamar-Mattis, A. (2014). Identifying transgender and other gender minority respondents on population-based surveys: Special considerations for adolescents, race/ethnicity, socio-economic status, and intersex status. In J. L. Herman (Ed.), *Best practices for asking questions to identify transgender and other gender minority respondents on population-based surveys* (pp. 29–43). Los Angeles, CA: The Williams Institute.

Gunter, C. (2013). Science: It's a role model thing. *Genome Biology*, *14*, 105.

Hancock, A., & Haskin, G. (2015). Speech-language pathologists' knowledge and attitudes regarding lesbian, gay, bisexual, transgender, and queer populations. *American Journal of Speech Language Pathology*, *24*(2), 206–221.

Hehman, E., Flake, J. K., & Calanchini, J. (2017). Disproportionate use of lethal force in policing is associated with regional racial biases of residents. *Social Psychological and Personality Science*, 1–9.

Henderson, S., Horne, M., Hills, R., & Kendall, E. (2018). Cultural competence in health care in the community: A concept analysis. *Health and Social Care in the Community*, *26*(4), 590–603.

Honest Accomplice Theatre Group. (2019). *The trans literacy project*. Retrieved from http://honestaccomplice.org/the-trans-literacy-project/

Hook, E. B., & Warburton, D. (1983). The distribution of chromosomal genotypes associated with Turner's syndrome: Livebirth prevalence rates and evidence for diminished fetal mortality and severity in genotypes associated with structural X abnormalities or mosaicism. *Human Genetics*, *64*, 24–27.

Intersex Society of North America. (2019). *What is intersex?* Retrieved from http://www.isna.org/faq/what_is_intersex

James, S. E., Herman, J. L., Rankin, S., Keisling, M., Mottet, L., & Anafi, M. (2016). *The report of the 2015 U.S. Transgender Survey*. Washington, DC: National Center for Transgender Equality.

Kattari, S. K., & Hasche, L. (2016). Differences across age groups in transgender and gender non-conforming people's experiences of health care discrimination, harassment, and victimization. *Journal of Aging and Health*, *28*(2), 285–306.

Kattari, S. K., Walls, N. E., Whitfield, D. L., & Langenderfer, M. (2017). Racial and ethnic differences in experiences of discrimination in accessing social services among transgender/gender non-

conforming people. *Journal of Ethic and Cultural Diversity in Social Work, 26*(3), 217–235.
Kelly, R. J., & Robinson, G. C. (2011). Disclosure of membership in the lesbian, gay, bisexual, and transgender community by individuals with communication impairments: A preliminary Web-based survey. *American Journal of Speech-Language Pathology, 20*, 86–94.
Kerry, S. C. (2014). Sistergirls/brotherboys: The status of indigenous transgender Australians. *International Journal of Transgenderism, 15*(3-4), 173–186.
Kosenko, K., Rintamaki, L., Raney, S., & Maness, K. (2013). Transgender patient perceptions of stigma in health care contexts. *Medical Care, 51*(9), 819–822.
Kumas-Tan, Z., Beagan, B., Loppie, C., MacLeod, A., & Frank, B. (2007). Measures of cultural competence: Examining hidden assumptions. *Academic Medicine, 82*(6).
Lai, C., & Banaji, M. R. (in press). The psychology of implicit intergroup bias and the prospect of change. In D. Allen & R. Somanathan (Eds.), *Difference with domination*. Chicago, IL: University of Chicago Press.
Leaper, C., & Ayres, M. M. (2007). A meta-analytic review of gender variations in adults' language use: Talkativeness, affiliative speech, and assertive speech. *Personality and Social Psychology Review, 11*(4), 328–363.
Leaper, C., & Robnett, R. D. (2011). Women are more likely than men to use talkative language, aren't they? A meta-analysis testing for gender differences and moderators. *Psychology of Women Quarterly, 35*(1), 129–142.
Lee, P. A., Houk, C. P., Ahmed, S. F., & Hughes, I. A. (2006). Consensus statement on management of intersex disorders. *Pediatrics, 118*(2).
Lev, A. (2004). *Transgender emergence: Therapeutic guidelines for working with gender-variant people and their families*. New York, NY: The Haworth Clinical Practice Press.
Levesque, J., Harris, M., & Russell, G. (2013). Patient-centred access to health care: Conceptualizing access at the interface of health systems and populations. *International Journal for Equity in Health, 12*(18), 1–9.
Lewis, O. (1941). Manly-hearted women among the north Piegan. *American Anthropologist, 43*(2), 173–187.
Majumdar, B., Browne, G., Roberts, J., & Carpio, B. (2004). Effects of cultural sensitivity training on health care provider attitudes and patient outcomes. *Journal of Nursing Scholarship, 36*(2), 161–166.
Margolies, L., Joo, R., & McDavid, J. (n.d.). *Best practices in creating and delivering LGBTQ cultural competency trainings for health and social service agencies*. Retrieved from https://cancer-network.org/wp-content/uploads/2017/02/best_practices.pdf

Mayer, K. H., Bradford, J. B., Makadon, H. J., Stall, R., Goldhammer, H., & Landers, S. (2008). Sexual and gender minority health: What we know and what needs to be done. *American Journal of Public Health*, *98*(6), 989–995.

Nanda, S. (1999). *The hijras of India: Neither man nor woman* (2nd ed.). Belmont, CA: Wadsworth.

National Academies Press (U.S.). (2011). Conducting research on the health status of LGBT populations. In Institute of Medicine (U.S.) Committee on Lesbian, Gay, Bisexual, and Transgender Health Issues and Research Gaps and Opportunities (Eds.), *The health of lesbian, gay, bisexual, and transgender people: Building a foundation for better understanding*. Washington, DC: National Academies Press.

National Center for Cultural Competence. (n.d.). *Curricula Enhancement Module Series*. Retrieved from: https://nccc.georgetown.edu/curricula/culturalcompetence.html

National Center for Cultural Competence. (n.d.). *Curricula Enhancement Module Series*. Retrieved from: https://nccc.georgetown.edu/bias

National Prevention Information Network. (2015). *Cultural competence*. Retrieved from https://npin.cdc.gov/pages/cultural-competence

Nielsen, J., & Wohlert, M. (1990). Sex chromosome abnormalities found among 34,910 newborn children: Results from a 13-year incidence study in Arhus, Denmark. *Birth Defects Original Article Series*, *26*, 209–223.

Paoletti, J. (2012). *Pink and blue: Telling the boys from the girls in America*. Bloomington, IN: Indiana University Press.

Phelps, E. A., O'Connor, K. J., Cunningham, W. A., Funayama, E. S., Gatenby, J. C., Gore, J. C., & Banaji, M. R. (2000). Performance on indirect measures of race evaluation predicts amygdala activation. *Journal of Cognitive Neuroscience*, *12*, 729–738.

Poteat, T., German, D., & Kerrigan, D. (2013). Managing uncertainty: A grounded theory of stigma in transgender health care encounters. *Social Science and Medicine*, *84*.

Roberts, T. K., & Fantz, C. R. (2014). Barriers to quality health care for the transgender population. *Clinical Biochemistry*, *47*(10–11), 983–987.

Roughgarden, J. (2009). *Evolution's rainbow: Diversity, gender, and sexuality in nature and people*. Oakland, CA: University of California Press.

Russell, S. T., Pollitt, A. M., Li, G., & Grossman, A. H. (2018). Chosen name use is linked to reduced depressive symptoms, suicidal ideation, and suicidal behavior among transgender youth. *Journal of Adolescent Health*, *63*(4), 503–505.

Saraswat, A., Weinand, J. D., & Safer, J. D. (2015). Evidence supporting the biologic nature of gender identity. *Endocrine Practice*, *21*(2), 199–204.

Sawyer, J., Perry, J. L., & Dobbins-Scaramelli, A. (2014). A survey of the awareness of speech services among transgender and transsexual individuals and speech-language pathologists. *International Journal of Transgenderism*, 15(3–4), 146–163.

Shivayogi, P. (2013). Vulnerable population and methods for their safeguard. *Perspectives in Clinical Research*, *4*(1), 53–57.

Smith, B. A., Murib, Z., Motta, M., Callaghan, T. H., & Theys, M. (2018). "Gay" or "homosexual"? The implications of social category labels for the structure of mass attitudes. *American Politics Research*, *46*(2) 336–372.

Sojourn (2015). *More than just male and female: Genders in classical Judaism*. Retrieved from http://www.sojourngsd.org/blog/sixgenders

Stern, K. (2009). Queers in History: The comprehensive encyclopedia of historical gays, lesbians, bisexuals, and transgenders. Dallas, TX: BenBella Books.

Stryker, S. (2008). *Transgender history: The roots of today's revolution*. New York, NY: Seal Press.

Stryker, S. (2017). *Transgender history: The roots of today's revolution* (2nd ed). New York, NY: Seal Press.

Tervalon, M., & Murray-Garcia, J. (1998). Cultural humility versus cultural competence: A critical distinction in defining physician-training outcomes in multicultural education. *Journal of Health Care for the Poor and Underserved*, *9*(2), 117.

Testa, R. J., Bliss, W., Balsam, K. F., Michaels, M. S., Rogers, M. L., & Joiner, T. (2017). Suicidal ideation in transgender people: Gender minority stress and interpersonal theory factors. *Journal of Abnormal Psychology*, *126*(1), 125–136.

Testa, R. J., Habarth, J., Peta, J., Balsam. K., & Bockting, W. (2015). Development of the gender minority stress and resilience measure. *Psychology of Sexual Orientation and Gender Diversity*, *2*, 65–77.

Vedantam, S. (2018). The mind of the village. *Hidden Brain*. Retrieved from https://www.npr.org/templates/transcript/transcript.php?storyId=591895426

West, C., & Zimmerman, D. H. (1987). Doing gender. Gender and Society, 1, 125–151.

Winter, S., Diamond, M., Green, J., Karasic, D., Reed, T., Whittle, S., & Wylie, K. (2016). Transgender people: Health at the margins of society. *Lancet*, *388*, 390–400.

Winter, S., Settle, E., Wylie, K., Reisner, S., Cabral, M., Knudson, G., & Baral, S. (2016). Synergies in health and human rights: A call to action to improve transgender health. *Lancet*, *388*, 318–321.

Wisniewski, A. B., Migeon, C. J., Meyer-Bahlburg, H. F., Gearhart, J. P., Berkovitz, G. D., Brown, T. R., & Money, J. (2000). Complete androgen insensitivity syndrome: Long-term medical, surgical, and psychosexual outcome. *Journal of Clinical Endocrinology and Metabolism*, *85*(8), 2664–2669.

World Health Organization (WHO). (n.d.). *Gender and genetics: Genetic components of sex and gender.* Retrieved from http://www.who.int/genomics/gender/en/index1.html

World Professional Association for Transgender Health (WPATH). (2010). *WPATH De-psychopathologisation statement* [Press release]. Retrieved from https://www.wpath.org/newsroom/policies

World Professional Association for Transgender Health (WPATH). (2011). *Standards of care for the health of transsexual, transgender, and gender nonconforming people.* Retrieved from https://www.wpath.org/publications/soc

World Professional Association for Transgender Health (WPATH). (2017). *WAPTH identity recognition statement* [Press release]. Retrieved from https://www.wpath.org/media/cms/Documents/Web%20Transfer/Policies/WPATH%20Identity%20Recognition%20Statement%2011.15.17.pdf

Wylie, K., Knudson, G., Khan, S. I., Bonierbale, M., Watanyusakul, S., & Baral, S. (2016). Serving transgender people: Clinical care considerations and service delivery models in transgender health. *Lancet, 388*(10042), 401–411.

Yeager, K. A., & Bauer-Wu, S. (2014). Cultural humility: Essential foundation for clinical researchers. *Applied Nursing Research, 26*(4), 1–12.

APPENDIX 2-A
Resources Related to Cultural Considerations

CULTURAL FOUNDATIONS

An ally's guide to terminology (GLAAD)
http://www.glaad.org/sites/default/files/allys-guide-to-terminology_1.pdf

Glossary of terms from the Human Rights Campaign (HRC)
https://www.hrc.org/resources/glossary-of-terms

"Key terms and concepts in understanding gender diversity and sexual orientation among students" by APA divisions of school psychology and society for the psychological study of LGBT issues
https://www.apa.org/pi/lgbt/programs/safe-supportive/lgbt/key-terms.pdf

American Psychological Association (APA): Office on Sexual Orientation and Gender Diversity
http://www.apa.org/pi/lgbt/index.aspx

It's Pronounced Metrosexual
http://itspronouncedmetrosexual.com/#sthash.2zaTkpbd.dpbs

DOCUMENTARY FILMS

1996: "Transsexual Menace"

1999: "Boys Don't Cry"—about a 1993 rape and murder of a trans person AFAB.

2001: "Southern Comfort"—about the life of a trans man who died from ovarian cancer after he was unable to get health care due to his status.

2006: "Cruel and Unusual"—about the prison experiences of five trans women.

2008: "Be Like Others"—about young Iranians choosing to undergo gender affirmation surgery.

2009: "Two-Spirits"—in Colorado, 16-year-old Fred Martinez, a Navajo (Dine) youth who identified as gay, two-spirit, and "Nadleeh" (nonbinary) was murdered by schoolmates.

2010: "Faces & Facets of Transgender Experience"—18 people and their families share their story, includes varieties of age, ethnicity, and backgrounds.

2010: "Trained in the Ways of Men"—Gwen Araujo's killers were found guilty of murder despite their "panic defense" of surprise upon discovery of her male genitalia.

2014: "Lady Valor: The Kristen Beck Story"—a U.S. Navy SEAL lives as a transgender woman.

BOOKS

1918: "The Autobiography of an Androgyne" by Jennie June

1995: "The Apartheid of Sex: Manifesto on the Freedom of Gender" by Martine Rothblatt

2004: "Becoming a Visible Man" by Jamison Green

2007: "Omnigender: A Trans-religious Approach" by Virginia Ramey Mollenkott

2013: "She's Not There: A Life in Two Genders" by Jennifer Finney Boylan

2014: "Trans Bodies, Trans Selves" by Laura Erickson-Schroth

RADIO, PODCASTS, AND VIDEOS

2010: "Middle C"—a trans man and a soprano vocalist undergo hormone and surgical interventions. http://www.abc.net.au/radionational/programs/360/middle-c/3106624

2017: "Hidden Brain: Nature, nurture, and our evolving debates about gender"
https://www.npr.org/2017/10/09/556116385/nature-nurture-and-our-evolving-debates-about-gender

"The Accidental Gay Parents"—series of episodes on "The Longest Shortest Time" podcast
https://longestshortesttime.com/podcast-60-accidental-gay-parents

"The Science of Being Transgender" on Science Vs podcast
https://www.gimletmedia.com/science-vs/the-science-of-being-transgender

How to be a Girl
http://www.howtobeagirlpodcast.com/

Transgender Scientist
https://player.fm/series/the-transgender-scientist

Gender Reveal
https://www.genderpodcast.com/

TED TALKS

Jackson Bird at TED Residency (n.d.)
"How to talk (and listen) to transgender people"
https://www.ted.com/talks/jackson_bird_how_to_talk_and_listen_to_transgender_people

Geena Rocereo at TED 2014
"Why I must come out"
https://www.ted.com/talks/geena_rocero_why_i_must_come_out?referrer=playlist-the_gender_spectrum

Lee Mokobe at TEDWomen 2015
"A powerful poem about what it feels like to be transgender"
https://www.ted.com/talks/lee_mokobe_a_powerful_poem_about_what_it_feels_like_to_be_transgender

Karissa Sanbonmatsu at TEDWomen 2018
"The biology of gender, from DNA to the brain"
https://www.ted.com/talks/karissa_sanbonmatsu_the_biology_of_gender_from_dna_to_the_brain

CONFERENCES

Southern Comfort (Atlanta, GA)
https://sccfla.org/

WPATH (ANZPATH, CPATH, USPATH)
https://www.wpath.org/

Trans Wellness Conference (Philadelphia)
https://www.mazzonicenter.org/trans-wellness

MULTIPLY MARGINALIZED COMMUNITIES

Directory of LGBTQ People of Color Organizations and Projects in the United States
https://www.lgbtfunders.org/wp-content/uploads/2016/05/FLGI_POC_Dirctry_2009.pdf

Human Rights Campaign Resources: Communities of Color
https://www.hrc.org/resources/topic/communities-of-color

TransLatina Coalition
https://www.translatinacoalition.org/

National Queer Asian Pacific Islander Alliance (NQAPIA)—a network of Asian, South Asian, Southeast Asian, and Pacific Islander LGBTQ organizations
http://www.nqapia.org/wpp/

Network on Religion and Justice (NRJ) for Asian Pacific Islander LGBTQ people
http://www.netrj.org/index.html

National Resource Center on LGBT Aging
https://www.lgbtagingcenter.org/about/index.cfm

Mariposas Sin Fronteras: Supporting LGBTQ People in Immigration Detention
https://mariposassinfronteras.org/

Southerners on New Ground (SONG)—people of color, immigrants, undocumented people, people with disabilities, working class, and rural and small-town LGBTQ people
http://southernersonnewground.org/

Trans Student Educational Resources
http://transstudent.org/

GUIDES FOR LEADING CULTURAL TRAININGS

2009: "Teaching Transgender"—A resource from the National Center for Transgender Equality
https://transequality.org/sites/default/files/docs/resources/NCTE_Teaching_Transgender.pdf#overlay-context=press/releases/transgender-equality-and-federal-government

2017: "Best practices in creating and delivering LGBTQ cultural competency trainings for health and social service agencies," authors from the National LGBT Cancer Network
https://cancer-network.org/wp-content/uploads/2017/02/best_practices.pdf

PROFESSIONAL ASSOCIATIONS

American Medical Association
https://www.ama-assn.org/delivering-care/policies-lesbian-gay-bisexual-transgender-queer-lgbtq-issues

American Psychology Association: Transgender people, gender identity, and gender expression
http://www.apa.org/topics/lgbt/transgender.aspx

World Professional Association for Transgender Health (WPATH)
https://www.wpath.org/

Gay Lesbian Medical Association (GLMA): Health Professionals Advancing LGBT Equality
http://www.glma.org/

American Speech-Language-Hearing Association (ASHA): Providing Transgender Services
https://www.asha.org/Practice/multicultural/Providing-Transgender-Transsexual-Voice-Services/

POLICY AND LAW

Lambda Legal
https://www.lambdalegal.org/

National Center for Transgender Equality
https://transequality.org/

Transgender Law Center
https://transgenderlawcenter.org/

U.S. Department of Health and Human Services: Recommended actions to improve the health and well-being of LGBT communities
https://www.hhs.gov/programs/topic-sites/lgbt/enhanced-resources/reports/health-objectives-2011/index.html

ADVOCACY, EDUCATION, AND SUPPORT[6]

Trans Lifeline (run for and by trans people)
U.S.: 877-565-8860
Canada: 877-330-6366

National LGBTQ Task Force
http://www.thetaskforce.org/

GLAAD (formerly Gay & Lesbian Alliance Against Defamation)
http://www.glaad.org

Parents, Families, and Friends of Lesbians and Gays (PFLAG) Transgender Network (TNET)
http://www.pflag.org

Tyler Clementi Foundation: Advice on bullying, harassment, and humiliation
https://tylerclementi.org/

The Trevor Project: Crisis intervention and suicide prevention for LGBTQ youth
http://www.thetrevorproject.org

[6]Available on companion website for easy use of hyperlinks.

Out for Health
http://www.outforhealth.org/

INCLUSION PRACTICES

"A Guide for Being Inclusive of Transgender"
http://transvivor.com/transgender-inclusion.html

Trans-Inclusive Environments
http://www.the519.org/education-training/training-resources/trans-inclusion-matters

"Making Primary Care Trans-Friendly" (*The Atlantic*, 2017)
https://www.theatlantic.com/health/archive/2017/04/trans-medicine/523731/

"LGBTQ Inclusive Curriculum and Classroom Climate," Center for Ethics Education at Fordham University (a Jesuit, Catholic university)
https://www.fordham.edu/info/25663/education_and_research_ethics_resources/6346/lgbtq_inclusive_curriculum_and_classroom_climate

Center of Excellence for Transgender Health (Learning Center page)
http://transhealth.ucsf.edu/trans?page=lib-00-00

Georgetown National Center for Cultural Competence
https://nccc.georgetown.edu/

RELIGION AND FAITH
(with grateful acknowledgment to Oneida Chi)

Institute for Welcoming Resources
http://www.welcomingresources.org/transgender.xml

The LGBT Religious Archives Network
https://www.lgbtran.org/

Center for Lesbian and Gay tudies in Religion and the Ministry (Pacific School of Religion)
http://clgs.org

Human Rights Campaign Resources: Religion and Faith
http://www.hrc.org/resources/topic/religion-faith

Gender Diversity in Jewish Tradition
https://reformjudaism.org/jewish-lifesocial-justice-advocacy/jewish-views-on%E2%80%A6/health-wellnesscivil-rights/gender-diversity?

The Reformation Project
https://www.reformationproject.org/

QChristian
https://www.qchristian.org/

Transforming: The Bible and the lives of transgender Christians by Austen Hartke (audiobook read by the author, a transgender person AFAB)

CHAPTER 3

Practical Planning

After preparing ourselves to receive clients with some understanding of their cultural context, we are almost ready to think about assessment and intervention approaches. But first, you may be wondering:

Who is going to come?

Will they stay?

What will they want?

Disparities in health care access will not improve if we only learn about the clients we have. In addition to practical ways to serve our clients, we can consider practical ways to reach more individuals and open avenues of access to quality and timely health care. We should also wonder:

Who isn't coming for services? Why not?

Why might clients discontinue services?

How do I engage clients to participate in decisions about their care?

This chapter will address those practical questions. The ideas in this chapter are largely borne out of our disposition to notice and remedy areas in which we could improve our own practices. Connecting with colleagues to learn what they have noticed and tried in response to their local community's needs is another source of inspiration. Throughout this chapter we will highlight thoughtful and innovative colleagues who model ways to overcome some of the common barriers to voice services experienced by trans and gender-diverse populations.

WHO HAS ACCESS TO YOUR CARE?

Our voice clinic at the Speech and Hearing Center of George Washington University tends to serve Caucasian trans women, ranging in age from 20 to 60. The majority of our clients, but not all, are employed. We noticed this is not particularly representative of the trans people in our local urban surroundings. Careful not to make assumptions, we wondered why our clientele was not more diverse in race, ethnicity, and socioeconomic status. A dedicated team of student clinicians volunteered to search the literature for information about disparities in health care delivery and outcomes (see Chapter 2 for some of the disparities we found). We quickly noticed populations described as *multiply marginalized*, or identifying within intersections of minority statuses, were often reported to be facing multiple barriers. For example, trans people of color are more likely to live in poverty, be unemployed, and have greater health disparities than their Caucasian counterparts (James, Herman, Rankin, Keisling, Moffet, & Anafi, 2016). However, the type and degree of barriers to voice and communication services specifically is not apparent from the available literature.

In conceptual models of how people access health care (or don't), several barriers are proposed, ranging from financial and socioeconomic to discrimination and lack of competent providers (Safer et al., 2016). Additionally, barriers are identified at the individual, household, community, and population levels and are influenced by health systems, organizations, and individual providers. Levesque, Harris, and Russell (2013) synthesized several published frameworks to create a model of access to health care that considers both the provider and consumer perspectives. In their model, five dimensions of health care access correspond to various consumer abilities to progress through potential barriers and obtain positive economic, satisfaction, or health outcomes (Figure 3–1).

- Approachability: Does the person know the service exists and understand how it can impact them?
- Acceptability: How do the person's cultural and social factors influence their decision to seek care?
- Availability and accommodation: Do resources (i.e., providers) exist in adequate number and proximity? Are they able to be reached even by those needing accommodations for age, physical ability, and logistical feasibility (e.g., unable to access during typical working hours, availability of Internet access for telehealth)?
- Affordability: Can the person spend time and money to use appropriate services?
- Appropriateness: What is the quality of the technical and interpersonal aspects of the service? Is the client empowered to choose the service and participate fully in treatment decision making?

Guided by this model of access and barriers to care (Levesque et al., 2013) and in collaboration with students and local LGBTQ-focused health and wellness centers, we

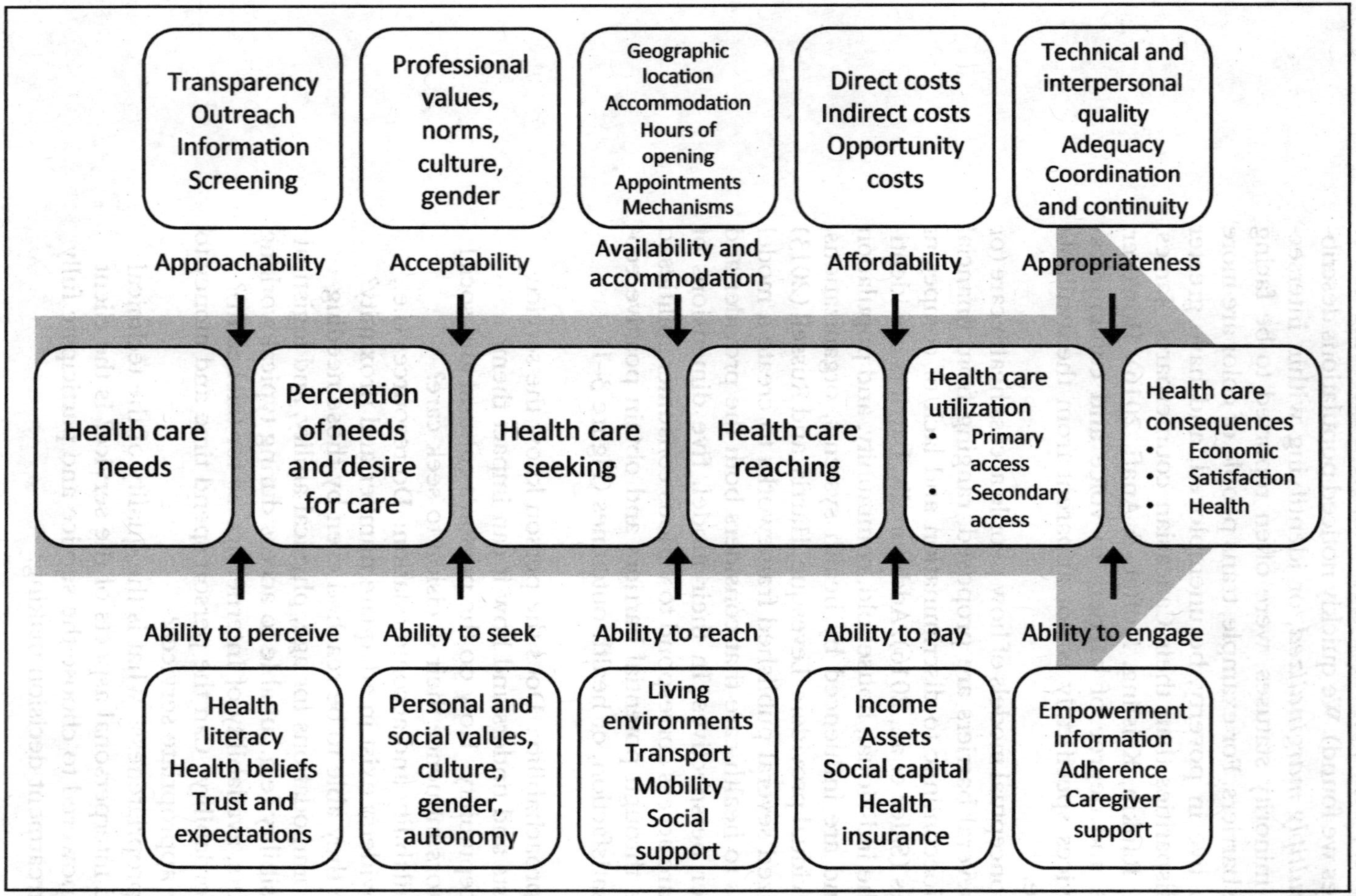

Figure 3–1. Model of Barriers to Positive Health Care Consequences from Provider (top) and Client (bottom) Positions. *Source:* Levesque, J-F., Harris, M. F., and Russell, G. (2013). Patient-centred access to health care: conceptualizing access at the interface of health systems and populations. *International Journal for Equity in Health*, *12*(18), 1–9.

conducted two focus groups to explore the specific reasons for our clientele's demographics. We wondered what gender-diverse people of color in our local community felt or knew, if anything, about voice and communication interventions for gender presentation. The quotes below represent some of the major themes that emerged.

> *" . . . you get ridiculed if what you look like doesn't match your voice."*
>
> *—Female AMAB, African American, 47 years of age*

> *"It can also be a struggle when you're trying . . . to come out of sex work and get a job . . . cuz* [sic] *when you get a job presenting like to the public, like when you're trying to get a job as a cashier or as a receptionist or as a nurse's aide even . . . front line stuff where you work in public, it can cause difficulty . . . it's really sad."*
>
> *—Female AMAB, African American, 60 years of age*

> *"I just feel like I would be phony."*
>
> *—Female AMAB, African American, 58 years of age*

> *"I don't think it's being phony."*
>
> *—Female AMAB, African American, 60 years of age*

> *"When I had heard about voice training in the past, I mostly only heard about it in the context of like, testosterone or a tracheal shave."*
>
> *—Third gender AFAB, Pacific Islander, 22 years of age*

> *"My understanding is that there aren't any [speech-language pathologists] for FtMs, and also that good ones which are trans-friendly are hard to find."*
>
> *—Male AFAB, African American, 38 years of age*

> *"For me, it's how much would it cost, do I have to pay with the Medicaid, if Medicaid would pay for it? Then a lot of people would go take that step."*
>
> *—Male AFAB, African American, 38 years of age*

APPROACHABILITY AND ACCEPTABILITY

From the focus groups, we learned almost immediately that the sample of gender-diverse people of color lacked information to make an informed decision, corresponding to the very first barrier in the model by Levesque et al. (2013). Even though there was strong consensus that voice played a significant role in self-satisfaction as well as desired gender attributions in personal and occupational roles, the focus group participants were generally unable to accurately describe the effects or availability of behavioral, medicinal, or surgical options to modify their voice. Obviously, before a consumer would desire to receive services, they would need to know about them and know what to expect from them. Yet professionals may take this step for granted because we typically only meet people who are seeking our services, or are at inquiring about the cost and availability of services.

Feedback within a person's social circles, including family and work, may influence prospective clients' opinions about services. For example, some cultures would not consider it acceptable for a cisgender female physician to see a cisgender male patient. Similarly, some family members may not be supportive of voice changes; acceptability barriers can mirror the barriers for transition in general. One of our AMAB clients was asked not to use her feminine-sounding voice at home around her wife and children until they were more comfortable with the idea of transition. Other clients are motivated to sound feminine at work for the sake of their coworkers and feel pressure to conform to gender stereotypes. These examples highlight how surrounding perceptions of acceptability influence the client's ability to achieve optimal outcomes. The acceptability factor is particularly relevant for people with low autonomy, such as adolescents or anyone dependent upon others for basic needs of housing, food, transportation, money, or employment.

According to the model by Levesque et al. (2013), if informed people decide they may benefit from such services, and it is conducive to their personal and cultural values, they will seek to approach an "acceptable" provider. Perceptions of a provider's acceptability are influenced by their professional values, personal statements and actions, and their own sociocultural positionings (e.g., gender, sexual orientation). Therefore, increasing the visibility of yourself and your services —particularly to those multiply marginalized such as trans people of color—is one important way to improve equitable access. Kevin Dorman, a speech-language pathologist (SLP) in North Carolina (USA), gave considerable thought to this issue when they decided to open a private practice largely devoted to transgender vocal training (see their story in Box 3–1). Consider what you can do to diminish barriers at this level.

Box 3–1

Kevin Dorman, MS, CCC-SLP (they/them/theirs)
Prismatic Speech Services

As a nonbinary SLP, advocacy for my community is central to my private practice, Prismatic Speech Services. I share my personal and professional expertise by leading discussions of transgender culture for businesses and student groups. Increasing awareness and understanding of LGBTQ needs in my local and professional circles is good for my community and good for my business. I'm involved in a local transgender-specific support group, the Southeastern Transgender Ally Initiative (SETAI), as well as the local chapter of PFLAG, a national nonprofit that support LGBTQ people and their families. I also volunteer as a voice teacher at Queer Oriented Radical Days of Summer (QORDS), a music- and activism-centered camp for queer and trans youth.

Many features of where I live and practice contribute to why people who want professional help modifying their vocal gender expression have limited options, including many rural areas and strict anti-LGBT laws (e.g., bathroom bills, voter ID requirements). Thus, telepractice is crucial for my practice. It provides access for the community I aim to serve, as well as financial sustainability by broadening my potential client base. Telepractice allows people to reach me from hours away, from the comfort and safety of their own home, and without time and money spent on transportation. I am currently licensed to provide services to clients in three U.S. states. The portion of my caseload receiving my services online has ranged from 50% to 90%.

I typically see people for 12 to 14 individual sessions, weekly at first then at increasing intervals as they become more independent and confident with technique. Occasionally people work with me for up to a year, particularly if they come to me with very little initial vocal flexibility (e.g., they have difficulty changing pitch or perceiving pitch change). These factors are typically detectable at the initial assessment, so if a client falls into this outlying group, we are able to discuss it upfront before they fully commit to this ongoing process. Most of my clients are white and middle-aged, though ages have ranged from 17 to 65 years. I have a couple transmasculine nonbinary clients, but most are transfeminine. When I started this practice, I offered discounted rates, as neither myself nor my practice had much of a reputation with the trans community and telepractice was fairly new to me. My clients appear to enjoy working with me, in person and remotely, as I receive a solid number of referrals from previous clients. Word of mouth is a powerful advertisement!

People who are still unable to access my resources include those with low income, not enough time to commit to the daily homework, and low emotional energy or motivation due to dysphoria or other factors. With these factors in mind, I decided to offer two free group sessions each month: one for beginners and one more advanced for clients who are discharged or close to discharge. I also develop and share educational material for free on my business' website.

My hope for this area of speech-language pathology is to incorporate more collaboration with professionals who are not SLPs but do this work (e.g., those who approach this work from an acting or singing background). I also hope the experience and expertise of trans and nonbinary practitioners can be highlighted as particularly valuable.

The examples below are not exhaustive, nor intended to be implemented only as described. Be creative and consider who you are trying to reach. Consider the following actions:

- Post educational material on your website, or links to information.
- Articulate your values and intentions in writing or in a video recording of yourself. Have this available on your website as well as upon entry to your workspace.
- Network with other voice specialists and other professionals who serve trans and nonbinary clients. Include voice and gender presentation whenever you describe—either verbally or in written material—your available services. Volunteer for professional organizations or local trans and gender-diverse support and advocacy groups.

- Provide educational material to local support groups. If invited to do so, give a guest presentation about voice or communication concepts.
- Get the attention of media outlets. Inform them about events, openings, human interest stories (with client permission of course). Make yourself available as an information source via programs such as "Help A Reporter Out" (https://www.helpareporter.com).[1]
- Use social media (e.g., Facebook, YouTube, blog, Twitter). Ventola (2014) describes the benefits, risks, and best practices for health care professionals using social media.

It is important to note that barriers may need to be addressed more than once, and new barriers may emerge after your initial inventory of them. Even after a client has attended sessions, they may reconsider their decision before they reach their desired outcomes. Efforts to create inclusive environments that respect and welcome diversity will keep the process open for them. Consider adopting transgender-affirming policies, such as those articulated with explanations by the Human Rights Campaign (HRC), Lambda Legal, and the LGBTQ Rights Committee of the New York City Bar Association (HRC, 2016). The Human Rights Campaign also developed 10 benchmarks of LGBTQ cultural competency and 3 levels of recognition for participating agencies (HRC, n.d.). Benchmarks generally relate to nondiscrimination policies, inclusive language on forms and reports, staff and consumer trainings and resources, and partnerships with community members and affirming organizations.

A Toronto-based group, The 519, is an abundant source of information and material useful for developing an inclusive environment. Practical actions include:

- Provide reading material (i.e., magazines, brochures) in the waiting area that reflects interests for people of a variety of ages, races, genders, and sexual orientations.

[1]The authors have never done this, but have been found by reporters nonetheless. Useful, brief tips for communicating with the media are available from: Center for Public Engagement for Science and Technology (https://www.aaas.org/pes/working-reporters), the American Association of University Professors (https://www.aaup.org/article/faculty-and-fourth-estate#.W2sWmdhKhE5), and the National Council for Behavioral Health (https://www.thenationalcouncil.org/wp-content/uploads/2016/11/Tips-for-Talking-with-Reporters.pdf).

- Post nondiscrimination policies in prominent locations in the facility, website, and marketing materials.
- Require all team members, including staff and volunteers, to have routine education about inclusive practices, particularly use of positive language.
- Use forms that acknowledge variation (i.e., write-in line for gender identity) and awareness of appropriate accommodations (i.e., legal name and another name).
- Implement and communicate practices that allow concerns to be acknowledged and addressed.

Routine review of your efforts and client satisfaction will guide continued improvement to accessibility. After Bockting, Robinson, Benner, and Scheltema (2004) conducted patient satisfaction surveys in their transgender health services center for 7 years, they were able to target three areas for improvement fairly easily:

- therapist caring and warmth (therapists made efforts to increase empathy),
- therapist promptness (pagers were introduced and each office got a clock), and
- staff friendliness and courtesy (new staff were hired with emphasis on customer service and comfort with gender and sexuality).

AVAILABILITY, ACCOMMODATION, AND AFFORDABILITY

A provider's visible commitment to cultural competency and considerate services can alleviate initial barriers of provider approachability and acceptability. Unfortunately, just knowing about and desiring the services doesn't mean people can reach the services. As the number of trans and gender-diverse people who feel comfortable enough to seek our services increases, more providers are needed.

Many SLPs are willing to provide services but want more guidance on evidence-based practices to follow. The interprofessional standards published by WPATH in 2011 added standards for voice and communication care. Now, the field is flourishing with more empirical evidence and opportunities to learn via presentations and written material. Graduate professional programs in the U.S. are beginning to incorporate gender issues in cultural training and gender presentation services in coursework and practicum experiences (Hancock & Haskin, 2015). Tricia Thomas is an SLP serving the trans community in many ways, including through her training of SLP students and colleagues (see Box 3–2 for her story).

Until qualified practioners are more prevalent, you may find yourself searching within your professional network on behalf of someone seeking services. Word of mouth is a powerful tool, particularly in marginalized communities wary of untested providers, so as you work with more clients you may get more inquiries. Even if someone is within a reasonable proximity, you may already have a full caseload, or may not be able to accommodate their work/school schedule or their insurance. Credentialing organizations may have searchable databases (e.g., ASHA's ProFind) or listservs that are helpful when searching outside of your local area.

Referral among trans-friendly providers is a common way access to services is gained. When a psychologist at Lurie Hospital's Gender and Sex Development program noticed a flyer for voice services nearby at the Northwestern University

Box 3–2

Tricia Thomas, MA, CCC-SLP (she/her/hers)
Portland, Oregon

I started my career as a school SLP in 2013, but I also have a background as a singer and voice coach. I have transgender people in my life and know that voice may be a huge barrier to safety and happiness. In 2014, I started to train speech-language graduate students from a local university to develop the skills needed to coach trans people to produce a voice that would be perceived as matching their gender. In January 2016, I contracted with the university to supervise two graduate students per year in order to give the students enough time to develop the production and perceptual skills necessary. Initial outreach to the transgender community left us with a waitlist so during summer term I invited two additional students.

When university space in downtown Portland was no longer available, I reached out to number of community organizations and eventually found a spot at Outside In, a center for marginalized people and homeless youth. Outside In agreed to provide a free, HIPAA-compliant space one night weekly. Collaboration with Kaiser Permanente's Gender Pathways Clinic and other medical and service providers frequented by transgender individuals have provided a steady stream of clients. In the meantime, I have trained university faculty to provide transgender voice services, and now they supervise graduate students in their program work with voice as well.

Student training focuses on cultural aspects, voice basics, forward resonance, and other elements of voice training pertinent to altering perception of gender. Because most students typically have no experience with voice work, a large part of their training comprises learning basic exercises used with clients and honing the perceptive skills essential to voice work. My students also agree to complete a project to support the program, including compiling a list of referrals, collating research data on client-reported outcomes, and professional presentations.

Resonance is the primary focus of my training and program, although students adjust the protocol based on the client's wishes. When the client and clinician reach a place of satisfaction, the client stops coming weekly and may check back in every 6 weeks or so. Additionally, near the end of the term, clients and clinicians may partner up for small group sessions in the clinic or out in a public space, in which the clinicians use preagreed-upon signals to indicate that their client should slow her speech, adjust resonance, and so on.

Clients have ranged in age from 15 to 78, and most are in their 20s. Some have good support systems but many are not as lucky. Because my program does not charge a fee, clients' most frequent barriers to care include mental health issues and unstable housing and/or job situations. These barriers manifest in a variety of obstacles including poor attitude, incomplete practice, missed sessions, and dropping out. Not surprisingly, clients who are able to commit to practice and who struggle less with getting basic needs met demonstrate greater satisfaction with results of coaching.

Center for Audiology, Speech, Language, and Learning, he invited SLP Nathan Waller to give a presentation about voice intervention options to the team there. Be Heard, a voice program specifically for trans youth, developed from this collaboration (see Box 3–3 for his story).

Not surprisingly, focus group participants asked about the costs of services. Coverage by government-supported health plans in the U.S. (i.e., Medicare, Medicaid, the military, and veteran's affairs) varies. Laura Cord, an SLP for the U.S. Department of Defense, has trans people on her caseload for

Box 3–3

Nathan Waller, MM, MA, CCC-SLP (he/him/his)
Northwestern University

A growing segment of the trans and nonbinary populations is under 18 years of age. In recent years, a growing number of programs in the U.S. have been established to specialize in providing gender-affirmative medical and mental health care to trans and nonbinary adolescents. Dr. Marco Hidalgo, Northwestern faculty and a psychologist at Ann & Robert H. Lurie Children's Hospital of Chicago, contacted me for information about available voice interventions for patients in the Gender and Sex Development program. I shared evidence and options for voice modifications, and I learned about the unique aspects of trans and nonbinary youth. Over time, a collaboration developed and now a Be Heard voice modification program is offered to youth each year through the Northwestern University Center for Audiology, Speech, Language, and Learning and the Gender and Sex Development program at Lurie Children's Hospital.

Small groups of five to nine youth are guided in learning and exploring vocal care and techniques by me and Sarah Penzell, MA, CCC-SLP, who supervises two graduate students who assist in the program. Over time we have determined that a 6-week program, with 90-minute sessions each week, is an appropriate and a logistically ideal commitment for our clientele. Evenings seem to be better, scheduling around school, extracurricular activities, and other health-related appointments. Every client is first individually assessed using standard auditory-perceptual and acoustic measures, and a discussion of their personal goals is held privately. We sometimes all work together, such as when discussing vocal care, and other times we separate into smaller groups for practice. We may invite them to go to one room if they want to explore lower pitches, another room for higher pitches, or yet another room for conversation-level work. Small groups based on target communication behaviors fosters a few of the many valued features of Be Heard:

- a nonbinary, inclusive environment,
- semi-individualized practice,
- engagement in decisions about their communication goals, and
- autonomy in gender expression.

Although not the case for all adolescents in the marginalized populations, most of our clients have supportive parents and are attending school. This may be due to our partnership and referral source. We get parental permission for treatment, HIPAA agreements, and charge our center's rates, though on a sliding scale. For clients without these supports and resources, we've partnered with Groupon to fundraise for scholarships. We find that most clients didn't realize professional services for voice modifications existed, let alone could facilitate such a degree of vocal change.

This time frame just allows for basic vocal care and exploration with techniques, but some vocal changes start and can be developed if and when the client is ready. Psychosocial outcomes see the greatest improvements. Participation in Be Heard is sometimes the first, or one of few, opportunities for clients to be in a peer group. As voice and communication are very social, the tenderness of using and changing voice can be experienced in this type of safe space.

(In 2018, Dr. Hidalgo joined the faculty of the Center for Transyouth Health and Development at Children's Hospital Los Angeles and is assistant professor of clinical pediatrics at the University of Southern California's Keck School of Medicine.)

voice modification services (see Box 3–4). Other health care systems, such as in Sweden, Canada, and Australia, appear to have more services available to a wider population. The

Box 3–4

Laura Cord, MS, CC-SLP (she/her/hers)
Walter Reed National Military Medical Center

In June 2016, Former Secretary of Defense Ashton Carter announced transgender persons could serve openly in the military and receive medical care and interventions for transition (Department of Defense Instruction 1300.28). As this policy was unfolding, Walter Reed National Military Medical Center (WRNMMC) was one of the primary military treatment facilities preparing to provide care for transgender service members from all branches of the U.S. military. A multidisciplinary team, including myself, was assembled and a monthly support group was established for service members.

To prepare for providing clinical services to this special population, I utilized internal WRNMMC resources and attended a continuing-education webinar. I also prepared by reaching out for advice and instruction from speech-language pathology colleagues experienced with this topic. My colleague and I even brought a service member to another local colleague for consultation. That's the beauty of this discipline: In addition to helping our patients, we help each other.

Communication assessment and intervention techniques at WRNMMC are comparable to those used in nonmilitary (civilian) settings. The person's communication behaviors and perceptions are assessed prior to intervention and reassessed upon program completion. I create activities to facilitate achievement of patient-developed goals. A variety of feedback is provided—initially by me, through a software application or even unfamiliar listeners. Eventually, we engage in more realistic interactions such as phone calls or even trips to the WRNMMC coffee shop.

Intervention is dynamic and patient centered, so the type and schedule vary. Typically, I start with 45- to 60-minute individual sessions on a weekly basis until target behaviors generalize to daily life. Then, I schedule treatment sessions as needed to tackle specific areas of desired focus. The total program runs for approximately 10 sessions, although I have seen patients for as few as three and as many as 20 sessions. The 1:1 approach allows the plan to be individualized and time to be fully devoted to the patient. In addition, our monthly WRNMMC support group seems to provide a support network and camaraderie that our patients really appreciate. I believe that the patient's comfort with the clinician and within the setting creates a foundation for success. Overall, I find these sessions to be fun and comfortable. For example, we allow ourselves to feel vulnerable while trying out a variety of voice productions and communication styles and usually end up laughing!

Some barriers to access to care and desired outcomes are similar between civilian and military settings (e.g., schedules, work demands, available support). However, the military setting presents other unique challenges. Some service members experience extended time away from home, resulting in gaps between practice sessions and a reduced support network. They may feel pressured to meet requirements for promotion to the next rank. There are often high vocal demands, such as background noise on a ship or airfield or maintaining the perception of leadership by using a "command voice." Service members must also adhere to appearance and grooming standards according to the sex assigned at birth until their gender marker is changed in their electronic medical records, which occurs when the medical care plan is completed. These include appearance and grooming standards (uniform, hair length, nail length, physical readiness [scores on physical fitness tests], and other gender-specific standards. These gender-binary standards may hinder the use of voice techniques in the work environment.

Access and quality of gender-transition care in the military has improved since 2016. However, congressionally mandated policies can shift abruptly, limiting clinical services, and may contribute to our patients' overall psychological stress.

The views expressed in this spotlight are those of the author and do not reflect the official policy of the Department of Army/Navy/Air Force, Department of Defense, or U.S. government.

politics of this is beyond the scope of this text, but nonetheless the availability and affordability of services in your area are worth considering.

If cost is a significant barrier, think creatively about ways to at least alleviate the burden. Some settings permit sliding scales according to income. Discounts according to student status, age, or in celebration of LGBTQ Month may provide an opportunity for someone otherwise unable to afford services. Some service delivery models can reduce costs for the providers, which translates to savings for the consumer.

Traditionally, clients are seen individually for a 45- to 60-minute session each week (Hancock & Garabedian, 2013; Mészáros et al., 2005; Söderpalm, Larsson, & Almquist, 2004). However, treatment effectiveness research has included a variety of schedules and durations of varied lengths; there is not yet evidence of a superior service delivery model. There are many options.

Oneida Chi and Judy Jewett developed a completely online program for groups of gender diverse people across California working to modify the communication aspect of their gender presentation. Participants log-on to the HIPAA-compliant platform weekly; the agenda alternates weekly between instruction with guided practice from an SLP, which has a sliding-scale fee, and group practice led by an experienced peer who completed a previous offering of the program, which has no fee (see Box 3–5 for their story).

One single-subject experimental design study with four trans women demonstrated impressive effectiveness using a pitch-monitoring app to supplement 10 to 11 weekly individual sessions of just 30-minute durations each, essentially reducing the cost for the SLP's time by half (Hawley, Hancock, & Simpson, in review). Additional research to directly compare the efficiency of models supplemented with technology, such as apps or telehealth, could guide us to more affordable methods.

Group sessions may reduce costs in that each session of multiple clients with one service provider might be less expensive than individual attention, but it is unknown whether the pace of progress would slow given presumably less practice and feedback compared to a one-on-one session. On the other hand, realistic practice settings may improve learning and generalization. After group sessions twice per week for eight weeks, five "male-to-female" clients were perceived as less masculine-sounding, and perception as female increased from 1.9% to 50.8% in this short time (Gelfer & Tice, 2013).

Box 3–5

Oneida Chi, MS, CCC-SLP (they/them/theirs)
Bay Area OUTspoken Speech Services

Judi Jewett, MS, CCC-SLP (she/her/hers)
Jewett and Associates, Inc.

The program began when Judi's family member explained that she was transitioning and that she had gender dysphoria regarding her voice. She had hoped Judi would be her speech therapist. After working on her voice for some time, there was not the progress she and Judi had hoped for. Simple book learning regarding gender presentation of voice was insufficient, and they needed a way to practice with safe practice partners.

Judi and Oneida teamed up to offer an online group program. The group meets online once a week for 45 to 60 minutes; each session begins with a privacy agreement. Every other week the sessions are led by the two SLPs; alternate weeks are led by group practice leaders, who are often participants from previous groups who want more practice. The program runs for three months, so the SLPs lead six sessions, which are billed individually because a lump sum was prohibitive for some people, and the practice group leaders lead six sessions, which are free. SLP sessions cover pitch, intonation, resonance, articulation, nonverbal communication, communication style, and content. When the SLPs teach a skill at a beginning or word level, then the group practice covers these skills at the next level, such as sentence or conversational level. The free group sessions are available to clients who have been through the program before, or clients that therapists are seeing individually. As it turns out, participants in one city know each other and practice when they get together. Participants in another city have also met up occasionally for pizza or coffee. The current group has seven people working toward a more feminine-sounding voice: Three are new regularly-attending members and others have enrolled in prior groups or drop-in sessions.

Judi and Oneida split the cost of the Zoom platform with encryption and a business associate's agreement. Participants have two apps, if possible: the equivalent of Pitch Perfect and Voice Analyst, so they can get a cue for the intended pitch and have a way to analyze their productions. It is recommended, if possible, to pay for the version that enables them to keep the recordings to track and take responsibility for their progress. Many clients come to the clinic for an evaluation prior to starting the group, but if that is not possible, they at least have an online consultation.

The group model helps people be accountable and provides safe conversation partners, proving to be an invaluable component of success for these clients. In-person groups have some advantages, but in some areas it can be difficult to recruit enough people and schedule sessions. The evening, online delivery appears particularly useful for reducing financial burdens of transportation and time off work, and for relieving the anxiety of going out in public, sitting in a waiting room, and practicing with cisgender people. While most clients present as themselves in the group, some still present as their assigned gender at work or even still at home. For people who do not have a safe place to practice or access to Internet, the clinic is offered as a place to come and participate. Participants have been very happy with the group, one even calling the opportunity to learn and connect "a dream."

Group settings seem to be most beneficial for clients toward the end of their program, when they need to practice with a variety of people but still in a safe space. However, groups can be particularly challenging when clients are not yet comfortable with the space and the clinicians or are still learning techniques and finding their voice. In these instances, pairs or triplets may be more appropriate.

The voice clinic at the Speech and Hearing Center of George Washington University has experimented with intensives. During one 4-hour program, clients are paired with student clinicians for a brief initial assessment, followed by a group orientation to the techniques, two individual treatment sessions and, finally, elective stations tailored to skill levels and practice needs. We have been able to serve discharged clients requesting a "tune up" but not needing to occupy a session spot for an entire semester, as well as clients on the waitlist who wanted something to work on until a semester spot became available, and clients who couldn't commit to weekly sessions through a semester for a variety of reasons (e.g., financial cost, schedule, readiness). From just one intensive session, a sample of nine transwomen demonstrated a median gain of 2 semitones (ST) in reading and 3 ST gain in conversational speech (Hancock, Siegfriedt, Goldstein, & Friedman, 2016). Progress varied greatly by individual, with gains in semitones and listener perceptions correlated with fewer years presenting in full time female role and less time in previous voice treatment. In other words, the intensive format was most useful for the people from the waitlist, possibly because they had more to gain. This conclusion is consistent with motor learning theory, in that blocked practice and consistent feedback is most beneficial during the initial, acquisition stage of motor learning.

In an effort to respond to what we learned about barriers to care from our review of the literature and the local focus groups, we offered a free, modified intensive workshop for vocal feminization at the LGBTQ-friendly health center (Giegerich, Davis, Griffiths, & Hancock, 2018). Nine adult transgender and gender nonconforming individuals (all AMAB) learned and practiced adjusting vocal characteristics of pitch, resonance/quality, and intonation in small groups led by six graduate SLP students and supervised by the authors. As these were all people naive to voice services, the workshop began with education about the process and testimony from a transwoman who had finished voice services. Again, group orientation to the techniques was followed by guided practice in small groups. Speaking fundamental frequency (F0) increased by a mean of 2.8 ST, although there the range of improvement varied from .9 ST to 4.6 ST. Participants went home with practice material and audio recordings of their practice and target productions. At the conclusion of the workshop, and in follow-up phone calls two weeks later, participants were very satisfied with the experience. They desired a longer workshop, and most felt they would continue to improve with practice. They reported that resonance was particularly challenging to practice on their own at this stage of the process.

Further research is needed to determine long-term outcomes of intensive formats and compare to traditional service delivery models. It is of note that the authors' experiences with intensives are made possible by available and eager student clinicians who have completed a semester of supervised practicum with a trans client already. Even with the personnel, financial flexibility, and local collaborations, the university can only manage to offer one or two intensives per year. After these intensives, clients, students, and all feel rewarded by the experience. Every barrier that is overcome matters and brings trans people closer to accessing high-quality desired outcomes.

APPROPRIATENESS

After a client has sought, found, and committed to your services, the final barrier to accessing desired health outcomes is "appropriateness" (Levesque et al., 2013). Described as the degree of fit with the client's need and the quality of care spent in assessing and planning treatment, appropriateness of care is dependent on your clinical competency. The following chapters are all designed to support clinical competency in the technical sense. Information and prepatory practices described in the first three chapters of this book, however, are integral to interpersonal aspects of clinical competency. Having both will strengthen the chances that client will be engaged and ultimately access optimal care.

In the final barrier category of the Levesque et al. model (2013), appropriateness is evaluated by the degree to which the client is choosing and participating fully in the interventions. Unfortunately, the psychomedical perspective in trans health care positions the provider as significantly more powerful than the client because they are the so-called gatekeeper to accessing medical care. A social perspective, however, appreciates society's limited conceptualizations of sex and gender and does not view the client as pathological or incapable of discerning their own identity. A survey of 415 trans-identified individuals confirmed clients' desire for opportunities to communicate and provide feedback to their health care providers. A vast majority (96.5%) want high decision-making power in treatment-associated decisions (Eyssel, Koehler, Dekker, Sehner, & Nieder, 2017). Thus, a client-centered approach is most appropriate for working in this area of gender and communication (Figure 3–2; Hancock & Azul, 2017).

In a client-centered approach, the client's needs and wants remain central to all services. Assessment and interventions are guided by empirical evidence and clinical expertise, but the client's role in decision making is central. This requires assessment of not only the biological integrity and function of the voice, but also the cultural factors involved in constructing gender and the impact on the client's well-being.

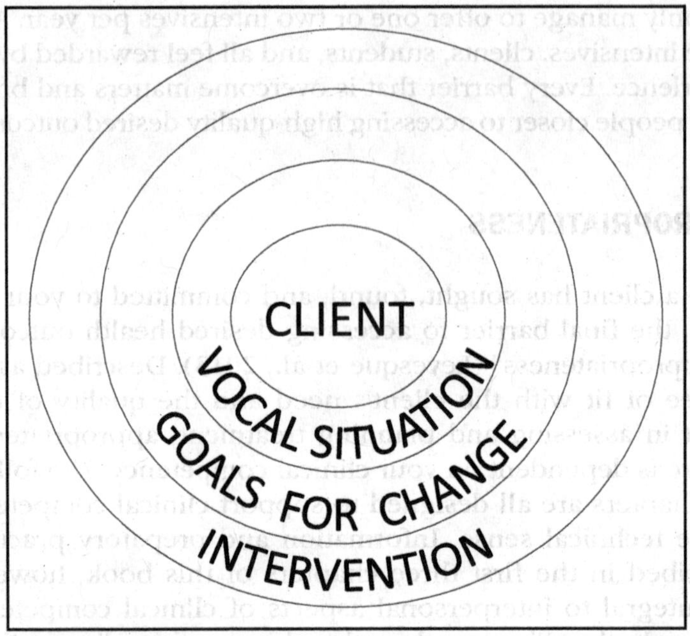

Figure 3–2. Client-Centered Care Model for Voice and Communication Services. *Source:* Hancock, A., and Azul, D. (2017). *Cultural and clinical considerations for EBP with transgender and gender nonconforming people*. ASHA presentation, Los Angeles, CA.

This assemblage has been described as the "vocal situation" (Azul, 2015; Hancock & Azul, 2017) and assessment of it is described in Chapter 4. Informed by the assessment results, as well as understanding of the scope and limits of the client and clinician's capacity to contribute, goals are determined in a collaborative manner (see Chapter 5). Finally, intervention(s) are selected. The competent clinician is equipped to support the client in their physical, emotional, and mental marathon toward ultimately accessing the desired outcomes.

CONCLUSION

Access and barriers to care are serious concerns for trans populations. Providers have a professional and social obligation to mitigate barriers to our services. This could take many forms, from education and advocacy to investment in your clinical competency and donation of services. After considering the barriers and practical solutions described in this chapter, take time to write down your action-oriented responses to the questions opening this chapter:

Who is going to come?

Will they stay?

What will they want?

Who isn't coming for services? Why not?

Why might clients discontinue services?

How do I engage clients to participate in decisions about their care?

REFERENCES

Azul, D. (2015). Transmasculine people's vocal situations: A critical review of gender-related discourses and empirical data. *International Journal of Language and Communication Disorders, 50*(1), 31–47.

Bockting, W., Robinson, B., Benner, A., & Scheltema, K. (2004). Patient satisfaction with transgender health services. *Journal of Sex and Marital Therapy, 30*(4), 277–294.

Department of Defense Instruction 1300.28. (2016). *In-service transition for transgender service members.* United States Office of the Under Secretary of Defense (Personnel and Readiness). Retrieved from Defense Technical Information Center: http://www.dtic.mil/

Eyssel, J., Koehler, A., Dekker, A., Sehner, S., & Nieder, T. O. (2017). Needs and concerns of transgender individuals regarding interdisciplinary transgender health care: A non-clinical online survey. *PLOS One, 12*(8), e0183014.

Gelfer, M. P., & Tice, R. M. (2013). Perceptual and acoustic outcomes of voice therapy for male-to-female transgender individuals immediately after therapy and 15 months later. *Journal of Voice, 27*(3), 335–347.

Giegerich, A., Davis, K., Griffiths, S., & Hancock, A. (2018). *Community partners facilitate access to voice and communication services for transgender and gender-diverse people.* Presented at GW Research Day, Washington, DC.

Hancock, A. B., & Azul, D. (2017). *Cultural and clinical considerations for EBP with transgender and gender non-conforming people.* Presented at the ASHA Convention, Los Angeles, CA.

Hancock, A. B., & Garabedian, L. (2013). Transgender voice and communication treatment: A retrospective chart review of 25 cases. *International Journal of Language and Communication Disorders, 48*(1), 54–65.

Hancock, A., B. & Haskin, G. (2015). Speech-language pathologists' knowledge and attitudes regarding lesbian, gay, bisexual, transgender, and queer (LGBTQ) populations. *American Journal of Speech-Language Pathology*, *24*, 206–221.

Hancock, A. B., Siegfriedt, L., Goldstein, N., & Friedman, R. (2016). *Transgender voice: Treatment outcomes from two service delivery models.* Seminar presented at the ASHA Convention, Philadelphia, PA.

Hawley, J., Hancock, A., & Simpson. (In review). *Effects of a voice treatment program including home practice using mobile technology on voice feminization.*

Human Rights Campaign (HRC). (n.d.). *All children—all families: Tiers of recognition.* Retrieved from https://www.hrc.org/resources/all-children-all-families-tiers-of-recognition

Human Rights Campaign (HRC). (2016). *Creating equal access to quality health care for transgender patients: Transgender affirming hospital policies.* Retrieved from https://www.hrc.org/resources/transgender-affirming-hospital-policies

James, S. E., Herman, J. L., Rankin, S., Keisling, M., Mottet, L., & Anafi, M. (2016). The report of the 2015 U.S. transgender survey. Washington, DC: National Center for Transgender Equality.

Levesque, J-F., Harris, M. F., & Russell, G. (2013). Patient-centred access to health care: conceptualizing access at the interface of health systems and populations. *International Journal for Equity in Health*, *12*(18), 1–9.

Mészáros, K., Vitéz, L., Szabolcs, I., Goth, M., Kovács, L., Görömbei, Z., & Hacki, T. (2005). Efficacy of conservative voice treatment in male-to-female transsexuals. *Foliz Phoniatrica et Logopaedica*, *57*, 111–118.

Safer, J. D., Coleman, E., Feldman, J., Garofalo, R., Hembree, W., Radix, A., & Sevelius, J. (2016). Barriers to health care for transgender individuals. *Current Opinion in Endocrinology, Diabetes, and Obesity*, *23*, 168–171.

Söderpalm, E., Larsson, A., & Almquist, S. (2004). Evaluation of a consecutive group of transsexual individuals referred for vocal intervention in the west of Sweden. *Logopedics Phoniatrics Vocology*, *29*(1), 18–30.

Ventola, C. L. (2014). Social media and health care professionals: Benefits, risks, and best practices. *Pharmacy and Therapeutics*, *39*(7), 491–499, 520.

PART II

Press On

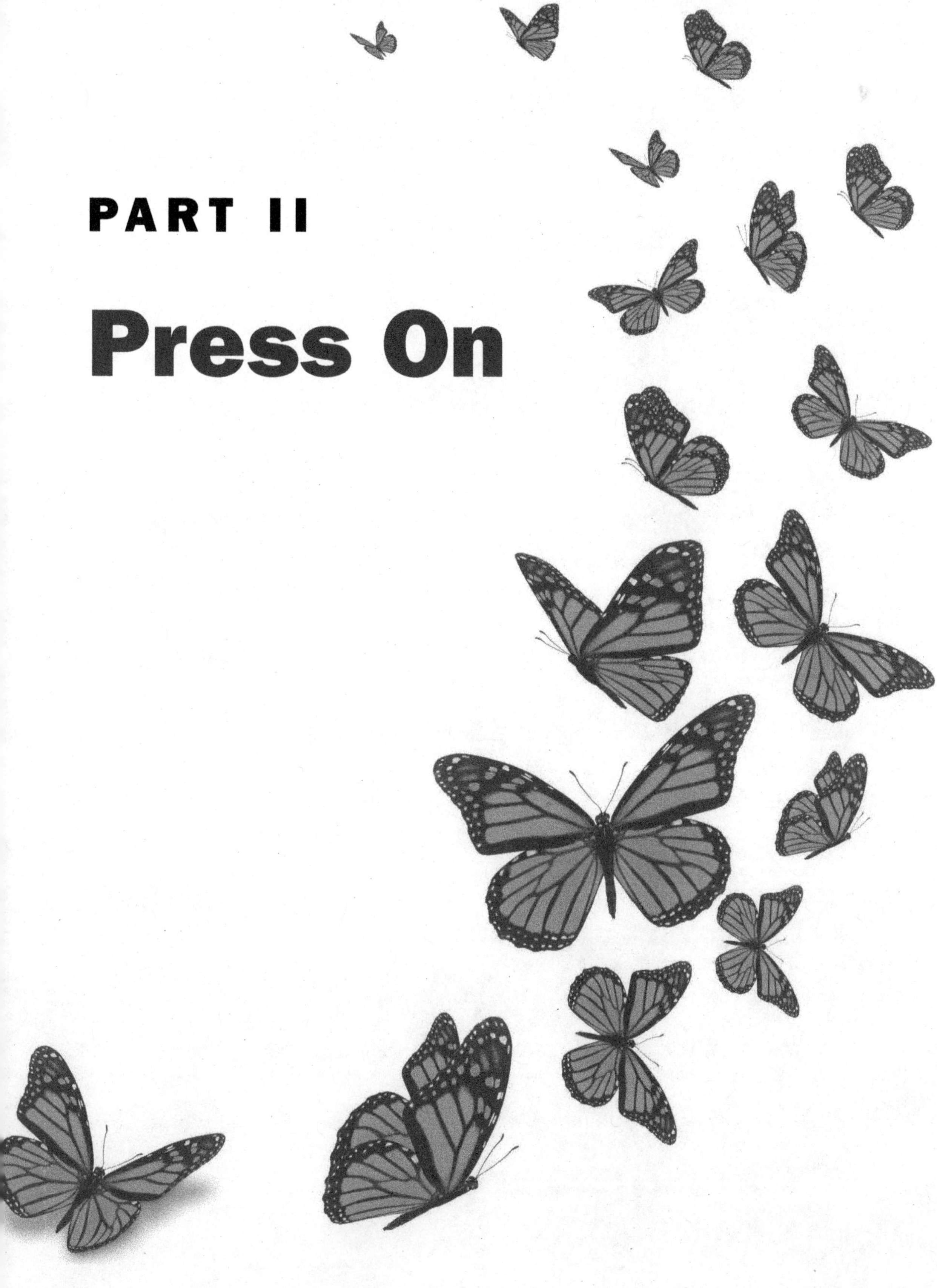

CHAPTER 4

Assessment

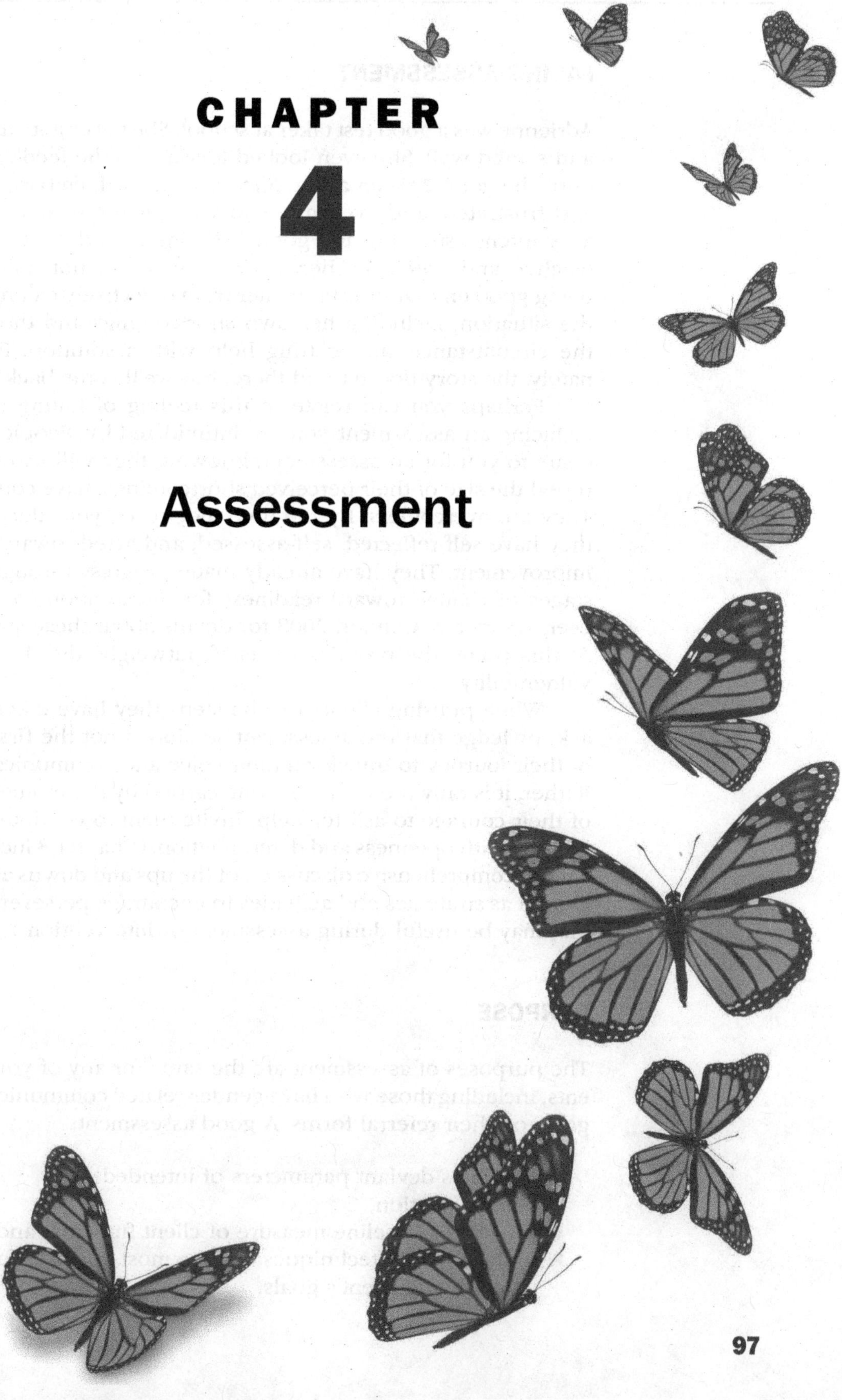

FACING ASSESSMENT

Adrienne was a good test taker at school. She never got anxiety, and scored well. She even looked forward to the feedback—until she got a 26% on a test. She was shocked, embarrassed, and frustrated, and even more so when she retook the test after intense studying and got a 35%. She cursed the test, the teacher, and especially herself. The shame of not doing or being good enough prevented her from objectively examining the situation, including her own shortcomings and those of the circumstance, and getting help with a solution. Fortunately, the story doesn't end there, but we'll come back to it.

Perhaps you can relate to this feeling of failing a test or facing an assessment you are intimidated by. People who come to you for an assessment, knowing they will learn and reveal the size of their perceived shortcomings, have courage. They are overcomers. By the time they reach your doorstep, they have self-reflected, self-assessed, and acted toward self-improvement. They have already made progress through the stages of change toward readiness for intervention (see Van Leer, Hapner, & Connor, 2008 for details about these stages). At this point, the promise of relief outweighs the threat of vulnerability.

When praising clients for the steps they have taken, we acknowledge that the assessment session is not the first day of their journey to transform their voice and communication. Rather, it is only the next step, one carried by the momentum of their courage to ask for help. Invite them to continue that journey with openness and determination. (Chapter 8 includes a more comprehensive discussion of the ups and downs ahead, as well as strategies and activities to encourage perseverance, that may be useful during assessment or intervention.)

PURPOSE

The purposes of assessment are the same for any of your clients, including those who have gender-related communication goals on their referral forms. A good assessment:

- identifies deviant parameters of intended communication,
- provides a baseline measure of client function, and
- indicates what techniques may be most effective for reaching the client's goals.

Assessing for the presence of a voice disorder—even when that is not the client's stated reason for coming—is important because it will greatly influence the rest of the assessment, let alone intervention planning. There are many wonderful references about traditional voice assessment that detail the use of various instrumentation and measures (Baken & Orlikoff, 2010; Colton, Casper, & Leonard, 2011; Ferrand, 2019). We assume readers of this book already have a basic level of knowledge and skills related to speech production, assessment, and intervention. It is beyond the scope of this book to cover diagnosis of a voice disorder, but we want to emphasize the importance of this competency when working with voice for any reason.

It seems reasonable to expect hyperfunctional voice disorder in a person habitually speaking in a new frequency range, especially a higher range. Desired changes can be achieved by straining the body—a maladaptive habit that will need to be addressed. For example, fundamental frequency (F0) is increased by tension in the internal laryngeal muscles and the supralaryngeal muscles. Articulating with forward tongue carriage to adjust resonance and raise the second formant (F2) is another common goal in voice feminization. One way to achieve this is to prolong contraction in the mylohyoid and anterior digastric muscles, which could also contribute to laryngeal tension problems.

Recent attention to the vocal function of "transmasculine"[1] people uncovered problems with voice quality, limited pitch range/variability, and vocal power (Azul et al., 2017). In the largest study of "trans men's" voice to date, 18% (nine out of 50) of participants self-reported vocal quality concerns, and voice range profiles revealed restricted pitch range in 31% (11 out of 36) and restricted volume range of 100% (36 out of 36). More research is needed to understand the severity and basis of these vocal restrictions (Nygren, Nordenskjöid, Arver, & Södersten, 2016).

Incidence of voice disorders in trans people varies widely in the literature from 0% to 100%. Perceptual, acoustic, and aerodynamic measures in descriptive studies of 25 (Holmberg, Oates, Dacakis, & Grant, 2010) and 13 (Gorham-Rowan & Morris, 2006) "male-to-female transsexual" people have not identified hyperfunctional voice or disorders. In contrast, in a study using stroboscopic examination, slight supraglottic

[1]As explained at the beginning of this book, we use quotation marks to indicate terms used by the authors of the cited study.

constriction of both ventricular folds was observed in nine (100%) "male-to-female transsexual" people, and approximation of epiglottis and arytenoids in eight of the nine. Only six of nine (67%), however, reported strain and/or fatigue, and no diagnoses of muscle tension disorder or other voice disorders were made (Palmer, Dietsch, & Searl, 2011). Another study using stroboscopy found that 13% of trans people[2] have pronounced constriction during their preferred phonation, 39% have moderate, and 48% have none. Only one patient had laryngeal pathology: a "minor sulcus on one vocal cord" (Söderpalm, Larsson, & Almquist, 2004, p. 21).

Most of the people in these studies of vocal function had not received professional voice treatment. Clients with voice disorders may have additional challenges and therefore may be more likely to come for our services. In a chart review of 25 trans women receiving voice treatment between 2006 and 2010, only one had a voice disorder diagnosis (bilateral sulcus vocalis), four (16%) were noted to have mild or mild-moderate dysphonia, and two others (8%) self-reported vocal strain (Hancock & Garabedian, 2013). This prevalence is greater than that of the general population, reported to be 1% to 7% (Cohen, Kim, Roy, Asche, & Courey, 2012; Roy, Merrill, Gray, & Smith, 2005).

In studies of gender-related intervention effectiveness, participants with concomitant voice disorders are typically excluded; therefore, we know little about the impact voice disorders have on our clients or on their prognoses. Still, all factors that need to be treated prior to or in conjunction with transforming habitual voice should be identified, as this process alone can be delicate. If there are findings that indicate underlying physical issues, a laryngologist must be consulted to assure the safest passage for the client, and optimal treatment. If a client does have a voice disorder, we don't want them to carry it into their new voice. See Box 4–1 for two case examples of this happening.

In the case of a client with a generally healthy speech mechanism but desiring transformation, we assess communicative function. Together, you and the client must figure out the current status and the desired status, and estimate the gap between these. More specifically, you can inventory[3] the client's communication behavior patterns associated with

[2]The sample in this study consisted of 22 "male-to-female" and three "female-to-male transsexuals."

[3]*Inventory* is a term we use for *examine* that sounds less clinical.

Box 4–1

A 45-year-old woman AMAB with an unremarkable medical history was seen for approximately eight months for voice feminization before she began to demonstrate changes in quality that were initially subtle but appeared to be progressing. Vocal quality was becoming less and less stable. We discussed it with her and referred her to a laryngologist. His examination revealed idiopathic unilateral vocal fold paresis. We had to treat this issue before we could proceed with the plan for a feminine-sounding voice. She was then able to finish the intervention and is now satisfied with her speaking and singing voice.

A 55-year-old trans woman arrived for her evaluation with a consistently rough, weak voice. She seemed to have low energy and moved as if she was working against resistance. Posture was slouched in both standing and sitting positions. Speech rate was reduced, intensity was reduced, and breathing was shallow. Her F0 was lower than most cisgender male normative data. Examination by a laryngologist ruled out laryngeal pathology. We asked her primary physician for a neurology consult to rule out a neurological disease, and to meanwhile grant permission for her to start working with an athletic trainer to increase muscle tone, improve posture, and general energy level. This helped enormously with her respiration and voice quality. In her case, elevating pitch for the feminization process contributed to additional dramatic improvements in her voice quality. Although the laryngologist did not report it, vocal characteristics were consistent with presbyphonia. Regular physical workouts and vocal exercises for changing pitch and resonance facilitated vocal function overall and enhanced the vocal feminization process for this client.

(Note: These clients had different preferences for how to be described: "woman AMAB" and "trans woman.")

production of gender within their culture. For this purpose, there are particular parameters of speech and language worth focusing on and additional considerations to include when interpreting the findings. We will go into more detail about these below. Also, see Appendix 4–A for an example of an assessment report for a client AMAB wishing to feminize their gender presentation. As with any assessment, initial measures identify baseline levels and inform direction of intervention. Rationales and research supporting the decision to address (or not) these various communication parameters in intervention is covered in depth in the next chapter.

We offer one final reminder before we get to specific protocols. In every facility we have worked in, whether it was a medical center, university, or private practice, the assessment protocol is different. Whatever your setting, you will have to be comfortable enough with the overall purpose and your protocol outline to be able to completely let go of the protocol once you are in the session so that you can be fully aware of what is going on in the session, and not be distracted by what has to happen according to your specific plan. As discussed in Chapter 1, your clinical intuition is a valuable part of client-centered care. Keep the client's well-being and purposes as your utmost priority.

EARLY CONVERSATIONS

Let the client know you want to honor them by addressing them as they wish while you get to know one another. It may help to give your own examples, such as, "Hi, I'm Dr. Hancock. Please call me Adrienne and use she/her pronouns." Cisgender people introducing themselves with pronouns makes trans people doing it normal rather than forcing them into a position as the "other" or the "exception" to the rule. If they don't follow suit after your self-introduction, it is okay to ask directly if they have thought about or decided what name you should use while you are in the room together. Assure them you intend to respect their privacy and honor their wishes, and that it is okay if the name used in the room is different than what they use outside—including in the waiting area or on the phone and email communication. You may be one of the few people in their lives that uses that name and pronoun. In other cases, the name given to them at birth—and still listed on the insurance account—is not used anymore and is now distressing for the client to hear. Make sure office staff and others seeing the client's birth name and current name are aware of when to use which name.

Acknowledge or inquire about several aspects of their whole identity before diving in with questions about why they are seeing you today. Look for topics to ask about in their history forms: relatives, occupation, locations where they want to use their voice, such as, "I see you are in finance. My father was in the mortgage business. I'm interested—what drew you to that work?" This builds rapport for therapeutic alliance and communicates that this is going to be about their whole person, not just the sound coming from their mouth. It also provides information about their communicative demands, available support, and general personality.

The client's sources of support may include other professionals, so request written permission to talk to those for coordinated care. The client is often, but not necessarily, seeing a psychiatrist, psychologist, or counselor to learn how to cope with experiences of gender dysphoria or distress, unsupportive people in their family or work environments, or obstacles navigating related health services. In addition to their general medical practioner, clients may have ongoing care from specialists such as endocrinologists for hormone therapy. You will work closely with a laryngologist if there is suspected voice disorder or if the client is considering, or has already had, voice surgery. Even interventions seemingly unrelated to communication, such as egg harvesting prior to testosterone therapy, may have an effect on their ability to allocate time or attention to voice change. Fortunately, some settings are designed to facilitate coordinated care and can serve as models for interdisciplinary care. Sweden, for example, has six specialized teams to serve every individual diagnosed with gender dysphoria in their national health care system (Södersten, Nygren, Hertegård, & Dhejne, 2015). Each team consists of psychiatrists, psychologists, and social workers who evaluate and diagnose by consensus, and then refer to endocrinologists for hormonal treatment, speech-language pathologists (SLPs) for voice and communication assessment, gynecologists for germ cell preservation, dermatologists for hair removal, and reconstructive plastic surgeons for gender confirmation interventions (Södersten et al., 2015). Collaboration with a local health or community center, as described in Chapter 3, can also facilitate coordinated assessment and goals for care.

INVENTORY

When following a client-centered model of care, it is imperative to understand the client. Everything else, including assessments during your first session, will be dependent on the clinician's understanding. Forms and standard surveys often begin this process. Example forms are provided in Appendix 4–B, but you are encouraged to modify as you see fit. Note the inclusive language used!

Asking clients to answer complete forms prior to arriving has a few advantages. Answering the questions at their leisure in a private space may allow the client to be less anxious and provide more thoughtful answers compared to a rushed job in a waiting room. They can consider their answers with their confidant, counselor, social worker, or other care team member. Seeing the questions in advance orients them to what will be covered in the session so they can begin increasing awareness of their voice and gender presentation if they have not already. Clients may feel more at ease about the upcoming appointment as they notice the inclusive and thoughtful language on the forms. For the clinician, having forms completed in advance allows more time in the session for you to review the information on the forms, including any questions that were skipped or answered vaguely.

Consider carefully which forms to assign in advance. While some forms cover standard billing or medical history information that would apply to anyone, others will be specific to the client's gender positioning and goals, which you may not know prior to meeting them. More general questions about their gender positioning, presentation, and attributions would be appropriate for presession forms if it is not yet clear what their goals are when they schedule the appointment. For example, ask them to make two lists: one describing who the client (use desired name) is, and one about who they aren't (Helou, 2017). These lists may include adjectives, adverbs, titles, metaphors, or even pictures. The following paragraphs will describe the development of more standard questionnaires tailored for clients with gender-related communication goals.

As with many clients seeking voice and communication services, the first assessment activity is the client providing information about their physical, functional, and emotional state. These categories may sound familiar because they are subsections of the Voice Handicap Index (VHI) (Jacobson et al., 1997). The VHI, however, is not ecologically valid for gender-related voice concerns. In other words, it does not capture the voice's impact on the health and well-being of a gender-diverse person. In one of the earliest efforts to document voice as a source of dysfunction for trans people, T'Sjoen et al. (2006) found no indication of disability or handicap according to VHI scores of 28 "male-to-female (MTF)" and 20 "female-to-male (FTM)" middle-aged people, most of whom were taking cross-sex hormones. Yet, scores on one extra question regarding how they were addressed in telephone conversations (i.e., when the listener evaluates gender based on speaker's voice alone) were quite high for the MTF group and more consistent with the clients' reported experiences and feelings of disability.

With the need for a customized tool evident, Davies adapted the VHI for use with trans people. This adaptation, the Transgender Self-Evaluation Questionnaire (TSEQ), was printed in the first edition of Adler, Hirsch, and Mordaunt (2006) and again in the second edition (2012). Of the TSEQ's 30 items rated by the client as occurring on a 1 (never) to 5 (always) scale, some are identical to the VHI (i.e., "People have difficulty hearing me in a noisy room"), some are altered (i.e., "I am less outgoing because of my voice" instead of "voice problem") and some are completely unique (i.e., "When I laugh, cough, or sneeze I sound like a man [MTF]/woman [FTM]"). The TSEQ can be used with trans men or women. A small (n = 14) study of trans women indicated the TSEQ has concurrent validity with the VHI and Voice-Related Quality of Life (V-RQOL), and has good test-retest validity (Hancock, Krissinger, & Owen, 2011). That exploratory study also found that scores on the TSEQ correlated with speakers' perceptions of their vocal femininity and likability, as well as with listeners' perceptions of the same (Hancock, Krissinger, & Owen, 2011). These findings provided rationale for feminizing vocal quality to impact well-being, and motivated practitioners to include self-evaluation measures when documenting and quantifying intervention outcomes. You may notice the TSEQ used as an outcome measure in studies documenting effectiveness of voice intervention (e.g., Hancock & Helenius, 2012).

As the TSEQ was reviewed and tested over the next decade or so, it was refined and evolved into a questionnaire distinct enough to warrant its own title: the Transsexual Voice Questionnaire for Male-to-Female Transsexuals (TVQ^{MTF}). In an excellent example of community involvement in research, the initial review and revision of the TSEQ was a collaboration involving two SLPs and two "MTF individuals" comparing the TSEQ to themes extracted from interviews with 14 "MTF transsexuals" at LaTrobe University in Australia. Key changes included improved item clarity and specificity in instructions for trans women to complete the questionnaire "based on your actual experience of living as a female" and the addition of items to capture the effect of emotion and mood on voice, vocal quality problems, and discrimination because of voice (Dacakis, Davies, Oates, Douglas, & Johnston, 2013, p. 314).

Currently, the TVQ^{MTF} is the standard and recommended measure of the trans female client's self-perception of their physical, functional, and emotional voice function. It has demonstrated content and construct validity, internal consistency, and reliability (Dacakis et al., 2013; Dacakis, Oates, & Douglas, 2017; Davies & Johnston, 2015). Authorized translations of the TVQ^{MTF} in a dozen languages are available for free download (http://www.shelaghdavies.com/questionnaire/questionnaire.html). A limitation of the TVQ^{MTF} is that it is specific to people desiring a female presentation. The TSEQ remains the tool of choice for trans men. There are no formal tools designed for nonbinary people, though select items or adaptations of items on these questionnaires could be useful.

With a slight shift in focus from the health and impairment target of the VHI-like questionnaires to an objective that is more helpful for identifying and prioritizing specific areas of (dis)satisfaction for the client, clinical researchers developed an alternative/complimentary measure to the TSEQ or TVQ^{MTF}: the Functional Communicative Satisfaction Questionnaire (FCSQ). Clients rate both their satisfaction with and importance of 30 items on a scale of 1 to 11. Items were developed based on five themes derived from focus groups of 12 middle-aged "MTF transsexuals" living full time in the female role in Victoria, Australia (Pasricha, Dacakis, & Oates, 2008).

The five themes identified by Pasricha, Dacakis, and Oates (2008) are informative for understanding and exploring areas of importance to women of similar circumstance. The major themes from the focus groups were communicative situations, groups of people, emotions, other contributing factors, and features of communication. Communicating in situations involving the telephone, shopping, and noisy environments were commonly discussed, and the importance placed on maintaining "female communication patterns" was much greater if talking to strangers compared to their friends and family. Participants also discussed that any emotional expression, whether positive or negative emotions, interfered with their effort to use those patterns. There were several other factors for satisfaction that varied more by individual, including self-perception and confidence in their being able to be perceived as a woman by others. Perhaps most important is what concerned the participants about their communication the most and least: their voice was most likely to betray their birth gender, and their body language was already satisfactory because it came naturally to them, and in fact was sometimes the reason others perceived them to be a gay man before they transitioned. It is important to note the trans women in the focus groups desired to be, and put effort toward being, perceived by others as female, which is typical but not necessarily what all clients are seeking.

There are no normative data available for any of these questionnaires, so no threshold or severity ranges have been determined yet.[4] In our opinion, the most appropriate uses of these questionnaires are to compare comparing pre- and post-intervention status, and to be a starting point for a face-to-face interview. There are some questions that clinicians like to ask in the interview, rather than on a form, so as to begin to develop a rapport and to be able to go into depth for certain kinds of information. This gives the clinician a better sense of the client and their issues, and how the client relates to those issues. There is value to witnessing how a client responds to certain kinds of questions.

VOCAL SITUATION

Next in the assessment, you will explore the client's vocal situation, described by Azul (2015a) and Azul et al. (2017) as including voice production, vocal behaviors, meanings others attribute to the voice, and the cultural context in which this all occurs. The term *vocal situation* rather than *voice* or even *voice function* is apt because we are not exploring a static object or even event. Rather, as presented in the ASSEMBLE model (Chapter 3), the client's positioning of gender and other aspects of their sociocultural belonging is shaped by ongoing and dynamic forces including, but not limited to, vocal anatomy and physiology.

As discussed in Chapter 2, we cannot assume to know the client's gender identity/positioning, goals of gender presentation, and desired gender attributions. We certainly can't assume their level of satisfaction with each of these, or what contributes to it. Box 4–2 contains categories of questions with follow-up questions to use if the jargon terms get in the way. Experiment by answering them about yourself—it may be more difficult than you think! Appreciate the vulnerability and trust required for a client to share this information with you.

---

[4]Dacakis, Davies, Oates, Douglas, & Johnston (2013) report descriptive statistics for each item of the TVQ^{MTF}, based on their 35 participants from Australia and Canada.

Box 4–2

Gender Positioning

How do you describe your gender?

- Are you comfortable using terms like man, woman, masculine, feminine? What terms do you like?
- Can you describe how you position your gender identity in various ways, perhaps depending on the place or people around you?

How do you wish to present your gender identity?

- What style of clothing or shoes to do you like wear?
- What steps have you taken to change your presentation? (electrolysis, clothing, hairstyle, makeup, cosmetic surgeries, binding)
- What do you like about how you look and sound?
- Is there anyone you'd like to look or sound like? What is it about them?

Is there a gap between current and desired gender presentation?

- How would you like to look and sound to yourself?
- On a scale of 1 to 10, how satisfied are you with your gender presentation?

Gender Attribution

How do others tend to classify your gender?

- Do people call you ma'am or sir?
- Does it vary by context (phone, strangers, coworkers)?

How do you wish to be perceived and addressed by others?

- Do you have a preference for what pronoun people should or shouldn't use when referring to you?

- What do you do now that you think makes it more/less likely that you get the correct attribution?

Is there a gap between current and desired gender attribution by others?

- How often do you get misgendered?
- What do people misunderstand when they see or hear you (incorrect age, sexual orientation, or other types of social categories)?

One's gender positioning is not necessarily indicative of how they want to be addressed (Azul, 2015b). For example, they may identify as genderqueer but request he/him pronouns. In a study of 14 transmasculine people in Germany, there were six different positions among the participants (male, queer male, bigender, nonbinary, agender, ambivalent), but the majority wanted others to attribute male gender to them, and some had no preference or a slight preference hierarchy. Never assume!

It will be useful to gauge the client's psychosocial well-being, that is, view of their self and how they respond to stress caused by social misgendering (Hancock & Azul, 2017). How far are they from their goal, and how do they feel about that? What effects does that shortfall have on their relationships and participation in life activities? What is their response when they are misgendered, and is it harmful or helpful? Describing and analyzing specific instances is most informative (Azul, 2015b). Their answers to these questions influence the direction and pace of intervention. This is a good time to introduce the idea that a comprehensive approach to functional communication includes learning how to advocate and negotiate for one's desired gender attributions from others. You could present it as interpersonal communication skills. While you hope and expect this skill will become less and less necessary as their communicative behaviors transform, it might be unreasonable for them—or you—to expect a time when they will never be misgendered or misidentified in some way, particularly by people who knew them before they began modifying their gender presentation. Offering this for consideration early in the relationship and with the assurance of support and intention to address it is a kind way to begin setting reasonable expectations.

VOCAL FUNCTION

Assessment of the function aspect of vocal situation, also thought of as vocal ability, involves the areas and measures considered with every voice client and not specific to gender-related goals (Azul et al., 2017). The inventory collected with a form such as Appendix 4–B includes relevant medical and voice history. Information is relevant if it could influence diagnosis, prognosis, or intervention decisions. Common notable medical concerns for these populations include anxiety and depression, smoking, reflux, neck or shoulder muscle pain/tension, and thyroid function. Body modification practices, such as chest binding, can impact respiratory and phonatory function. Onset and extent of stress can impact the physical and emotional foundations necessary for voice work. We are particularly interested in any changes within the last year, such as events, surgeries, and illnesses, that could impact the speech system. Type, dosage, and initiation date of medications should be noted, especially those related to gender presentation such as cross-sex hormones.

Understanding how the person has already tried to change their vocal presentation is helpful for two main reasons. First, it provides insight on the level of knowledge and skills the person has for perceiving and producing sometimes subtle vocal changes. Ten years ago, clients came with no knowledge of the term *resonance*. Perhaps due to the proliferation of peer tutorials on the internet, many clients now come not only familiar with the term but have also attempted to modify their resonance. Second, it provides insight on what techniques work for the person—or don't. Without a professional guiding measured voice change, it is easy to habituate behaviors of vocal strain, particularly when elevating vocal pitch. Some techniques or behaviors may have to be unlearned before healthy vocal change can begin.

Box 4–3 has a brief list of the common measures for clients who do not exhibit signs of a voice disorder. Visualization of the larynx, via laryngoscopy or stroboscopy for example, is currently not required in the WPATH Standards of Care or best-practice literature (Davies, Papp, & Antoni, 2015). This is because our clients do not inherently have a voice disorder. If the clinician, via perceptual or instrumental measures, suspects a voice disorder, then a full evaluation including visualization of the larynx and exam by a laryngologist is needed prior to commencing gender-related communication intervention. It is

Box 4–3

Subjective Measures

- Breathing and posture
- Tension or asymmetries
- Musculoskeletal exam
- Oral mechanism screening and hearing screening
- Vocal quality, including resonance
- Prosody (rate, intonation, pitch) and articulation during standard reading passage and monologue

Acoustic Measures

- F0, F0sd of sustained vowel
- SFF and ST range used during connected speech
- Maximum phonation frequency range (MPFR)
- First–Third formants (F1, F2, F3) during corner vowels, at least /i/ and /a/
- Cepstral peak prominence
- Habitual pitch level (HPL)
- Maximum dB SPL range

important to refer the client on the basis of suspected voice disorder—rather than a gender-related issue—to be consistent with the standards of practice and for billing accuracy.

Elicitation Tasks

Protocols for collecting all these measures are beyond the scope of this book, but there are a few special considerations for application with gender diverse people. Realize and respect the difficulty of these tasks for some people. Explain to the client that you are checking to verify[5] overall health but also seeing what there is to work with, so you want to know all about their voice, including the parts they might be embarrassed about or not like right now. Still, do not be surprised if it takes a few sessions for them to truly feel comfortable using and showing all parts of their vocal ability.

[5] ***Checking to verify*** is another phrase that can replace ***examining*** to provide a less clinical atmosphere.

Speaking—even just a sustained vowel—at a frequency level they have been avoiding (e.g., trans men producing their highest pitch) often elicits an emotional reaction. This can range from surprise to discomfort to outright anxiety. There is no need to distress the patient beyond reason; simply note the limitation in your final interpretations.

If the client is using more than one voice—one masculine and one feminine, for instance—you should assess all of them for a voice disorder. It is possible only one of the voices will exhibit hyperfunction, which will bring complications later. For example, the feminine-sounding voice will not improve if the client keeps using a disordered masculine-sounding voice during the day.

Samples of connected speech, whether it be reading sentences or providing monologues, may vary in vocal parameters depending on the topic or even the other people in the room (Hancock & Rubin, 2015; Leaper & Ayres, 2007; Palomares, 2004). Therefore, select gender-neutral material for assessment so you can make comparisons over time. Material used in practice, however, can be stereotypically gendered if it is highly relevant for the client's goals.

Acoustic Parameters

The acoustic parameters most likely to be addressed and show change will be fundamental frequency during sustained phonation (F0), speaking fundamental frequency (SFF), maximum phonation frequency range (MPFR), habitual pitch level (HPL), and the first and second formants (F1 and F2, respectively). Indicators of vocal quality (e.g., voice turbulence index, cepstral peak prominence), vocal power or effort (e.g., intensity), and vocal stability (e.g., pitch breaks) should also be monitored. Appropriate intervention target ranges for these measures will be covered in the next chapter; for now, the focus is on accurate measure of baseline function. Recognize that coaching and encouragement to reach the boundaries of the client's abilities will influence the results, so develop a protocol you feel comfortable with and be consistent.

For all frequency measures, data should be reported in hertz (Hz) as well as semitones (ST). Hertz seems familiar and comfortable because most of us can remember that cisgender adult males speak near 100 Hz, whereas cisgender adult females speak near 200 Hz. Even clients, especially those who consult the internet before your intake appointment, may come to you with a single goal of "I want to be as close to 200 as I can get!" If you are only measuring one speech sample, using hertz to describe it is fine, but usually you are measuring at least two samples. If you compare a before- and after-intervention sample or calculate the range between the lowest and highest frequencies (i.e., MPFR), using hertz is deceptive. Perception of frequency (Hz) is logarithmic, not linear, while perception of difference between each ST is linear. The difference between 100 Hz and 105 Hz is 0.84 ST, but the difference between 200 Hz and 205 Hz is 0.43 ST. Therefore, increasing SFF by 5 Hz is a larger feat—almost twice the difference—for someone speaking at the low end of the scale compared to someone speaking at the higher end. Perhaps more importantly, the 5 Hz difference at the low end of the scale sounds like a bigger difference to our ears. Figure 4–1 is a graph of SFF measured three times prior to intervention (baseline) and once every 10 weeks of intervention. Each week the SFF increased by 10 Hz, but the slope of that change is quite different by the last week. According to the Hz measure, progress is steady at 10 Hz per week. However,

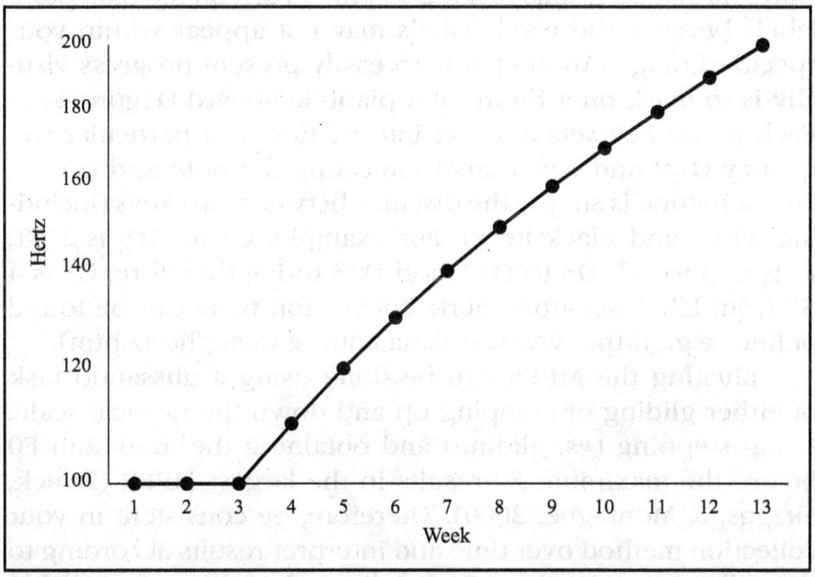

Figure 4–1. Graph of SFF measured three times prior to intervention (baseline) and once every 10 weeks of intervention. Gain, as measured by semitones, is diminishing despite a consistent 10 Hz gain each week of intervention. Semitones correspond to our auditory perception and are therefore a valid measure to describe change.

the ST measure and auditory perception show that progress is in fact slowing. Therefore, it is necessary to track progress using the ST measure.

Calculating the range between notes, required for the MPFR measure, must also be done with ST. The 20 ST range from G2 to D4 is 196 Hz. The 20 ST range from G4 to D6 is 782 Hz because it is much higher on the scale. According to the ST measure, these two people (or two occasions of the same person) are equivalent in their range. According to the hertz measure, the latter has a significantly greater range. Report MPFR in ST unit of measure, but also include the minimum and maximum to indicate where on the scale the range covers. For example, it is not unusual for trans women to have similar MPFR at the beginning and the end of intervention, but reaching new high notes and no longer reaching the lower notes of her original range (Mesaros et al., 2005; Gelfer & Tice, 2013; Gelfer & Van Dong, 2013). Trans men, on the other hand, are quite variable as to whether the MPFR will have an overall increase or decrease as it shifts downward on the scale during the first year of testosterone treatment (Hancock, Childs, & Irwig, 2017).

If your hertz data is in Excel or similar spreadsheet software, format the y-axis to a log 10 scale. Turn on the data point labels because the y-axis labels may not appear within your specified range. Another way to easily present progress visually is to mark on a figure of a piano keyboard (Figure 4–2). Each piano key sets a string into motion at a particular frequency (Hz) and has a label indicating the note and octave. One semitone is simply the distance between two keys (including white and black keys). For example, C3 to C#3 is 1 ST, as is C#3 to D3, D3 to D#3, and D#3 to E3; therefore, C3 is 4 ST from E3. A semitone-hertz conversion table can be found online (e.g., http://www.indiana.edu/~emusic/hertz.htm).

Eliciting the MPFR can be done using a glissando task of either gliding or stepping up and down the musical scale. Using stepping (vs. gliding) and obtaining the minimum F0 before the maximum F0 results in the largest MPFR (Zraick, Skaggs, & Montague, 2000). Therefore, be consistent in your collection method over time and interpret results according to the collection procedure. Free online calculators are available for precise results of range in ST (e.g., Go to http://users.utu.fi/jyrtuoma/speech/semitone.html and enter 100 to 105 and click *calculate*. Next try 200 and 205).

HPL is a calculated measure, reported as the percentage of the total MPFR that SFF is above the minimum F0. For

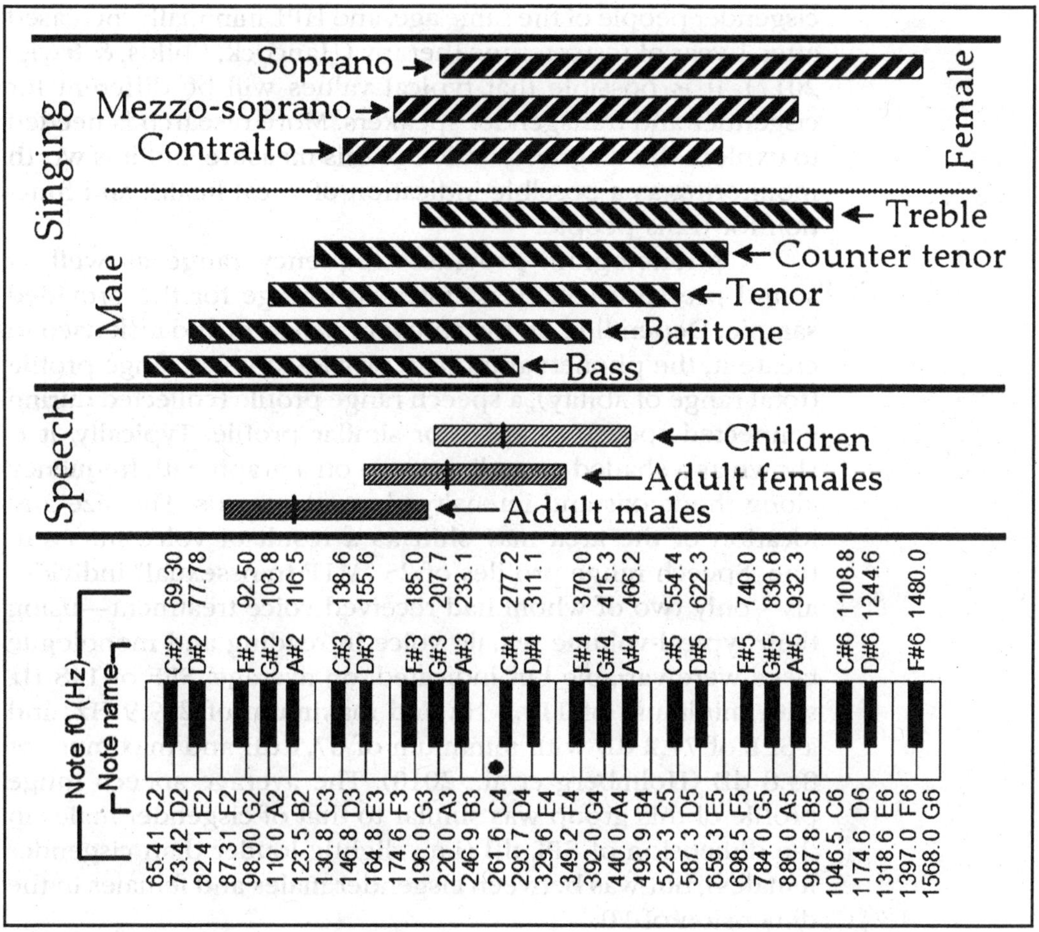

Figure 4–2. Frequencies and semitones along the scale. *Source:* Reprinted with permission from Howard and Murphy (2008). *Voice science acoustics and recording.* San Diego, CA: Plural Publishing.

example, if the client's MPFR is 40 ST and their SFF is 10 ST above the minimum F0, then they have a 25% HPL. Unlike SFF or MPFR, HPL is not different between cisgender men and women, singers and nonsingers, or young (age 20 to 35) and middle-aged (age 40 to 55) people. (Brown, Morris, Hicks, & Howell, 1993; Morris, Brown, Hicks, & Howell, 1995). Conventional wisdom cautions against speaking in the top of your range, although there is little empirical data to define a threshold or document consequence. Two studies in the early 1990s indicate habitual pitch for cisgender adults is approximately 13% to 20%, with elderly cisgender people (older than 65 years) tending to have the highest HPL (25% to 26%) (Brown et al., 1993; Morris et al., 1995). HPLs of seven trans men (i.e., 5% to 16%) were significantly lower than reported HPLs for cisgender people of the same age, and HPL minimally increased after 1 year of testosterone therapy (Hancock, Childs, & Irwig, 2017). It is possible that typical values will be different for cisgender and transgender speakers. More research is needed to explore the diagnostic value of this measure, but it is worth monitoring as a possible indication of vocal health and function for trans people.

A phonetogram provides frequency range as well as sound pressure level (i.e., intensity) range for the provided sample. Depending on the software program and task used to create it, the phonetogram may provide a voice range profile (total range of ability), a speech range profile (collected during connected speech sample), or similar profile. Typically, it is shown as a shaded or outlined area on a graph with frequency along the x-axis and intensity along the y-axis. The size and location of the area may shift as a result of voice intervention. Speech range profiles of 25 "MTF transsexual" individuals—only two of whom had received voice treatment—using their typical-volume female voice in reading and monologue tasks were variable but indicated, on average, SFF of 148 Hz with minimum of 110.3 Hz and maximum of 239.9 Hz, and a SPL of 77.2 dB with minimum of 67.1 dB and maximum of 84.8 dB (Holmberg et al., 2010). The average speech range profile of this group was similar to that of cisgender males in the dimension of SPL dB (i.e., slightly louder than cisgender females), but was between cisgender males and females in the dimension of F0.

Aerodynamic Parameters

Aerodynamic measures of gender-diverse people's voices have been reported in the literature but don't seem to play a large role in applied practice for gender-related interventions. You may collect these measures in assessment, however, if you suspect a voice disorder is present. Airflow, air pressure, and SPL as a collection can be useful for seeing changes across voice intervention toward a healthy voice production (Zeitels, Hillman, Desloge, Mauri, & Doyle, 2002). In two studies of aerodynamic measures of trans women, somewhat high airflow rates but no evidence of hyperfunction were found in these speakers. Importantly, the airflow values did not correlate with listener perceptions of the speaker's breathiness nor femininity. Airflow values slightly higher than those provided in cisgender norms appear to be typical for transfeminine speakers, but they do not need to be part of an outcome measure for goals related to perception of gender. Holmberg et al. (2010) evaluated 25 "MTF transsexual" adults and found a mean estimated transglottal pressure of 7.7 cm H_2O, glottal airflow of .272 L/s, SPL of 79 dB, and syllable F0 of 193.1 Hz.

COMMUNICATION, BROADLY DEFINED

Additional aspects of verbal and nonverbal communication may also be evaluated. Although there is very little evidence to support contribution to gender attribution, the client's language form and use, posture, hand gestures, and other nonverbal behaviors occasionally influence the overall communicative function. These are highly influenced by context and culture. This issue is discussed further in Chapter 5 in context of considering variables to target in intervention planning. Typically, if one of these presents an obstacle to the client's gender-related goals, you will notice it immediately during the interview. We have not felt it necessary nor valuable to dedicate much time to these factors during assessment.

STIMULABILITY

Stimulability testing—sometimes called dynamic assessment or a probe—guides us to techniques that may stimulate improved vocal function. To start this process, review your impression of the client and the assessment results and identify areas you can improve with some coaching and the appropriate technique (e.g., laryngeal massage, verbal cue or model) or treatment focus (e.g., elevate pitch, change resonance). The idea is to start with the simplest solution first. Once you identify which approaches are most effective, you have a place to start and can apply them during the first session.

Easy production of a clear voice without hoarseness or vocal fry will be a priority for every client, so we often start with simple semioccluded vocal tract exercises (Chapter 7; Guzman et al., 2018). Sometimes, this also facilitates a forward resonance and more precise articulation, both found to be associated with a feminine-sounding voice (see Chapter 5).

It is common to work on pitch directly; for example, elevating F0 for a transfeminine client. You will find that by elevating F0, the client's vocal quality sometimes completely clears. Remember that the body always wants to return to balance, so once the tension from speaking at an inappropriately low level is released, the rest may take care of itself.

People are different, and so will be each intervention. What works for one may not for another. Stimulability testing is a place to start. If it only alters one or two of the parameters, try a second and third technique. Most of the techniques used to improve production by people with voice disorders can serve gender-related goals. Chapters 6 and 7 will go into more details about techniques and targets to consider.

ANALYSIS

As you collect information through the various subjective and objective measures covered in this chapter, organize it by what it indicates about the client and their vocal situation. Compare to available cisgender or transgender data, or to data from studies about perception of gender (see discussion of these in Chapter 5). Distinguish normal from abnormal voice. Draw connections between findings that have the same indication. This breakdown process is analysis. Skilled clinicians do not wait until the assessment is over to start analysis because it may lead them to do more—or fewer—of the assessments described here. When you have enough information, you need to weigh and consider the raw ingredients as well as the analysis you have conducted.

EVALUATION STATEMENT

As appropriate for your professional and licensed scope of practice, you will need to provide an evaluative summary and prognosis statement. You may characterize the communication diagnosis as incomplete vocal feminization/masculinization, or perhaps more appropriate for nonbinary clients, vocal incongruence. *Gender dysphonia* has been defined in the literature as a condition in which the client's voice "is not consistent with the desired gender" (de Bruin, Coerts, & Greven, 2000, p. 221). The American Speech-Language-Hearing Association (ASHA) recommends using the ICD-10 code R49.8, "Other Voice and Resonance Disorders." You should also include any other physical or mental health diagnoses the client already has if they will impact service delivery or effectiveness (e.g., gender dysphoria in the F64 series, a voice disorder, respiratory disease).

Depending on what assessment you do, consider CPT code 92524 for evaluation and 92507 for treatment. Demonstrating medical necessity is key to insurance coverage in the United States. Coverage varies by carrier, and changes are likely in the coming years. Considerations and resources for billing and reimbursement in the U.S. can be found on ASHA's website (on.asah.org/trans-tx). Information about U.S. Medicare coverage can be found here: https://transequality.org/know-your-rights/medicare and for services in the U.S. Veteran's Health Administration check here: https://transequality.org/issues/resources/veterans-health-administration-transgender-health care-directive

PROGNOSIS

Most assessment is focused on characterizing the client's current status, perhaps relative to desired goals. The client will likely also want to know what they can expect in terms of extent and pace of progress but unfortunately we cannot know the results in advance. Research and clinical reports indicate that the rate of change is extremely variable. There is some information to guide our best guess, but we should be careful to make no promises.

Some people will transform quickly but have a difficult time stabilizing and habituating the new voice. Others will struggle until one day they sail through several levels in one session—often around the time they have a progress spurt in their emotional and mental well-being as well. Progress can also take a sawtooth pattern of ups and downs but overall improvement. In other cases, one parameter may lag in progress and hinder the overall effect. In a case study of one female "transsexual," F0 of vowels increased from 110 to 205 Hz in 4 months, but it was not until her resonance (F2) increased that she was consistently called "ma'am" on the telephone—11 months and 88 sessions after starting intervention (Mount & Salmon, 1988). In our experience, progress depends more on what is happening in the individual's life than on their anatomy or starting level.

Duration and Type of Intervention as Factors

Clients taking testosterone will mostly likely see few vocal changes after the first year, although in one study of seven trans men there were four different patterns of F0 change in response to testosterone: all within the first 6 months, within months 3 to 9 only, gradual over 12 months, and no significant change (Irwig, Childs, & Hancock, 2017). Whether a trans-feminine client is on cross-sex hormones does not appear to directly influence prognosis for behavioral voice intervention.

In a retrospective chart review of 25 trans women, the number of sessions averaged 22 but ranged from 2 to 77. The person requiring 77 sessions over 2.5 years began with an SFF of 80 Hz and MPFR of only 14 ST. Furthermore, this was in a university clinic, so intervention was conducted by supervised graduate clinicians and was interrupted by semester breaks. Spacing out or condensing sessions over time likely has an influence, but it is unknown whether it is a help or a hinderance. Other reports of fewer cases vary in schedule: weekly 45- to 60-minute sessions for three to more than 45 sessions, with an average of 17 sessions (Söderpalm et al., 2004); weekly sessions for 8 to 19 months, or approximately 32 to 76 sessions (Mészáros et al., 2005); and twice-weekly small group sessions for 8 weeks, or 16 sessions (Gelfer & Tice, 2013). Of course, the variability of vocal change across participants in these studies is large, but it is not entirely explained by the variation in duration of intervention.

Number of treatment sessions may predict a trans woman's overall increase of SFF, but it does not predict final SFF, nor whether listeners will perceive her voice as feminine sounding (Hancock & Garabedian, 2013; Holmberg et al., 2010). In other words, people continue to make progress with each session, but some take longer than others to reach their highest/best SFF because people start and end at different levels. It is important not to get too focused on SFF, though. After three "MTF transsexual" clients attended sessions twice per week for 6 weeks (12 sessions) and also performed vocal function exercises twice per day at home, SFF increased to an average of 177 Hz and listeners' femininity ratings of their voices indicated they sounded significantly more feminine, yet the percentage of listeners identifying each client as female was only 14.8%, 7.4%, and 0% (Gelfer & Van Dong, 2013).

Intervention target also does not result in consistent outcomes across participants. Ten "MTF transsexuals" followed a limited protocol focused on articulation to advance oral resonance for just five 45-minute sessions. On average, they increased F0, formants, and self-perceptions of feminine voice quality. Listener perceptions of feminine-sounding voice, however, varied greatly, with seven (70%) improving to some degree but two (20%) actually becoming more masculine sounding. This is a good illustration of the variation of responses to a single intervention, as well as the occasional weak link between acoustics and listener perception.

Client Characteristics as Factors

Client features and circumstances unrelated to gender may affect interpretation of data as well as intervention plans and prognosis. Research shows the voice is impacted by age, occupation, voice demands, general health and physical condition, neurological diagnoses such as ALS, systemic hydration, personality, and stress (Roy, Bless, & Heisey, 2000; Roy et al., 2005; Verdolini, Titze, & Fennell, 1994).

There is some indication that trans women of a younger age are more likely to have a feminine-sounding voice (i.e., a group averaging 43 years old vs. a group averaging 56 years old) (Palmer et al., 2011). One report of an adolescent in the literature showed excellent improvement in 15 sessions over 7 months (Hancock & Helenius, 2012). However, in another study, SFF, MPFR, and intensity did not correlate with age for 25 trans women (Hancock & Garabedian, 2013).

Portion of time using the techniques may be related to progress, based on simple principles of practice frequency. The client's mental health, stability, and general commitment to the work should be factored in to the prognosis and intervention planning (Davies, Papp, & Antoni, 2015). If the person doesn't have the opportunity or motivation to use and practice their gender presentation, they may be slower to habituate it. It is not uncommon for transfeminine clients to enroll in voice treatment as they are preparing to come out at work, as this is typically the last setting they are presenting as their sex assigned at birth and the one in which they are most concerned about gender attributions from others. In our chart review of 25 trans women, four came for initial assessment already in female presentation 100% of the time, nine presented female 50% to 99% of the time, and 12 presented female less than 50% of the time. The causal influence of this variable has not been investigated, but exploratory analysis found no correlation between the time spent in female presentation and SFF, MPFR, or intensity (Hancock & Garabedian, 2013). Sometimes clients with lunch-hour appointments for voice sessions arrive in clothes appropriate for their birth-assigned gender presentation and will change clothes or put on jewelry to help shift into their new communication style. These circumstances seem to slow the process if it is difficult to mentally and physically switch. As it is fundamentally a motor skill, adopting new vocal behavior requires practice. If the client is only using their new voice occasionally, they will not be practicing as often as someone who can have a more consistent gender presentation. This is not to say a person who does not want to use their feminine-sounding voice all the time should not enroll in intervention, just that they should be informed that it may impact the rate or extent of change possible.

In summary, intervention duration is highly individual and difficult to predict in advance. Variables related to intervention or client characteristics may be considered. Progress made in the first few sessions may provide clinical insight to estimate a reasonable pace for the client.

FINAL NOTES

The general purpose and procedures of voice and communication assessment are not drastically impacted by the motivating reason for attendance. Nonetheless, we have focused this chapter on the aspects that do require modification or special attention. Below are a few other general considerations to aid in your preparedness.

Typical Assessment Obstacles

Not unlike patients who are referred for suspected voice disorder, clients with gender-related voice issues may be nervous. They don't know what to expect and are literally being judged with every breath. Given the historical and cultural experience with health care providers (Chapter 2), there are additional reasons for the client to be hesitant and guarded. You have already invested time and effort in establishing an inclusive and welcoming environment (Chapter 3)—continue that vibe with a relaxed, steady pace. As covered extensively in Chapter 1, your own presence is influential here.

Record and assess their natural and full voice. When you give instructions, limit the verbiage and use a good model. They will do what you do, not what you say. Make a mental note of their natural voice during the initial stages of assessment so you can compare their recorded productions to that. For some reason the presence of a microphone and recording can cause the client to change their speech.

It is unlikely you will learn everything you need to know during the first session. Sometimes we cannot explain some observations or reports from the client, and circumstances become clear only later as treatment begins. Several medical, psychological, and emotional aspects of a client, as well as how they interact with the clinician and the planned intervention, can contribute to the voice. Assessment is an ongoing activity and does not end when you have finished the initial report.

Triggering Negative Emotions

Whether you elicit their maximum phonation frequency range using a glissando or stepping task or software for a phonetogram (e.g., voice range profile), clients may avoid some frequencies. Many trans men are at least uncomfortable if not unwilling to glide their pitch up to falsetto range. This requires sensitivity and assurance that you are interested in learning the full capability and flexibility of the voice. Some clients have experienced such extreme gender dysphoria that they disassociate from their body and have to learn how to connect and experience their body in a healthy way again. Let them know it is okay and normal for the voice and emotions to be connected. In fact, it can even be considered a good sign that they are responsive.

Related to body sensitivity and self-consciousness, clients may react negatively to your visual, auditory, or tactile observations. They may not assume the best when they realize you are looking at their abdomen and chest (to assess breathing patterns) or when you start rubbing their neck, face, and shoulders (to relieve tension and stimulate clearer vocal production). Conduct these activities after establishing some rapport and state observations aloud as you make them. For example, "I noticed you are slouching a bit. Do you mind if I stand behind you and position your shoulders and head while you say that again?" The client may be able to provide information to supplement your observation, such as a back problem contributing to slouching.

Sharing the Assessment Results

If you need more time to interpret and consider all the collected information before making definitive recommendations and writing a professional report, just a brief review of your findings and likely recommendations will be appropriate to end the assessment. Maintain a tone of respect and even admiration for completing tasks that may have been uncomfortable as you explain the overall health status of the speech mechanism as well as particular areas related to gender presentation that can be addressed with intervention.

Clients are typically very concerned with the hertz number. It can be helpful to tell them, as it relieves anticipation and anxiety. However, understanding change in a nonlinear measure like hertz is difficult, so mapping the hertz measures from their speech samples on a graph or using a piano keyboard with notes (semitones) as described above is advised. It is tempting to focus on something concrete, like increasing the hertz number, but the process is more about how they feel physically, emotionally, and socially. Circling back to the TSEQ or TVQ^{MTF} discussed at the beginning of the session can remind you both of the big picture as you adjourn the formal assessment portion and look toward goal setting.

Possible Referrals

In the event that your client is not already connected with a provider for their mental health, hormones, electrolysis, or other members of your typical interdisciplinary team, discuss the reasons why and make referrals as appropriate. Laryngologists, also known as voice-specialized otolaryngologists or ENTs, can tell us if there is normal vocal function neurologically, medically, and behaviorally. If there are questions beyond their scope, they will make a referral for further specialist consults such as a gastroenterologist, neurologist, allergist, and so on.

Your client will be grateful for a list of LGBTQ-friendly practitioners. WPATH maintains a member directory, searchable by location and specialty (including "vocal therapist"). Some professions maintain searchable databases on their websites. In ASHA's ProFind (https://www.asha.org/profind/), for example, ASHA members can select "transgender voice" as an area of expertise. However, these types of databases often operate by self-designations. You can also take note of practitioners your clients use and recommend. Seek and ask about trans services when you attend local health events and professional meetings.[6]

[6]Don't forget to distribute your own contact info with LGBTQ-friendly indicated so that even and especially if practitioners you meet aren't comfortable or competent treating trans clients, they can refer to you.

ONE LAST PURPOSE OF ASSESSMENT

At the conclusion of the initial assessment, you and your client will get ready to press onward by developing an intervention strategy using considerations outlined in the next chapter. This strategizing is the link between assessment and intervention. Adrienne wasn't always interested in developing strategies, but she is now. Can you guess what facilitated her learning of this invaluable skill? She attempted something challenging and came up short in an assessment. Only about 26% of the way there, as mentioned at the opening of this chapter. That shame of failing a test on statistical probability had to be overcome in order to later enroll in a PhD program requiring five courses of research and statistical methods. There was some test anxiety involved, but also courage found. Adrienne reflected on the assessment results, took action, and strategized, asking for help from caring and knowledgeable colleagues. Each time she finished a statistics course test, she marked her progress with celebration. Now doing and teaching statistics is a part of her career, and shame has given way to pride.

Adrienne's shortcoming, reaction, and resilience story about statistics is silly in comparison to the story most of our clients have lived, but it illustrates how assessment can play a role in such a story. You may have to help clients who fear assessment, possibly because they experience shame from it, to shift perspective and find courage. They can be proud of the progress they have made and will make on this transformation toward satisfaction with their voice and communication. Use the information in this chapter to regularly assess and chart their change for them. You will be honored to celebrate those progress markers along the way as you press on together.

REFERENCES

Adler, R. K., Hirsch, S., & Mordaunt, M. (2006). *Voice and communication therapy for the transgender/transsexual client: A comprehensive clinical guide*. San Diego, CA: Plural Publishing.

Adler, R. K., Hirsch, S., & Mordaunt, M. (2012). *Voice and communication therapy for the transgender/transsexual client: A comprehensive clinical guide* (2nd ed). San Diego, CA: Plural Publishing.

Azul, D. (2015a). Transmasculine people's vocal situations: A critical review of gender-related discourses and empirical data. *International Journal of Language and Communication Disorders*, *50*(1), 31–47.

Azul, D. (2015b). On the varied and complex factors affecting gender diverse people's vocal situations: Implications for clinical practice. *Perspectives of the ASHA Special Interest Group 3, 25*, 75–86.

Azul, D., Nygren, U., Södersten, M., & Neuschaefer-Rube, C. (2017). Transmasculine people's voice function: A review of the currently available evidence. *Journal of Voice, 31*(2), 261.e9–261.e23.

Baken, R. J., & Orlikoff, R. F. (2010). *Clinical measurement of speech and voice* (2nd ed). Clifton Park: NY: Delmar Cenage Learning.

Brown, W. S., Morris, R. J., Hicks, D. M., & Howell, E. (1993). Phonational profiles of female professional singers and nonsingers. *Journal of Voice*, *7*(3), 219–226.

Cohen, S. M., Kim, J., Roy, N., Asche, C., & Courey, M. (2012). Prevalence and causes of dysphonia in a large treatment-seeking population. *Laryngoscope, 122*, 343–348.

Colton, R. H., Casper, J. K., & Leonard, R. (2011). *Understanding voice problems: A physiological perspective for diagnosis and treatment* (4th ed). Philadelphia: PA: Lippincott Williams & Wilkins.

Dacakis, G., Davies, S., Oates, J. M., Douglas, J. M., & Johnston, J. R. (2013). Development and preliminary evaluation of the transsexual voice questionnaire for male-to-female transsexuals. *Journal of Voice, 27*(3), 312–320.

Dacakis, G., Oates, J., & Douglas, J. M. (2017). Further evidence of the construct validity of the Transsexual Voice Questionnaire (TVQ^{MTF}) using principal components analysis. *Journal of Voice, 31*(2), 142–148.

Davies, S. M., & Johnston, J. R. (2015). Exploring the validity of the transsexual voice questionnaire for male-to-female transsexuals. *Canadaian Journal of Speech-Language Pathology and Audiology, 39*(1), 41–51.

Davies, S. M., Papp, V. G., & Antoni, C. (2015). Voice and communication change for gender nonconforming individuals: Giving voice to the person inside. *International Journal of Transgenderism, 16*, 117–159.

De Bruin, M., Coerts, M., & Greven, A. (2000). Speech therapy in the management of male-to-female transsexuals. *Folia Phoniatrica et Logopaedica, 52*, 220–227.

Ferrand, C. T. (2019). *Voice disorders: Scope of theory and practice* (2nd ed.). New York, NY: Pearson.

Gelfer, M. P., & Tice, R. M. (2013). Perceptual and acoustic outcomes of voice therapy for male-to-female transgender individuals immediately after therapy and 15 months later. *Journal of Voice, 27*(3), 335–347.

Gelfer, M. P., & Van Dong, B. (2013). A preliminary study on the use of vocal function exercises to improve voice in male-to-female transgender clients. *Journal of Voice, 27*(3), 321–334.

Gorham-Rowan, M., & Morris R. (2006). Aerodynamic analysis of male-to-female transgender voice. *Journal of Voice, 20*, 251–262.

Guzman, M., Acuña, G., Pacheco, F., Peralta, F., Romero, C., Vergara, C., & Quezada, C. (2018). The impact of double source of vibration semioccluded voice exercises on objective and subjective outcomes in subject with voice complaints. *Journal of Voice, 32*(6), 770.e1–770.e9.

Hancock, A. B., & Azul, D. (2017). ***Cultural and clinical considerations for EBP with transgender and gender non-conforming people.*** Presented at the ASHA Convention, Los Angeles, CA.

Hancock, A. B., Childs, K., & Irwig, M. (2017). Trans male voice in the first year of testosterone: Make no assumptions. *Journal of Speech, Language, and Hearing Research, 60*(9), 2472–2482.

Hancock, A. B., & Garabedian, L. (2013). Transgender voice and communication treatment: A retrospective chart review of 25 cases. *International Journal of Language and Communication Disorders, 48*(1), 54–65.

Hancock, A. B., & Helenius, L. (2012). Adolescent male-to-female transgender voice and communication. *Journal of Communication Disorders, 45*, 313–324.

Hancock, A. B., Krissinger, J., & Owen, K. (2011). Voice perceptions and quality of life of transgender people. *Journal of Voice, 25*(5), 553–558.

Hancock, A. B., & Rubin, B. (2015). Influence of communication partner's gender on language. *Journal of Language and Social Psychology, 34*(1), 46–64.

Helou, L. (2017). Crafting the dialogue: Meta-therapy in transgender voice and communication training. *Perspectives of the ASHA Special Interest Group 10, 2*(2), 83–91.

Hillenbrand, J., Getty, L. A., Clark, M. J., & Wheeler, K. (1995). Acoustic characteristics of American English vowels. *Journal of Acoustical Society of America, 97*(5), 3099–3111.

Holmberg, E., Oates, J., Dacakis, G., & Grant, C. (2010). Phonetograms, aerodynamic measurements, self-evaluations, and auditory perceptual ratings of male-to-female transsexual voice. *Journal of Voice, 24*(5), 688–698.

Irwig, M. S., Childs, K., & Hancock, A. B. (2017). Effects of testosterone on the transgender male voice. *Andrology, 5*, 107–112.

Jacobson, B. H., Johnson, A., Grywalski, C., Silbergleit, A., Jacobson, G., Benninger, M. S., & Newman, C. W. (1997). The Voice Handicap Index (VHI): Development and validation. *American Journal of Speech-Language Pathology, 6*, 66–70.

Leaper, C., & Ayres, M. (2007). A meta-analytic review of gender variations in adults' language use: Talkativeness, affiliative speech, and assertive speech. *Personality and Social Psychology Review, 11*(4), 328–363.

Mészáros, K., Vitéz, L., Szabolcs, I., Goth, M., Kovács, L., Görömbei, Z., & Hacki, T. (2005). Efficacy of conservative voice treatment in male-to-female transsexuals, *Foliz Phoniatrica et Logopaedica, 57*, 111–118.

Morris, R. J., Brown, W. S., Hicks, D. M., & Howell, E. (1995). Phonational profiles of male trained singers and nonsingers. *Journal of Voice*, *9*(2), 142–148.

Mount, M. H., & Salmon, S. J. (1988). Changing the vocal characteristics of a post-operative transsexual patient: A longitudinal study. *Journal of Communication Disorders*, *21*, 229–238.

Nygren, U., Nordenskjöld, A., Arver, S., & Södersten, M. (2016). Effects of voice fundamental frequency and satisfaction with voice in trans men during testosterone treatment: A longitudinal study. *Journal of Voice*, *30*(6), 766.e23–766.e34.

Palmer, D., Dietsch, A., & Searl, J. (2011). Endoscopic and stroboscopic presentation of the larynx in male-to-female transsexual persons. *Journal of Voice*, *26*(1), 117–126.

Palomares, N. A. (2004). Gender schematicity, gender identify salience, and gender-linked language use. *Human Communication Research*, *30*(4), 556–588.

Pasricha, N., Dacakis, G., & Oates, J. (2008). Communicative satisfaction of male-to-female transsexuals. *Logopedics Phoniatrics Vocology*, *33*, 25–34.

Roy, N., Bless, D. M., & Heisey, D. (2000). Personality and voice disorders: A multitrait-multidisorder analysis. *Journal of Voice*, *14*(4), 521–548.

Roy, N., Merrill, R. M., Gray, S. D., & Smith, E. M. (2005). Voice disorders in the general population: Prevalence, risk factors, and occupational impact. *Laryngoscope*, *115*, 1988–1995.

Söderpalm, E., Larsson, A., & Almquist, S. (2004). Evaluation of a consecutive group of transsexual individuals referred for vocal intervention in the west of Sweden. *Logopedics Phoniatrics Vocology*, *29*(1), 18–30.

Södersten, E., Nygren, U., Hertegård, S., & Dhejne, C. (2015). Interdisciplinary program in Sweden related to transgender voice. *Perspectives on Voice and Voice Disorders*, *25*, 87–97.

T'Sjoen, G. et al. (2006). Impact of voice in transsexuals. *International Journal of Transsexualism*, *9*(1), 1–7.

Van Leer, E., Hapner, E. R., & Connor, N. P. (2008). Transtheoretical model of health behavior change applied to voice therapy. *Journal of Voice*, *22*(6), 688–698.

Verdolini, K., Titze, I. R., & Fennell, A. (1994). Dependence of phonatory effort on hydration level. *Journal of Speech Language and Hearing Research*, *37*, 1001–1007.

Zeitels, S. M., Hillman, R. E., Desloge, R., Mauri, M., & Doyle, P. (2002). Phonosurgery in singers and performing artists: Treatment outcomes, management theories, and future directions. *Annals of Otology Rhinology, and Laryngology*, *12*(Suppl. 190), 21–40.

Zraick, R. I., Skaggs, S. D., & Montague, J. C. (2000). The effect of task on determination of habitual pitch. *Journal of Voice*, *14*(4), 484–489.

APPENDIX 4–A

Initial Assessment Report Example

REFERRAL INFORMATION

B. H. is a 64-year-old retired army colonel self-referred to the center. Assigned male at birth, B. H. identifies as a trans woman. She comes to us with a 2-year history of her desire to change her voice to sound feminine.

MEDICAL, EDUCATIONAL, AND OCCUPATIONAL HISTORY

Overall Health

The client describes her health as excellent. She exercises three to four times each week and is diagnosed with high blood pressure (HBP) for which she takes medication (see below). She has never had surgery, has not had serious illness in her past, and has an annual physical.

Transition Process

The client's gender positioning is female and prefers people use she and her pronouns when referring to her. Gender self-attribution is more male than female, although the desired attribution from self and others is female. She reports that gender attribution from others is currently almost always male.

She is at the beginning stages of her transition to present as female. She came out to her family 6 months ago and has had limited contact with them as they come to terms with her intention to transition. She began female hormones under the care of her endocrinologist 8 months ago. She wears feminine clothing in her home only, although she is willing to bring them to the center and change into them for voice training. She has not decided about feminization surgeries at this time because of the considerations for family acceptance and support of this process. In her judgment, she feels that she will have time to practice her new voice and can move fully forward in all aspects of her transition once they have had time to process this, whether she learns that they can be supportive or not.

She says that she does not "pass vocally" in person or on the phone. While she acknowledges that it is distressing, she feels there is light at the end of the tunnel now that she has come out to her family. She is not attending support group meetings because she feels that there was too much going on that was not her philosophy at the first meeting she went to. Specifically, she felt she was being pulled into a situation where she was encouraged to be a part of the trans culture, versus integrating into the world as herself.

Specialists

The client is seeing a gender therapist weekly, and endocrinologist every 3 months for monitoring, and a primary care physician who has seen her for many years and is supportive of her transition.

Medications

Estradiol and spironolactone, starting 6 months ago, and Avapro for high blood pressure (HBP), starting 3 years ago.

Occupational and Domestic Status and Vocal Demands

The client is retired and lives alone. She has a sister who lives in Florida who she keeps in touch with; however, she is estranged from her wife and two sons aged 31 and 35 and feels "they need time to understand." Her typical day at this time is very quiet. She enjoys working in her woodshop, tending to the home, reading, and daily walks. Her current vocal situations involve greeting her neighbors, attending occasional get-togethers with a friend who knows about her transition, answering the phone, and making approximately five to six calls each week. She sees and greets her neighbors approximately twice a week. She estimates that she uses her voice 5% to 10% of the time. While she presents as female, she is using her birth voice. She is aware of the disconnection of her voice from her true female self and feels that this is one reason she prefers to live a quiet life.

Vocal Hygiene History

At this time, she does not speak in high background noise, to an audience, sing, or use her voice in an abusive manner situationally. She does not experience vocal fatigue, discomfort, or strain. She has two glasses of wine with dinner approximately three times a week. She drinks three to four glasses of water daily. Her HBP medication is a diuretic and drying.

Prior Speech, Language, and Voice Treatment

She has not participated in voice training or had a voice disorder or difficulties with her voice in her past. She is aware of some YouTube videos and CDs available to train the transfemale voice but reports that she wants to work with someone who can "guide me directly."

VOICE ASSESSMENT RESULTS

Transsexual Voice Questionnaire (TVQ^{MTF})

B. H. completed this 30-item self-assessment instrument to examine the impact of the perceived vocal incongruence and vocal difficulties on her life. She scored 82 out of 120. Results revealed that the voice problem negatively affects her life to a significant degree. Statements that she most strongly agreed with included "my voice makes it hard for me to be identified as a female, I feel my voice does not reflect the 'true me,' and I feel self-conscious about how strangers perceive my voice."

CAPE-V Results	
OVERALL SEVERITY	15/100
Roughness	20/100
Breathiness	0/100
Strain	9/100
Pitch	70/100 [reduced]
Loudness	25/100 [excessive]

OTHER: Auditory Perceptual Observations	
Resonance	Laryngeal
Glottal Fry	Mild to mild-moderate present
Speech Rate	WNL
Intonation	Mildly reduced
Respiratory Patterns in Connected Speech	
Mix of abdominal/diaphragmatic and upper thoracic	
Other Respiratory Characteristics	
Shallow inspiration	
Abdominal effort during phonation	
Speech/voice on reserve air	
Associated Tension Sites	
Postural Misalignment	Rounded posture
Shoulder Tension	Bilaterally rounded
Neck Tension	Forward hyperextension
Mandibular Tension	Restricted mandibular range
Presence of Discomfort	Mild tenderness on palpation
Laryngeal Tension	Moderate on L., mild on R.
Suprahyoid Hypertonicity	Moderate
Oral-Motor Screening	
Oral motor structure and function was judged to be within normal limits. No further action to be taken at this time. Client will be screened annually.	
Hearing Screening	
Hearing screening was WNL. No further action to be taken at this time. Client will be screened annually.	

B. OBJECTIVE VOICE ANALYSIS		
Measure	**Results (male voice)**	**Cisgender Male Normative Data***
Mean fundamental frequency		
Sustained /a/ Mean Hz/Semitone	124 Hz B2	138 Hz[3]
Reading Rainbow Passage Mean Hz/Semitone	97 Hz G2	112 Hz[1]
Conversation Mean Hz/Semitone	89 Hz F2	127 Hz[1]
Habitual Pitch Level	34%	25%[2]
Conversational Frequency Range		
F0 Min (ST)	85 Hz F2	
F0 Max (ST)	115 Hz E3	
***Total Conversation Frequency Range**	5 ST	6-12 ST
Max Phonation Frequency Range (MPFR)		
Fundamental Freq. Range: F0 Min (ST)	74 Hz D2	83 Hz[1] E2
F0 Max (ST)	350 Hz F4	443 Hz[1] A4
***Total Frequency Range**	27 ST	29 ST[1,2]
Intensity Range		
Min (dB SPL)	55	
Max (dB SPL)	80	110 dB[1]
Formants		
F1 /i/	380	342[3]
F2 /i/	2450	2322[3]
F3 /i/	3100	3000[3]
F1 /a/	813	768[3]
F2 /a/	1401	1333[3]
F3 /a/	2604	2522[3]

Measure	Results (male voice)	Cisgender Male Normative Data*
Cepstral Peak Prominence		
Reading	3.5	Threshold: 4.0
Sustained Phonation		
Maximum Duration (best of 3)	20 Seconds	25 Seconds[1]

**Normative data based on cisgender males as reported in (1) Colton, Casper, and Lenoard (2011); (2) Morris, Brown, Hicks, and Howell (1995); and (3) Hillenbrand, Getty, Clark, and Wheeler (1995).*

STIMULABILITY

Diagnostic stimulability testing revealed improved vocal quality and resonance when volume was reduced and frequency elevated to optimal levels. B. H. also reported her sensation of vocal effort was reduced during this production. Respiratory patterns were enhanced with more aligned posture. The establishment of the initial frequency target near 150 Hz revealed ease of function and client satisfaction in the lower gender-neutral range.

SUMMARY OF RESULTS

B. H. presents with a masculine-sounding voice 100% of the time but rates it as a 3 on a scale of 1 to 10 for congruence with her desired gender positioning and attributions from others. Subjectively, she presents with a mild vocal imbalance characterized by mild roughness and strain, laryngeal and chest resonance, narrow frequency range during speech (i.e., toward monotony), and low fundamental frequency (pitch) compared to cisgender males and females. Volume was excessive for the environment. Vocal imbalance appears to be related to laryngeal tension, excessive volume, mandibular restriction, rounded postural alignment, hyperextension of the head, restricted diaphragmatic excursion accompanied by chest expansion during inspiration prior phonation, and speaking through the end of the expiratory reserve.

Objectively, when compared to cisgender male normative data, maximum phonation frequency range was WNL. Her speaking fundamental frequency was reduced when compared to normative data and was significantly below a frequency level that elicited clear vocal quality. Voice quality improved significantly during sustained vowels.

The client presents with incomplete voice feminization characterized by significantly lowered pitch, narrowed intonation range, and laryngeal and chest resonance. There is a significant gap between desired and current gender presentation.

PROGNOSIS

Prognosis to improve voice quality and function as described appears to be excellent based on motivation, mild severity of symptoms, and high response to stimulability testing. Potential to improve congruency between present and desired vocal presentation appears to be good given her full-time presentation, medical history, absence of a voice disorder, and vocal responsiveness to stimulability for oral resonance, intonation, and pitch elevation trials. Other factors include high motivation and weekly counseling support. There may be some challenges related to age, low fundamental frequency, mildly restricted total pitch range, and unknown family support in this early phase of care. As long as there is consistent monitoring of laryngeal tension, the above vocal imbalance should not affect the vocal feminization process given that elevation of pitch appeared to relieve symptoms.

RECOMMENDATIONS

1. Voice and communication training once a week for 60-minute sessions until goals are reached.
2. Daily home program based on the weekly treatment results.

Goal

The client will produce voice that feels congruent with their desired gender presentation.

Behavioral Objectives

1. The client will demonstrate understanding of their vocal mechanism and other factors (physical, mental, and emotional issues; management of stressors; vocal hygiene issues) that may affect the voice by describing them to the clinician in her own words.

2. The client will reduce barriers to activities and participation in life initially by:
   a. developing a support system network within her family;
   b. creating a network of safe speaking partners in her neighborhood, with her sister, and a friend that she trusts; and
   c. open discussion as to how to comfortably negotiate gender attribution both on the phone and one-on-one.
3. Client will heighten self-awareness via self-assessment of overall vocal severity, vocal effort, throat discomfort, and home practice effectiveness each session.
4. Client will improve posture for head and neck, shoulder, hip alignment, and hyperextension of the head and neck for progressively longer and more complex vocal tasks and a variety of functional contexts.
5. Client will reduce general body tension during the session using deep breathing relaxation exercises and carry this or other stress management method into her home life.
6. Client will reduce general laryngeal tension via laryngeal and suprahyoid musculature tension massage.
7. Client will improve respiratory support by increasing diaphragmatic breathing during progressively longer and more complex tasks in a variety of clinical and functional contexts.
8. Client will reduce conversational volume to appropriate levels for the environment and a variety of functional contexts.
9. Client will elevate pitch to target frequencies as deemed appropriate by clinician and client during progressively longer and more complex utterances, and while gradually merging skill with intonation and oral resonance and a variety of functional contexts.
10. Client will increase feminine vocal expression through use of intonation training for progressively longer and more complex utterances and a variety of functional contexts.
11. Client will increase oral resonance through forward focus approach for progressively longer and more complex utterances and a variety of functional contexts.

____ ____________________

Clinician Date

APPENDIX 4-B
Inventory Form

Date: ______________________________

Legal Name: ______________________________

Preferred Name: ______________________________

Pronouns: ______________________________

When should I use your preferred name?

___ Always (except for billing needs)

___ Only when talking to me directly or via my voicemail and email address

___ Only at the center, in person (not voicemail or email)

___ Other instructions about name:

Please provide the following contact information and star your preferred method of contact.

Phone Number: ______________________________

Email: ______________________________

Mailing Address: ______________________________

____

The following questions will be discussed at our first appointment. Please review these questions and consider your answers. Some people find it helpful to write notes or answers to the questions in advance. If you do not feel comfortable answering or are uncertain about what the question is asking, just leave it blank.

GENERAL AND VOCAL HEALTH

1. Describe your overall health (diseases/disorders, surgeries, injuries, exercise, stress, alcohol use, smoking).

2. What other health practitioners do you see (primary care, endocrinology, psychiatry, social worker, ENT, acupuncture, etc.)?
3. What medication(s) do you take?
4. Describe your vocal health and demands.
   a. How do you use your voice during the day (work/home/social)?
   b. It is important to note if different voices are used according to setting or people (e.g., with husband at home, but not with extended family or at work).
5. Do you ever experience vocal fatigue, throat discomfort, vocal strain, hoarseness, or other changes related to when you use your voice?
6. Have you had to change your way of speaking because it wasn't feeling easy or sounding clear?
7. Voice care (how much fluid do you drink? caffeine? alcohol? long or loud voice use? coughing?)
8. Have you done voice training or therapy previously?

GENDER-RELATED INFORMATION

9. How do you describe your gender?
10. How do you want to present your gender (how you look, sound, move, etc.)?
11. Where or when are you able to present as you want? If not 100%, how to you present the other times? (Trans-masculine clients: is chest binding involved?)
12. How satisfied are you with your current gender presentation (scale: 1 = not at all, 10 = very)?
13. How do others tend to classify your gender?
14. How do you want to be perceived and addressed by others?
15. What happens when others misgender you (your feelings, thoughts, actions)?

GOALS

16. Why are you interested in changing your voice and communication?
17. Describe your support system. Who are (or aren't) you comfortable practicing your new voice with?
18. Do you have any concerns, hesitations, or questions about changing your voice and communication?

5

Intervention Phase 1: Get Ready . . .

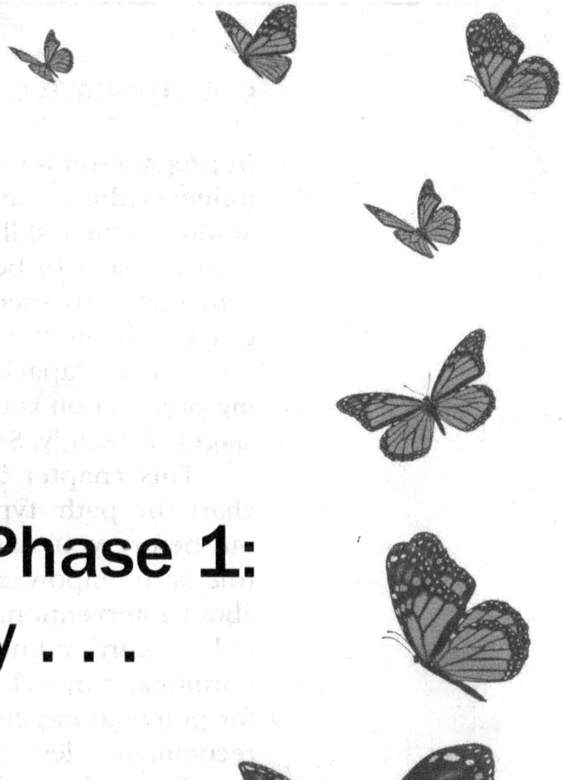

COLLABORATIVE GOAL SETTING

In preparation for a race, a runner considers factors that will influence their strategy. An important component of this preparation is their skilled collaborators. Serious runners partner with a coach to benefit from the support and guidance of someone with specialized knowledge. Together, runner and coach evaluate the distance and path of the course as well as the runner's capacity to train and perform. Collaboration during preparation is crucial to the first of the three intervention stages of "Ready, Set, Go!"

This chapter is about taking time with your client to chart the path, typically after you have assessment results but before you start voice work. A large part the provider's role is to empower the client to engage and make decisions about intervention. Your role as informer is a major reason to have current knowledge of intervention options, including hormonal, surgical, and behavioral avenues, and the rationales for potential targets of voice training. Do you know why we recommend elevating fundamental frequency in speaking, or how far to elevate it? What about the safest and most permanent way to elevate it? The rest of this book is intended to help you learn and explain what you know so you can teach your clients.

Knowing the intervention options is not as important, however, as acknowledging that interventions are only a part of what contributes to the production of gender. When developing a plan for the path forward, both the client and provider must recognize there will always be factors beyond their control. The cultural setting, the client's intentions and capacity to change, and the provider's clinical and cultural competence will significantly influence the strategy plan for intervention. Synergy of these elements has enabled the process to come this far, but there are important limitations to acknowledge to set reasonable goals. Agency is a term used to describe "capacity to act" or, in this case, capacity to contribute to communication (Ahearn 2010, p. 28). Most humans don't like to admit it, but there are limits to our agency. This is largely because several "agents" are constantly involved. These include not only the speaker, listener, and practitioners' actions, but also aspects individuals have even less capacity to influence: biophysiological process, sociocultural settings, and material forces (e.g., room acoustics, amplification devices). Furthermore, the ongoing interaction among these factors must be taken into account. Hancock and Azul's (2018) critical analysis of the literature resulted in the transdisciplinary ASSEMBLE approach, which is used to guide work in the crux of voice and gender:

Acknowledgment of ongoing and dynamic agency of:

Speaker's practices (e.g., self-presentation, lifestyle choices, self-attribution, responses to attributions from others)

Sociocultural mediation of meaning-making practices (e.g., linguistic rules and standards, normative forces, socialization practices)

External **M**aterial forces (e.g., physical, chemical, biological, technical)

Biophysiological processes (e.g., genetic, hormonal)

Listening practices (e.g., perceptions, interpretations, attributions)

Elected professional interventions (e.g., behavioral, surgical, medicinal)

The view of gender as continuously and flexibly constructed is critical in the ASSEMBLE model. We cannot expect nor aim for a single particular outcome of voice training, even at the individual level. While the speaker can modulate several contributions—these are the basis of much of the current research literature guiding our practice standards today—it is just as important to be aware of and develop a response to the contributions we are unable to control.

Explain and consider the elements of the ASSEMBLE model with your client in context of their wants and needs. Gender attribution from others, a common goal for many of our clients, is largely mediated by the listener's perception and processing, which are influenced by sociocultural factors and even external material factors such as the physical environment they are listening in. For example, large rooms require the speaker to raise their loudness, which may cause difficulty for maintaining the high pitch that cues listeners to attribute female gender to the speaker. Advances in science and medicine have enabled some influence on biophysiological processes in collaboration with our professional colleagues in endocrinology and surgical medicine, and the client should be well informed about those options as elected professional interventions.

One of your primary roles as practitioner during the goal-setting stage is to educate the client on the complexity of the process of gender production and what they can and cannot expect to influence via various interventions. Selecting interventions and goals does not have to been seen as an effort to manage or reduce expectations and thereby completely deflate the enthusiasm of starting. Encourage the client to select goals with a very broad and well-informed perspective. Many clients underestimate the richness of communication and during this discussion find relief in the freedom to find a unique voice all their own, as opposed to a highly specified sound they hope will be "good enough." Areas that seem to be commonly misunderstood, or not considered at all, by clients include:

- the varied and dynamic communicative elements influential in the production of gender,
- the various approaches to changing voice and communication, and
- the nature of voice and communication change as a process.

A discussion of these three topics may begin during the assessment session, especially if discussing your impressions and prognosis in person, or may be the bulk of your first intervention session. Whenever goal planning is discussed, stay true to a client-centered plan of care by educating the client about all their options and the factors to weigh when selecting interventions or when setting goal behaviors and target levels. The remainder of the chapter will provide information for consideration by you and the client as you collaborate and "get ready."

COMMUNICATION BEHAVIORS TO CONSIDER

The following sections will focus on the speaker practices that can, and do, influence how gender is attributed. In other words, what aspects of our communication help our communication partners attribute our gender as we do? An excellent peer-reviewed research literature review and meta-analysis of the voice, articulation, and prosody factors purported to contribute can be found in Leung, Oates, and Chan (2018). Another important reference is the entry for "Gender Issues in Intergroup Communication" in the Oxford Research Encyclopedia of Communication (Wingate & Palomares, 2017).

Although we focus in this chapter on the empirical evidence, we fully expect and advise that the practitioner and client will incorporate this information with their own knowledge and intuition when making decisions about interventions.

In the domain of gender and communication, the empirical evidence and rationale for what to target in intervention are generally found in two bodies of research: studies of speaker production and studies of listener perception. In other words, how is the communication of cisgender men and women different? And, how do listeners use various communication variables to judge how feminine/masculine the speaker sounds? Those answers are not always the same, in which case the latter question seems more relevant. More recently, interventions with target behaviors selected on the basis of this research have been studied, and those studies of intervention effectiveness are used to further support which targets are recommended for changing how the speaker's voice is produced and perceived.

This all may sound very systematic and logical, but there are a few assumptions and limitations to keep in mind. To start, much of the available data on speech production are from cisgender adult speakers and listeners and may not be readily applicable to all your clients. Additionally, the premise that men and women communicate differently, all the time and for all time, is untenable and has not borne out in research. It is just not that simple even in a binary conceptualization of gender, let alone a nonbinary one. Social identity attributed to a person is informed not only by meanings of gender, but also the meanings others hold in regard to race, social class, and sexuality (see De Vries, 2012, for explanation of this in regard to trans people). This concept, called *intersectionality* in social science literature, illuminates the flaw of overgeneralized conclusions. What may be true of a white cisgender woman in middle-class Western culture (i.e., much of the research participant pool) is not necessarily true for people of other races, genders, socioeconomic classes, and other domains of sociocultural belonging. Finally—and this cannot be emphasized enough—gender is a production involving the speaker, listeners, practitioners, and other components difficult to measure, let alone influence. Even in the most comprehensive models, a large proportion of how gender is constructed in each encounter remains unalterable or even unexplained.

As we discuss communication variables potentially influential to perception of gender, we will intentionally point out the myriad of contextual factors besides speaker gender that are contributing to the conclusions. As you will see, pitch and resonance are relatively robust predictors of gender attribution and thus are frequently and strongly recommended as intervention targets. Verbal and nonverbal language, however, are rarely justified as factors in perception of gender without considerable caveat. Many other communication variables fall generally somewhere between those in the range of value for influencing gender attribution.

Fundamental and Formant Frequencies

Many people will guess pitch, the perceptual correlate of fundamental frequency (F0), is the most important and differentiating acoustic cue in vocal presentation of gender (see Box 5–1 for the physiological bases of F0 and formant frequencies). This opinion is usually explained by the fact that cisgender men are reported to, on average, have much lower F0 than cisgender women do. Most cisgender adult males speak somewhere between 110 and 130 Hz and most cisgender adult females between 180 and 230 Hz (see Baken & Orlikoff, 2010, for tables of acoustic norms from multiple sources). However, listeners' perception of a speaker's gender:

- is often but not always predicted based on F0,
- can be predicted by select formant frequencies without F0, and F1–F3
- is predicted best when F0 and formants are both considered.

F0 and formant frequencies can lead to accurate distinction between the voices of cisgender men and women. In this context it is important to realize that accuracy does not mean 100%—it means better than chance. Results from a pattern recognition study of 45 men and 48 women (presumably cisgender) indicated a 96% accuracy level based on F0 alone and 92% accuracy for combination of formants 1 to 3 (Hillenbrand & Clark, 2009). In some studies, combinations of formants are more important for distinguishing speaker's gender than single formants or fundamental frequency (Childers & Wu, 1991; Gallena, Stickels, & Stickels, 2018). Accuracy above 90% is impressive, but computer recognition algorithms are not the same as human auditory perception.

Box 5–1. Physiologic and Acoustic Bases of Fundamental and Formant Frequencies

Speakers have some control over their fundamental frequency (F0) and formant frequencies. It is important to understand the physiologic and acoustic bases of these acoustic measures because they are strongly associated with gender expression and attribution and therefore are common targets of vocal training. Refer to a speech science book or tutorials on the National Center for Voice and Speech website (http://www.ncvs.org/ncvs/tutorials/voiceprod/index.html) for a more in-depth tutorial.

Fundamental Frequency and Pitch

During phonation, the glottis is repeatedly opened and closed by the vocal folds. This aspect of the voice can be likened to lip "raspberries" or "trumpeter's lips" (Baken, 1998). Unlike vibrating guitar strings, the vocal folds (or trumpeter's lips) make noise by producing bursts or pulses of air. The resulting pattern is referred to as the glottal wave, and the rate of the glottal wave is F0 measured in cycles/second, or hertz (Hz). F0's perceptual correlate is pitch although, as discussed in the text, they do not have a linear relationship, so intervals between two F0 are reported in semitones (ST) rather than hertz.

F0 is based on the length, density, and stress/strain of vocal fold tissue (Titze, 2011). Density and stress of the vocal fold tissues change as subglottal pressure deforms the shape of the vocal folds during phonation. Regardless of the starting/habitual F0, when the vocal folds are stretched and lengthened, shorter glottal cycles (i.e., higher F0) occur for two reasons: greater surface area of vocal folds allows subglottal pressure to be more effective in the opening phase of the cycle, and increased stiffness of vocal folds causes them to return to midline more quickly in the closing phase (Baken, 1998).

Keep in mind that this discussion of *lengthening* is useful for a within-subject application only. To say someone has a higher F0 because their vocal folds are *longer* than someone else's would be inaccurate. The determining factor of F0 in cisgender people is not the size of the person, nor the size of the larynx; it is the length of the part of the vocal folds that is actually oscillating, sometimes called the effective vocal fold length. Online tutorials available from the National Center of Voice and Speech explain this well (http://www.ncvs.org/ncvs/tutorials/voiceprod/tutorial/influence.html). On average, cisgender men have a 60% longer effective vocal fold length than women. With more of their vocal folds in motion, longer glottal cycles occur (i.e., lower F0). This difference in effective vocal fold length accounts for sex-based differences in F0.This information explains why both cricothyroid approximation surgeries (which fix the vocal folds in a lengthened state) and glottoplasty (which shortens the effective vocal fold length) can result in higher F0 post-surgery.

Formants and Resonance

Formant frequencies are the frequencies of sound waves that are amplified by a resonator. In speech, the vocal tract is the resonator and therefore controls the sound of the voice by allowing some frequencies to pass through better than others, effectively amplifying particular frequencies. Which frequencies are amplified depends on the size and shape of the vocal tract, which can depend on the person's size. In any resonator shaped like a tube closed at one end and open on the other, such as the vocal tract, the frequency resonating best is four times the length of the tube and is called the first formant (F1). The rest of the formant frequencies in this type of tube are the odd multiples of F1 (i.e., F2 = F1 × 3, F3 = F1 × 5, and so on). Changing the shape of the resonating tube is how speech sounds are produced and vocal quality shaped.

Vowels are produced with a relatively open (no constriction to airflow) vocal tract and differentiated by F1 (strongly influenced by mandible height) and F2 (influenced by tongue and lip placement). Vocal tract shape when you say "heed" and "hat" differs by your mandible height, so these vowels differ by F1. Whereas "heed" and "hood" differ by mostly by tongue shape/lip retraction, so they differ by F2. If resonance is going to be a target of the client's intervention (and it usually is), then it is important to understand that the basis for resonance is the shape of the vocal tract, and that the vocal tract is shaped by speaker's articulatory posture.

Normative formant frequency data for cisgender men, women, and children correspond to different vocal tract lengths. On average, cisgender men have longer vocal tracts (17 to 20 mm) than cisgender women (12.5 to 17 mm), and small children (5.5 mm) (Zemlin, 1998). How would you make a vowel sound more feminine? The short answer is: Shorten the vocal tract. The two main options for this are to raise F2 by retracting the lips as if smiling and/or raise F1 by raising the larynx, which occurs when you lower the mandible. In simple words: smile and overarticulate!

Conclusions from pattern recognition studies were dampened by follow-up studies with human listeners. In an orthogonal design with normalized values of F0 and F1–F13 to control for other voice features, Hillenbrand and Clark (2009) used a synthesizer to create four conditions of sentences originally spoken by groups of (presumably cisgender) men and women: only shift F0 toward norms for the other group, only shift formant frequencies, shift both, and shift neither. Listening tests showed that shifting both F0 and formant frequencies resulted in 82% of listeners perceiving the sentences spoken by the males as sounding spoken by females; this was significantly more than in conditions shifting only F0 (19% to 34% of listeners) or formants (12% to 19% of listeners).

Twenty-five individuals with "male-to-female gender identity" contributed reading samples to be acoustically analyzed and entered into a statistical model to determine if and how several acoustic variables might predict perception of vocal femininity ratings, in isolation or in context with one another (Hardy, Boliek, Wells, Dearden, Zalmanowitz, & Rieger, 2016). The potential variables included speaking fundamental frequency (SFF) and highest F0 during reading, highest and lowest frequency in total range task, relative average perturbation (%), shimmer (%), and first three formants of "ah" vowel. The F0 during reading was the best and only significant predictor of femininity ratings. However, these samples were collected from 25 trans women, 23 of whom were perceived to be men.

Inclusion of voices that were not definitely perceived as male sounding may shift the predictive model. In another analysis of picture descriptions by 20 trans women, five cisgender men, and five cisgender women, SFF was highly correlated with the listener's rating of femininity of the voice ($r = .881, p < .05$) as well as speaker's own rating of the femininity of the voice ($r = .766, p < .05$) (Owen & Hancock, 2010). This correlation means only 78% of the variation in listener's perception of femininity of voice could be attributed to SFF in a picture description task, which is similar to the 82% in Hillenbrand and Clark (2009).

The bottom line is that a minimum SFF is usually necessary but can be insufficient for a voice to be perceived as feminine-sounding. Formant frequencies, perceived as resonance, is also a major factor. Even studies purporting a F0 threshold for a voice to be perceived as feminine-sounding concede this point, and many examples can be found in the literature and our experience. For example, only two of the six "male-to-female" speakers with SFF above 170 Hz were identified as female by listeners in the study by Gelfer and Schofield (2000).[1] A "male-to-female transsexual patient" was able to sustain vowel at 210 Hz, but was only identified as a woman on the phone after she raised her F2 frequencies into the cisgender female range (Mount & Salmon, 1988). Some clients like this will report being perceived as a gay man, probably because of the stereotype that gay men are men with high voice pitch.[2]

One obvious indication from both production and perception research, then, is to modify one's pitch in the direction of the desired gender presentation. Details on techniques to do so safely are in Chapter 7, but before undertaking those, we should also consider a follow-up question: How much change to target?

It is important to factor the client's wishes into the decision about what SFF level to target. A nonbinary client may not want to change SFF significantly. However, very often our clients AMAB report that they want to sound "more feminine" or even "like a cisgender female," or to have others attribute female gender easily (i.e., use "she" pronouns). In this case, the change required would likely be a tremendous amount,

[1]As explained at the beginning of this book, we use quotation marks to indicate terms used by the authors of the cited study.

[2]This is likely untrue, but a stereotype nonetheless (Rendall, Vasey, & McKenzie, 2008).

at least compared to a cisgender case of poor vocal quality or glottal fry needing to come up just a few ST (Gelfer, 1999).

The numerous examples of speakers with high F0 still being perceived as male are clear cautions against aiming for a particular Hz value without context of other acoustic variables, yet there seems to be a fascination with getting past a so-called "gender-neutral range" of 145 to 165 Hz (Gelfer & Bennet, 2013), or 145 to 175 Hz (Davies, Papp, & Antoni, 2015). However, this range may only by applicable with speakers AMAB who are trying to have a more feminine-sounding voice, because in the Gelfer and Bennet study it was the cisgender males who began to be perceived as females when SFF was higher than 165 Hz; most cisgender female speakers were still perceived as female when speaking with F0 as low as 116 Hz. Even cisgender females using an electrolarynx to provide an F0 of 85 Hz could be feminine sounding (Coleman, 1971). As we increasingly see speakers who want to lower F0, testing the validity of that range would be valuable for them. It seems people who can lower their SFF *under* the gender-neutral range could still need to do more to influence other's perceptions (Hancock, Childs, & Irwig, 2017).

The upper limit of the gender-neutral range (i.e., 165 Hz) seems generally reasonable in light of other perceptual studies in which speakers were perceived as "female" when F0 was above 155 Hz (Wolfe et al., 1990), 164 Hz (Gelfer & Schofield, 2000), or 180 Hz (Gorham-Rowan & Morris, 2006). It is important to note that the threshold appears to increase as more situational and linguistic context is removed: 155 Hz was reported in a study of conversation samples, 164 Hz for read sentences, and 180 Hz for vowels. Therefore, it is important to educate the client about how to interpret their SFF in the context of the type of speech. Connected speech above 165 Hz with good forward resonance is typically an exciting benchmark for AMAB clients.

Though perceptual research may be more relevant for the client's presentation goals, current cisgender normative data can guide extent of change targeted. A variety of published norms exist, and should be applied with appropriate consideration for the measurement context and the client's demographic and lifestyle factors. It is not too early to explain to the client some factors that influence SFF, such as speech task, age, race, smoking, economic status, and currency of norms.

Clients may not be aware of factors beyond sex-linked differences of F0. It is true that adult cisgender males typically speak at lower frequencies than adult cisgender females do

(Berg et al., 2017; Stathopoulous, Huber, & Sussman, 2011). But it is also well documented that SFF during spontaneous speech will be slightly lower than SFF of the same person during reading—as much as 1.78 ST lower (Baken & Orlikoff, 2010). Additionally, in a study of 30 (presumably cisgender) women, speech directed to a superior had a lower F0 than speech directed to a subordinate (i.e., an average of almost 3 ST lower), this difference was statistically significant though there was some individual variation (Zraick, Gentry, Smith-Olinde, & Gregg, 2006).

Clients also may be unaware that puberty is not the only time in life the voice changes. As shown in Figure 5–1, after puberty F0 typically decreases for everyone very gradually until around age 50 to 60 years, but then F0 of cisgender men begins a noticeable steady rise into later years (Baken & Orlikoff, 2010; Stathopoulous, Huber, & Sussman, 2011).

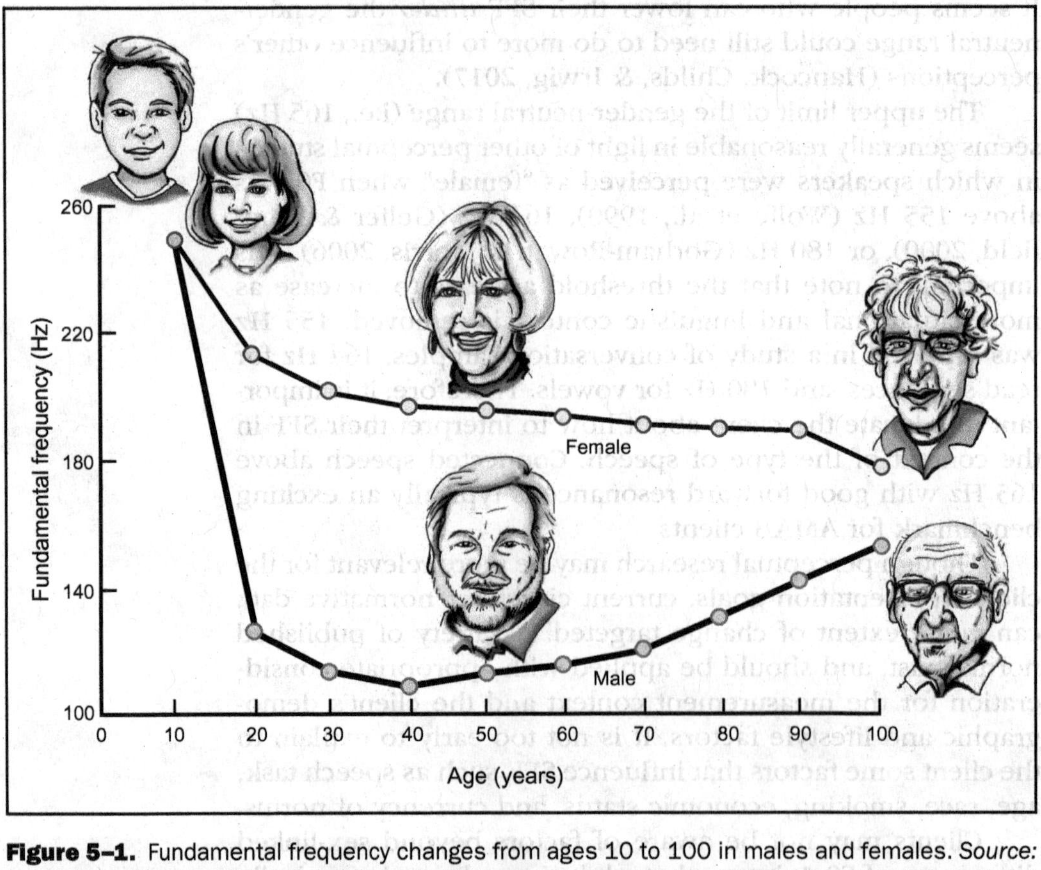

Figure 5–1. Fundamental frequency changes from ages 10 to 100 in males and females. *Source:* Reprinted with permission from Hixon, T., Weismer, G., and Hoit, J. (2020). *Preclinical Speech Science: Anatomy, Physiology, Acoustics, and Perception* (3rd ed.). San Diego, CA: Plural Publishing.

Though not as drastic as changes during cisgender male puberty or later stages of aging, hormone-related voice changes occur for most people AFAB during the menstrual cycle, pregnancy, and menopause (Kadakia, Carlson, & Sataloff, 2013; Hancock & Gross, 2015). The aging voice of trans speakers has not been adequately examined but could be influenced by their hormone treatment and levels.

Another demographic variable to consider when using normative voice data is race. Seldom is racial or ethnic information provided with normative voice data, but there is some indication that F0 may vary by race. Hudson and Holbrook (1982) measured F0 of 200 self-identified Black students, 18 to 29 years of age. The males' mean modal F0 value was 108 and 110 Hz for spontaneous speech and reading, respectively. The "females" mean modal value was 189 and 193 Hz for spontaneous speech and reading, respectively. A reasonable comparison for the reading values (i.e., modal F0 values collected from samples using the same instrumentation) is 117 Hz for white men and 217 Hz for white women (Fitch & Holbrook, 1970), which indicates a 1 ST difference for men and a 2 ST difference for women. These differences are small, but may warrant further investigation. Caution against assuming the normative data available, based largely on cisgender Caucasian volunteers, should be readily applied to gender-related voice goals without consideration of the source context. There is not good information about how other racial groups may compare to commonly used norms, at least not when using nontonal language such as English.

Lifestyle factors are associated with voice as well. People who currently smoke tobacco have significantly lower SFF in a counting task, compared to non- and former smokers (Berg et al., 2017). Speakers of higher economic status exhibited larger speaking voice frequency range (i.e., variable intonation) and dynamics (i.e., volume) (Berg et al., 2017).

A somewhat surprising finding from Berg et al. (2017) is that the SFF of female participants was lower than previous norms by almost 7 ST, which closes the gender gap by about half. Similar findings have been reported for Australian women 18 to 25 years of age speaking in 1993 compared to 1945 (Pemberton, McCormack, & Russell, 1998). Although still distinct from cisgender males, cisgender female speakers today appear to have a lower SFF than their cisgender female predecessors.

If you decide to address pitch, consider all these factors as you "get ready." Setting a specific SFF as a goal is convenient because it is tangible and quantitative, but it cannot be targeted too strictly or exclusively. After you find a starting SFF within the modal register and produced with a clear vocal quality (not breathy or strained), you will gradually work from there toward the goal. There is more than one right way to shift the SFF toward the goal. Chapter 7 contains useful techniques so you can experiment with cueing and strategies as they feel comfortable.

Prosody

While F0 and formants appear to contribute a large portion of the cues used by listeners to make judgements about speaker's gender, there remains some unexplained portion. A likely contributor is prosody, which includes suprasegmental elements of speech, such as intonation, tempo, and stress that convey meaning beyond what phonemes and vocabulary can (Leung, Oates, & Chan 2018). The unexplained portion in the series of experiments by Hillenbrand and Clark (2009) was larger for sentences than single syllables, perhaps because sentences can contain more prosodic features that could be contributing, although which prosodic features contribute remains unclear. When 19 cisgender males, matched for F0, were divided into groups of "less-masculine-sounding" (LMS) and "more-masculine-sounding" (MMS) by cisgender female listeners, the groups had similar numbers of rising and falling intonations, but MMS had intonation contours of smaller extent and slope compared to LMS (Avery & Liss, 1996). As for tempo, largely composed of articulatory rate, the MMS group had greater vowel reduction (i.e., smaller tongue and jaw movements) and less clear fricatives (i.e., smaller lip spreading) than the LMS group; there were no differences in speech rate (Avery & Liss, 1996). This is further evidence that changing F0 is not the only worthwhile goal; decisions about how to vary F0 and use articulators will influence perceptions of gender as well.

Intonation

Intonation is variation in F0, usually specified as within a phonation or utterance. Measures of interest include the pattern, degree, and rate of variation. Monotone pattern would have minimal F0 variation; some define this as a change less than 5 Hz (Wolfe et al., 1990), others as within 2 ST (Hancock,

Colton, & Douglas, 2014; Gelfer & Schofield, 2000).[3] Many other patterns exist and are described by the direction, extent, and duration of F0 shift (see Chapter 7 for examples). The latter two dimensions can be reported in a ratio (total SFF range divided by utterance duration) called the *pitch slope* or *pitch dynamism* (Henton, 1989).

Research about whether various intonation measures can differentiate speakers grouped by gender or correlate to listeners' perceptions of femininity and masculinity offers mixed results, which may be explained by the type of speech used or the measures of intonation. Analyses of trans speakers reading sentences (Gelfer & Schofield, 2000; Fitzsimons, Sheahan, & Staunton, 2001) suggest intonation does not differentiate perception of speaker's gender, whereas studies using picture descriptions (Hancock, Colton, & Douglas, 2014) and conversational speech may indicate otherwise (Wolfe, Ratusnik, Smith, & Northrop, 1990). Accepting that most intonation work should be done with and for generated speech, we will focus on those studies.

Wolfe et al. measured percentages of upward, downward, and level frequency patterns and "shifts" in conversation samples from 20 "male-to-female transsexuals." In this case a shift, occurring between utterances and sentences, is differentiated from an intonation pattern, which occurs over the utterance. The nine speakers perceived to be female used a higher percentage of upward intonation patterns and downward shifts and a smaller percentage of level shifts than the 11 speakers perceived to be male, although intonation and perception were not correlated. There was no analysis of the SFF range, extent, or speed of F0 change, nor control for variables known to be influential, such as F0.

Hancock, Colton, and Douglas (2014) analyzed picture descriptions by "male-to-female," "female-to-male," and cisgender males and females. As in Wolfe et al., speakers with larger percentages of upward intonation patterns were perceived as female sounding. Although it did not reach statistical significance, those with larger percentage of downward intonations were perceived as male sounding. Interestingly, there were not significant differences between the four speaker groups for these variables. That may have been a result of the small sam-

[3]Semitones, as a nonlinear, interval-preserving scale, are preferred for meaningful comparisons at different frequency areas on the scale (Graddol, 1986; Henton, 1995).

ple size in each group and the large within-group variation, or it could be another example of listeners making judgments based on stereotypes of feminine speech being "swoopy," even though those stereotypes are untrue (Henton, 1995).

An extensive review of speech production literature by Henton (1989) revealed that when published pitch range data were reanalyzed using the perceptually salient, nonlinear scale of ST, females have a slightly narrower SFF range than males. This is consistent with reports by Owen and Hancock (2011) but in contrast to the report by Hancock, Colton, and Douglas (2014), in which SFF range in feminine-sounding samples was slightly wider (median = 4.93 ST) than in masculine-sounding ones (median = 4.09 ST). This may be explained by a mediating variable of longer duration for pitch changes, which is accounted for in the pitch slope ratio. The pitch slope, or pitch dynamism, has not been found to be significantly different between cisgender males and cisgender females in spontaneous speech (Hancock, Colton, & Douglas, 2014).

In summary, the role of intonation in influencing listener's perceptions remains curious. Intonation pattern stereotypes might be used to mark speaker gender, but intonation measures accounting for degree and rate of pitch change do not appear to be accurate gender markers. At this time there is not enough evidence to strongly recommend adopting a particular intonation pattern or SFF range to sound more masculine or feminine, though there may be other reasons to attend to intonation in voice training.

In our experience, as clients AMAB transition their voice to higher levels of SFF they tend to become monotone and even lose what prosody they had in their initial voice session. This is perhaps a result of trying to maintain a new higher F0 by not speaking in a low voice at all, as well as not yet being comfortable with speaking higher than the new F0 as would be needed in an upward intonation (Hancock, Colton, & Douglas, 2014). When elevating SFF, Gelfer (1999) suggests staying 3 ST lower than the highest note produced with clear vocal quality to avoid falsetto and allow for upward inflections. A monotone pattern sometimes is problematic for gender attribution of female, but more importantly is problematic for the natural quality of the voice. The best predictor for how listeners will perceive naturalness of "male-to-female" voices is the lowest frequency in the speaker's total range (Hardy et al., 2016). Higher minimum frequencies predicted lower naturalness ratings.

In addition to aiding with naturalness, we suspect a wider SFF range may serve to keep the mechanism loose and flexible, facilitating extension of overall frequency range and SFF. In this sense, intonation tasks could be viewed as glissando exercises overlaid on a functional string of words. We also notice that as clients explore how intonation contours convey emotional messages, they naturally affect other prosodic features, such as loudness and rate, as well as nonverbal cues such as facial expression.

Presentation skills programs teach that vocal variety or speaking with greater expression creates emotional connection and excitement in a presentation. More specifically, broader and more varied intonation versus emphasis with volume alone can be highly effective in engaging an audience whether for a business meeting or as a professional story teller. Without intonation and other suprasegmental features superimposed on the intended message, the effectiveness of the presentation is reduced. It may not be a big leap to find that social communication with a speaker who uses vocal expression is engaging and interesting to listen to.

Until there is more research to clarify the role of intonation in voice training goals and indicate the frequency, direction, degree, and rate of pitch change that would be "enough," we simply encourage our clients to use variable intonation that matches the emotional and semantic content of the material. Of course, this means it is important to practice material with varied emotional content. Such material, starting simply and extending to more linguistic and cognitively complex speech, and visual cues that may be helpful for training are covered in detail in Chapters 6 and 7, and Appendix 6–C.

Stress and Tempo (Loudness, Rate)

We know of no studies directly investigating whether volume and rate in conversational speech contribute to gender attribution or degree of femininity or masculinity. Evaluation of vocal intensity as a factor in gender attribution is complicated by the inverse relationship between vocal intensity and breathiness, as well as the lack of investigations (Leung, Oates, & Chan, 2018). As for rate, few studies have investigated actual gender effects; those that have indicate either no gender differences or a faster speech rate in men than women (Van Borsel & De Maesschalck, 2008; Tsao & Weismer, 1997). However, the one study of conversational English speech that reported significant differences of median speech rate offered no statistical analysis and reported a range that indicates completely overlapping results from the two gender groups (Lutz & Mallard, 1986).[4] Even one of the rare studies including transgender speakers showed no significant differences in syllables per second for a read passage (Van Borsel & De Maesschalck, 2008).

A notable exception regarding rate as it relates to duration of phonemes is when the rate of speech is slowed by lengthening vowels, which may occur more with cisgender females and certain American dialects, such as Southern (Clopper, Levi, & Pisoni, 2006). Lengthening already long lax vowels of Southern male speakers makes them sound relatively more feminine (Shport, 2018).

Overall, there is hardly rationale for a hypothesis that the absolute volume or rate of a speaker contributes to perception of gender. And yet, there appears to be a belief or stereotype that women speak more quietly, slowly, and with "swooping" melody compared to men (Henton, 1995, p. 43). Two studies demonstrate this by examining what speech features change when a person is asked to switch their own vocal gender presentation from male to female. In one study, 11 speakers AMAB self-described as heterosexual cross-dressers read a standard passage in their typical masculine voice and again in their feminine voice. The feminine voice samples were consistently perceived as high (as opposed to low), breathy (not full), melodious (not raspy), and animated (not monotonous) (Andrews & Schmidt, 1997).[5]

In a similar design, six "male-to-female transsexual" speakers read material in a "female way" and a "male way," although perceptual measures were collected to validate the efforts for only two of the speakers (Gunzburger, 1995). There was individual variation among the speakers, but for the most part the "female way" samples were significantly higher pitched, quieter, and slower than the "male way" samples. Variation in pitch and volume was also different between the productions, but in opposite directions: The "female way" had greater SFF range, while the "male way" had greater intensity range. There was no further analysis of this difference, such as when and why the variations were used (i.e., emphasis for emotion, clar-

---

[4]Lutz and Mallard (1986) compared 25 cisgender males (median = 167.7 words per minute [wpm], range = 120.6 to 209.5 wpm) and 25 cisgender females (median = 151.2 wpm, range = 84.2 to 220.1 wpm).

[5]These terms and their opposing terms are what was used in the Andrews and Schmidt (1997) study.

ity, holding attention). It is also unclear which, if any, of these manipulations were conscious decisions by the speakers. If intentional, these choices may be based on unfounded stereotypes, genuinely useful cues, or strategy. It is possible that when the speakers made "extra effort to read in the female mode," as they admitted to doing, they were focused on pitch elevation and variation to such extent that the dynamism of their volume and rate decreased. We have observed something similar with clients: a capacity to focus on just one or two aspects of speech at a time, at least until they have some mastery.

Future research on suprasegmental speech features may clarify whether volume and rate are used for gender attribution, but it seems stereotypes associated with these variables, rather than genuine gender-based differences, would be the basis. We walk a fine line between capitalizing on stereotypes and perpetuating them.

As with discussions of other speech features, we do not mean to indicate goals for rate and volume are never worthwhile or justified. We have incorporated such goals with clients for various reasons. For example, in the case study of an adolescent AMAB, her self-cue mantra was "Up, slow, and strong" because her primary goals for a feminine—but also natural and age-appropriate—voice were pitch elevation, slowed rate, and confident-sounding communication (Hancock & Helenius, 2012). A speech rate of 280 wpm for the standard reading passage was too fast—even for a 15-year-old. This case is a clear example of person-centered goals, as opposed to femininity-centered goals.

Articulation

Articulation is entwined with the factors of resonance, rate, and even facial expression. As discussed above, articulator positions dictate resonant formant frequencies and first and second formant frequencies are associated with more feminine-sounding speech. Ergo, it is the articulator positions that place resonance more forward in the vocal tract (i.e., retracted lips as in "eat") and create larger space (i.e., open jaw as in "at") that serve clients targeting a more feminine sound. This appears to hold true even for speakers whose dialect already includes relatively fronted and long lax vowels, such as Southern Louisiana (Shport, 2018).

Derived using F1 and F2 of the corner vowels, vowel space area would also be dictated by articulatory positioning.

A larger vowel space area, created by exaggerated articulation, is associated with clearer speech, which can make cisgender men be perceived as feminine (Booz, 2016; Munson, 2006), though not necessarily (Avery & Liss, 1996). Clear speech via exaggerated articulation would conceivably also slow speech rate, albeit to a slight degree.

Finally, although speculative, retraction of the lips to advance F2 for resonance resembles a smile and may explain why smiles during speech are associated with women more than men in some contexts (Henton, 1995; LaFrance, Hecht, & Paluck, 2003).

Vocal Quality

Another possibility for the unexplained acoustic portion of how gender is attributed is vocal quality. Cisgender women tend to have a somewhat breathier vocal quality than cisgender men do (Klatt & Klatt, 1990; Södersten & Lindestad, 1990). This is associated with audible noise in the sound spectrum as a result of incomplete glottal patterns, which are found most often—but not always and not exclusively—in cisgender women.

An oft-cited test of breathiness' influence on perception of gender is a study by Van Borsel, Janssens, and De Bodt (2009), involving two experiments of "ah" vowels produced by seven cisgender women—one normal and one breathy but of a similar pitch (180 to 220 Hz) and intensity. Whether heard alone or in pairs, the breathy samples were always judged to sound more feminine than the nonbreathy samples. As the authors point out, because these were stimuli from cisgender women, any application to trans voice goals should be made as though other significant gender cues, such as F0 and formant frequencies of the vowel, were already in place. All the samples were perceived as belonging to women, but some to more feminine women. No acoustic analyses of the breathy samples in that experiment were provided. In another perceptual study using voice samples of mostly cisgender people, acoustic variables of voice turbulence index (VTI), soft phonation index (SPI), and the difference between the levels of first harmonic and peak of the third formant (L1 to LF3) in combination with F0 resulted in a significant predictive model for auditory perception of speaker gender (Porter & Dalhousie, 2012, as reported in Leung, Oates, & Chan, 2018), although this still only explained 67% of the variance and there is skepticism about whether these acoustic measures are valid indicators of auditory perceptions.

There are several reasons to hesitate when considering adding a breathy quality to the client's voice. First, there is no guide as to what degree of breathiness is necessary to elicit or facilitate particular gender attributions. Clients attempts to increase or decrease it could go too far, either way resulting in an inefficient phonation pattern (Berry, Verdolini, Montequin, Hess, Chan, & Titze, 2001). Also, breathiness is inversely related to volume and positively related to airflow (Södersten, Hertegård, & Hammarberg, 1995), so increasing breathiness may make adequate volume difficult. Finally, breathiness is a difficult goal to target for the same reason that its contribution is unclear: because it hard to measure. Perceptual ratings of breathiness have only low to moderate reliability as subjective measures and no clear acoustic correlate to measure objectively (Baken & Orlikoff, 2010; Zraick et al., 2011). A slightly breathy vocal quality, no more than "flow" voice (Berry, Verdolini, Montequin, Hess, Chan, & Titze, 2001), is probably just icing on the cake for transfeminine clients.

Language and Style

Gender-Linked Language Use

In the 1970s, Robin Lakoff proposed that men and women use different language according to their roles in society: Men are dominant and women are tentative. She had no empirical evidence of this but, to her credit, called for researchers to test this hypothesis and also consider context (Lakoff, 1973, 1975). Unfortunately, popular science and media did not wait for the results. Lakoff's hypotheses that women express uncertainty ("I'm not sure but I think . . . "), hedge ("kind of"), tag questions (" . . . isn't it?"), and intensifiers ("very," "so") more than men do morphed into a stereotype and solidified with confirmation bias.

Decades and scores of studies later, we know there is a kernel of truth to Lakoff's hypotheses. There are indeed some linguistic features that are used to different extents by cisgender men and women (Leaper & Ayres, 2007; Mulac, Bradac, & Gibbons, 2001; Mulac, Lundell, & Bradac, 1986), this is called *gender-linked language use.* Several meta-analyses have found a statistically significant but small effect of speaker gender on language use (Leaper & Ayres, 2007; Leaper & Robnett, 2011).

As more and more caveats were added to the lists of gendered language, the two popular explanations were found inadequate and overly simplistic (Palomares, 2016, p. 2). Assertions that differences were due to men's social power over women (dominance explanation, Lakoff, 1973, 1975) or early socialization of boys to be competitive and girls to be cooperative (gender-as-culture explanation, Mulac, Bradac, & Gibbons, 2001; Mulac, 2006) were not supported when even a few other factors were accounted for, particularly social context.

A More Accurate Basis for Language Use

Distinctions between gender groups appear to reflect cultural prototypes of men as assertive and women as affiliative. In meta-analyses the significance of moderating variables can also be tested. In other words, what else in addition to the speaker's gender is contributing to differences in how groups use language? As it turns out, there are many of these moderating variables. Aspects of the interactional context, data collection method, or even publication characteristics can influence whether or not men and women were found to use gender-linked language in controlled studies. Specifically, a large meta-analysis by Leaper and Ayres (2007) concluded:

- men are more talkative than women (significantly moderated by: operational definitions used, relationship between speakers, group size and gender composition, whether in a lab or natural space, activity context, and tier of journal that published the study);
- men use more assertive speech than women (significant moderators: operational definition, age of speaker, relationship and genders of speakers, presence of researcher in the room, whether in a lab or natural space, and activity context); and
- women use more affiliative speech than men (significant moderators: operational definition, age of speaker, familiarity and gender of speakers in lab or natural space, topic of conversation, publication year, and length of observed speech).

To illustrate the impact moderating variables can have on conversation, consider the variable of conversation topic. When discussing a stereotypically masculine topic (i.e., car repair), women use more tentative language than their male conversation partner does; however, with a stereotypically feminine topic (i.e., shopping), men use more tentative language than females do (Palomares, 2009; Wingate & Palomares, 2017). Tentative language in particular has received a lot of attention in research; meta-analyses have pointed out that despite statistical differences, "many men use tentative language with equal or even greater frequency than the average woman" (Leaper & Robnett, 2011, p. 139).

Sometimes a gender difference is not indicative of gender-based language. Just because the man and woman use different language does not guarantee that the difference is because of their genders (Palomares, 2016). Many variables involved in interactive contexts, such as conversation topic or relationship between speakers (strangers, classmates, friends, dating partners, spouses, parent-child pairs), contribute to what may at first glance seem like gender differences (Leaper & Ayres, 2007). Overall, current research demonstrates more similarity than difference between cisgender men's and women's language use. Popular science and media have not been as quick to catch on this time.

While men and women may tend to be assertive and affiliative, respectively, they are not exclusively so. Additionally, these are separate dimensions, not opposite ends of the same continuum. A person can be simultaneously highly assertive and highly affiliative at once, as in "Let's go get coffee together," or very unassertive and unaffiliative, as in "I need coffee; I can hardly keep my eyes open" (Wingate & Palomares, 2017). Of course, there is also assertive but not affiliative, such as "Go get me coffee," and unassertive but affiliative, such as "I'd love to get coffee with you." We are quick to confirm our bias that men are assertive and women are affiliative, but the empirical evidence indicates it is only sometimes true—much more often it is false. One implication of this is that the dimensions of affiliation and assertiveness, as opposed to a gendered dimension, are preferable for use when training clients to use language style that is authentic and effective.

It may be useful at this point to briefly describe an explanatory framework for why and how people decide what language to employ in any given situation. In short, it is based upon how they categorize themselves relative to the situation. Speakers choose what language features to use depending on their gender schema (i.e., their beliefs or stereotypes about gender as it relates to personal attributes and roles) and their gender salience in the given situation (Palomares, 2009).

Gender salience is the degree to which one's identity as a member of a gender group is cognitively activated. In other words, how much one's gender identity matters in a social context. For example, gender salience is greater among strangers than familiar people so speakers are more likely to use gendered language when communicating with strangers than friends (Leaper & Ayres, 2007). Even when gender salience is somewhat activated, it may take a back seat to other aspects of identity that influence language if they are more salient. For example, language differences between cisgender men and women disappeared when gender salience was low. Gender salience was lowered simply by being directed to think about being a student, as opposed to thinking about being a female or male (Palomares, 2008). Any gender-based language differences are dependent upon gender being salient to the speaker.

Gender salience stems from self-categorization theory, coupled with an intergroup perspective on social interactions, and is an improvement from the dominance and gender-as-culture theories because it can explain gender-linked language use while accounting for factors such as modality of language and social context (Palomares, 2016). Discussion of how the client categorizes themselves in various contexts—understanding it is and should be dynamic—will be important for any client wondering what to say. Shifting away from a *men-say-this-women-say-that* mentality can bring freedom to our clients who fear saying the wrong words, let alone the wrong way. Once again, the literature supports a person-centered view of communication rather than a checklist for binary gender presentation.

How Language Is Perceived

Our clients may be interested in choosing language for the purpose of their gender presentation, with hopes of influencing other's perceptions. We will now turn to discussion of if, when, and how that could happen.

That listeners can accurately predict speaker gender based on these language features is called the gender-linked language effect (GLLE) (Mulac, 2006). Will our clients using more directives, for example, be classified as men? Not necessarily. The GLLE is not direct (i.e., "They said x, so they are a man") but rather mediated by gender schemata, which again are essentially gender-based stereotypes of personal attributes (i.e., "They said x, and that makes them very dynamic, and men are more dynamic than women, so they must be a man"). Our clients using a lot of directives will be perceived as dynamic. If the listener's gender schemata is that men are more dynamic than women, then the client may be perceived as male in addition to dynamic.

The GLLE posits that language influences perceptions of the speaker attributes of sociointellectual status, aesthetic quality, and dynamism. In spontaneous natural language ranging from picture descriptions to public speaking, females rated higher on sociointellectual status and aesthetic quality and lower on dynamism, compared to males (Mulac & Lundell, 1982; Mulac, Lundell, & Bradac, 1986).

When the GLLE is considered in the big picture—termed the General Process Model of Speaker Evaluations—the situational input (i.e., context) is distinguished from the speaker and hearer's perception of context (Cargile & Bradac, 2001; Mulac et al., 2003; Mulac, Giles, Bradac, & Palomares, 2013). Both the speaker and listener have gender-linked language schemata and stereotypes that influence speaker's behavior and the listener's judgments and behaviors. This is consistent with the ASSEMBLE approach described at the beginning of this chapter, because it includes multiple factors, some unalterable by the speaker and provider, that contribute to communicative exchanges. In summary, the client's agency to use language to their advantage when constructing gender is limited.

Nonverbal Language

In studies comparing audio-only, video-only, and audiovisual modes of presentation, physical appearance influenced the audience's rating of "femaleness/maleness" of "male-to-female transsexuals" (Van Borsel, De Cuypere, & Van den Berghe, 2001) but not seven "female-to-male transsexuals" (Van Borsel, de Pot, & De Cuypere, 2009). This research has been used to demonstrate the role of noverbal behavior in gender attributions. Yet, this is based on reading a passage in Dutch, and only the participants' head and shoulders were shown. Although the participants in Van Borsel et al. (2009) were reported to be "dressed as women," aspects of the visible appearance (e.g., hairstyle, facial structure, clothing) and movement (e.g., head nodding, eye gaze, smiling) were not described nor analyzed. Further studies are needed to clarify which aspects of the video presentation were meaningful in these studies.

It is not disputed that meaning can be constructed from body position and movement, proxemics (i.e., distance between people), haptics (touching behavior), and other nonverbal behaviors and appearances. Nothing leverages this better than the arts; consider dance, silent movies, sculptures of people, and portraits. Social sciences examine subtle visual cues to a person's unspoken thoughts, feelings, and intentions (e.g., lie detection, threat assessment, attraction) with numerous personal and industrial applications (e.g., business, politics, healthcare decisions). Yet, most of the popular research claiming that a large portion[6] of communication is nonverbal is highly context specific to emotional topics. Furthermore, the gender-linked nonverbal behaviors and the power of nonverbal behaviors to influence how others attribute gender are routinely overgeneralized without caveat. In both the arts and in the sciences, it is clear that context can drastically shift the meaning. Gender-based differences in nonverbal behavior such as smiling, gaze, interpersonal distance, and touching are mediated by cultural gender norms and gender salience (Wingate & Palomares, 2017).

One of the more robust gender-linked findings is that cisgender women tilt and nod their head, and smile more often than cisgender men do (Boker et al., 2011; Krumhuber, Manstead, & Kappas, 2007). In a large meta-analysis, the size of this gender effect was low to medium (d = .41) but varied by nationality, ethnicity, age, and situational factors. For example, the effect diminished when gender or familiarity with the communication partner—which influence gender salience—are accounted for; women smile most with other women, men smile least with other men, and gender differences are very small with a familiar partner (LaFrance, Hecht, & Paluck, 2003). In a study of 740,984 participants from 12 countries, females smiled more than males did, with a much larger gender effect found in more individualist countries such as the U.S. and U.K., compared to Columbia, Peru, and China (McDuff, Girard, & Kaliouby, 2017).

In the vast sea of popular books on gendered body language—which generally ignore the pesky factor of context—there is some consensus of how cisgender men and women in Western cultures communicate with their bodies. One very popular axiom is that men position and move to take up more space than women do, typically explained by men's intention to assert control over the space. This has been

[6]Mehrabian (1972) reported messages communicating feelings and attitudes are conveyed by words (7%), vocal elements (38%), and nonverbal elements such as facial expression, gestures, and posture (55%). The series of studies involved perceptions of speakers of one-word utterances and has not been replicated in studies using paradigms disguising the purpose of the study (Trimboli & Walker, 1987).

studied in contexts from artwork (Davies, 2018) to airplanes (Hai, Khairullah, & Coulmas, 1982).

It is true that people with higher status display more open posture (i.e., limbs open instead of crossed) and take up more space (Hall, Coats, & LeBeua, 2005). Also, when people feel powerful, they stretch out, specifically with arms up and lifted chin, described as a "V" shape. This is referred to as the "power pose" and made popular in Cuddy's TED talk about this research (2012). Conversely, when people feel powerless, they hold their arms in, essentially making themselves smaller. Very importantly, this is done because of the person's social power or how the person feels—or perhaps is trying to feel. If men are taking up more space, it is because they are feeling more powerful. If women are not taking up space, it is because they are feeling powerless. The link between body language and gender is indirect, mediated by sociocultural power dynamics. Consider the implications for your client. If she learns to take up less space, she may or may not be perceived as more feminine—depending on whether her audience associated powerlessness with femininity—but research shows she will begin to feel more powerless.

Role Congruity Theory explains that traits associated with women and traits associated with power are often seen as incompatible to the extent that gender alone becomes a cue for power status. Anecdotally, trans clients have experienced this sexism from both sides and attest to the difference. However, in a study designed to directly investigate how power hierarchies are formed and maintained, the person's pose—not their gender—primed the perception of dominant versus submissive (Bailey & Kelly, 2015). This suggests that anyone of any gender can be perceived as more powerful if they have open posture and use more space when communicating. In this case, your marginalized, disadvantaged, fearful client may benefit from working on this nonverbal aspect of their communication.

By operating with a philosophy of person-centered intervention for communicative function and satisfaction, we are certainly within our bounds to address interpersonal communication affected by non-verbal behavior. We make it clear, however, that the best available evidence is about a person expressing feeling and conveying degrees of power or confidence in personal interactions. We acknowledge and navigate the socialized gender norms, but do not have to aim for them.

In summary, ascribing personality or motive to body language purely according to the users' gender meets the same downfalls that gendered language faced. Once again, we find that "people of this gender do that communicative behavior" is an inaccurate social stereotype based on culturally entrenched beliefs about gender roles. A more precise description is, "people of this gender tend to do that if *x, y, z*," or "people perceived as this attribute do that communication behavior." Correlations must be explored to identify underlying cause(s). Meanwhile, we refuse to perpetuate the overlay of gender-related absolutes where there is no evidence for it.

Implications for Including Language and Style in Intervention Plans

As scientists began to explore the communicator's behavior in context of the recipient, including their cultural, functional, and biological factors, the picture of gendered language became more complicated and nuanced, but allowed us to be less reliant on untested stereotypes. Practical activities to explore what works for the client are described in Chapter 7. Some general approaches for setting goals in this area are as follows:

- Address language style without attaching it to a gender group or norm. Linguistic research has described styles as being affiliative, assertive, talkative or indicative of a person with high sociointellectual status, aesthetic quality, and dynamism. Any gender can be any of these. These terms are descriptive and easier to understand than parts of speech for many clients. Most people can adopt a style of speaking without having to explicitly tally the number of adverbs or adjectives they're using. No need to add cognitive load!
- Frame the discussion to focus on effective interpersonal communication as the primary goal. The purpose and context of communication will dictate the appropriate language style. For example, all clients—not just trans men—should learn to communicate with high and with low assertiveness, and how to select appropriately based on purpose and context. Too often we hear trans women say they don't know how to be assertive as a boss anymore because they are only able to sound assertive by lowering their pitch. In these cases, training assertive language is an important goal and you can assuage their fears about "only men use

assertive language" by discussing the many moderating variables that make that statement only rarely true.

- Gender salience is a robust moderating variable in gendered language use and effects and is fairly easy to manipulate, so this would be a worthwhile target as a means to produce more gender-based language in contexts for which it could matter. This concept is applicable to any person regardless of sex assigned at birth or binary/nonbinary positioning. Since any person will use more gendered language more when their gender salience is high (Palomares, 2016), simply learn how to raise their gender salience (a frame of "lower their gender salience" might be better for some, especially nonbinary clients). Research studies have increased gender salience by choosing feminine or masculine topics for conversation (Palomares, 2009; Postmes & Spears, 2002) or reading a paragraph about being female, male, or student (for low gender salience) prior to a task (Palomares, 2004, 2008).
- Related to the interpersonal communication framework and gender salience, consider the genders of the client's communication partners. Gender salience, and therefore gendered language use, is greater in mixed-sex dyads than same-sex dyads and with strangers than familiar partners (Leaper & Ayres, 2007; Hancock & Rubin, 2015; Palomares, 2009). Thus, clients' language use during practice with familiar cisgender female providers may not correspond to their language use with unknown cisgender men in everyday social and occupational contexts. In general, design practice contexts to be similar to target contexts, including number and gender of conversation partners, topics and purpose of conversation, and setting (i.e., get out of the provider's office).
- When discussing these areas of visual communication with clients, guard against the great potential for your own aesthetics and biases to crowd out the client's desires and intentions. Guiding them to learn and become skillful with tools for how to communicate their sociocultural positioning visually follows the same person-centered approach we have discussed for doing it auditorily. The major difference is that there is much less research about how visual and nonverbal communication contribute to the construction of gender in

a cultural context, so we have relatively less to offer in this area. Given the current paucity of empirical research, it would be easy to inadvertently perpetuate an unfounded gender stereotype by telling clients exactly what to look, move, or be like.

INTERVENTION OPTIONS

At this stage, the practitioner and client are considering what behaviors to target and how. The client is likely most interested in a behavioral approach if they are in your office, but they may have questions about a hormonal or surgical approach, either concurrently or as a possibility for the future. Evidence for various intervention options will be organized here in terms of feminizing or masculinizing the sound of the voice to be consistent with the literature. Specific techniques used in a behavioral approach are presented in Chapters 6 and 7, where they are organized for facilitating vocal change in various aspects of voice and speech rather than organized by binary gender concepts.

Masculine-Sounding Voice

Years ago, the notion of transmasculine people receiving voice training would be generally dismissed, citing that testosterone therapy would largely meet the vocal needs of that population. However, the extent and rate of voice change to expect when starting testosterone varies widely. When F0 of just seven trans men was tracked over the first year of testosterone therapy, four different patterns of lowering were identified: minimal change (n = 1), change over first 6 months only (n = 2), change over months 3 to 9 only (n = 2), and gradual change over all 12 months (n = 2) (Irwig, Childs, & Hancock, 2016). The phonation frequency range of these patients all shifted down the scale, but three actually experienced a decrease in range (Hancock, Childs, & Irwig, 2017). A meta-analysis of testosterone therapy for masculinizing voice and trans patients specifically found that 21% of participants still had F0 above 131 Hz after 1 year on testosterone, 21% reported incomplete voice-gender congruence, 46% had voice problems, and 16% were unsatisfied with their voice (Ziegler, Henke, Wiedrick, & Helou, 2018).

In addition to acknowledgement of unpredictable effects of testosterone, potential for undesirable side effects of testosterone on the voice should not be ignored. Like cisgender women exposed for various reasons to high-levels of testosterone, our clients taking testosterone may experience detriments in vocal stability, power, and quality (Azul et al., 2017).

As transmasculine populations are studied it becomes clear that the vocal situations are far from unproblematic (Azul, 2015, 2016). In a review of 14 research studies and 10 expert opinion papers on transmasculine voice, the majority identified restrictions to vocal situations and function (Azul et al., 2017), including:

- voice quality,
- pitch range and variability,
- vocal control and stability,
- vocal power,
- vocal endurance,
- glottal function,
- singing voice (other than pitch range),
- respiration, and
- muscle tension and posture.

As an alternative or supplement to hormone therapy, transmasculine people may consider surgical or behavior interventions. A surgical approach to lower pitch would likely involve Type 3 thyroplasty. Most often used in cases of puberphonia, this surgery has also shown success for a few case reports of trans men but is not yet widely used or thoroughly investigated (Saito, Nakamura, Itani, & Tsukahara, 2018).

As described previously, pitch and resonance would likely be worthwhile targets for changing gender-related vocal presentation. Recall that speech with a low pitch may still sound feminine without adjusting resonance to balance the formant frequencies with the lowering F0. Therefore, even if hormonal or surgical intervention effectively addresses F0, behavioral interventions may be appropriate and even necessary to achieve voice-gender congruence as well as balance voice production to decrease vocal dysfunction reported by Azul et al. (2017).

There are very few empirical examinations of the effectiveness of a purely behavioral approach. Söderpalm, Larsson, and Almquist (2004) reported outcomes of 25 people referred to the voice clinic in Sweden, three of whom were identified as "female-to-male transsexuals," but data from only one of those was available at follow up. This person was able to decrease F0 from 148 to 113 Hz, improve vocal stability, and extinguish vocal fatigue. Information regarding the targets or techniques were not provided. At this time, clinical expertise based on knowledge and experience is guiding recommendations for this approach with people AFAB (Block, 2017; Davies, Papp, & Antoni, 2015).

Feminine-Sounding Voice

Estrogens, progestins, and/or antiandrogens may be included in endocrine treatment regimens of trans women or people wishing to feminize their presentation. In cisgender women, fluctuation in estrogens and progestins cause small changes in the voice during the menstrual cycle, pregnancy, and menopause (Abitbol, Abitbol, & Abitbol, 1999). Recommended dosages of these hormones for trans women are often two to three times the levels recommended for hormone replacement therapy in postmenopausal cisgender women, yet changes in voice are not evident (Moore, Wishniewski, & Dobs, 2003). This is likely attributed to the irreversible effects of testosterone on the voice. Therefore, the expectations for voice effects of endocrine treatment depend on the client's previous testosterone exposure. Clients who experienced deepening of the voice from testosterone may consider surgical, behavioral, or a combination of these approaches to feminize their vocal presentation.

Surgical Approach

Laryngeal surgery can elevate fundamental frequency (so-called "pitch-raising surgery") by either stretching the vocal folds or shortening them. Vocal folds are attached anteriorly to the thyroid notch (Adam's apple) so when the thyroid is tilted forward and down the vocal folds are stretched, increasing tension and resulting in a higher F0. Normal contraction of the cricothyroid muscle facilitates increased F0 this way (Figure 5–2). Cricothyroid approximation (CTA) surgery affixes the thyroid cartilage to the cricoid cartilage so that the vocal folds will be stretched without need for sustained contraction of the cricothyroid muscle (Figure 5–3).

Surgically shortening the length of the vocal folds (called glottoplasty) is typically achieved by removing some anterior

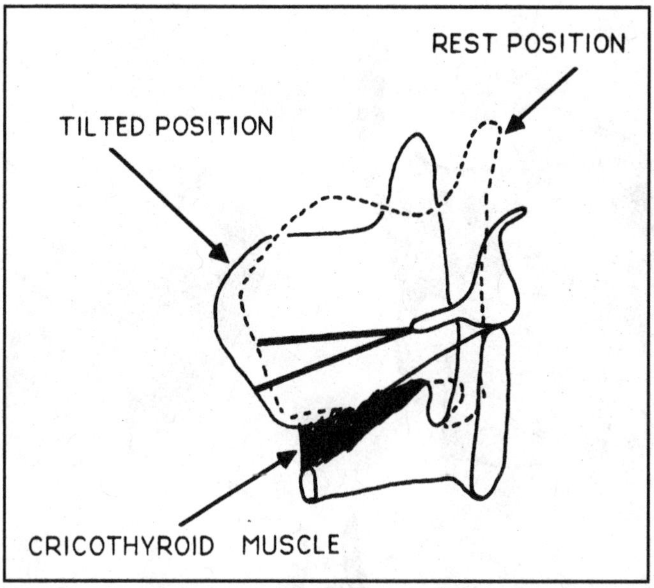

Figure 5–2. Normal function of cricothyroid muscle. *Source:* Reprinted with permission from Baken, R. J. (2017). An overview of laryngeal function for voice production. In R. T. Sataloff (Ed.), *Voice science* (2nd ed., p. 153). San Diego, CA: Plural Publishing.

portion of the vocal folds and connecting the folds anteriorly to form a new anterior commissure posterior to the original (Figure 5–4). Variations of this approach include Wendler glottoplasty, feminization laryngoplasty, and vocal fold retrodisplacement and advancement of the anterior commissure.

Attempts to increase F0 by decreasing the mass of the vocal fold have also been described in the early literature but are infrequent, or done in conjunction with other methods. Titze (2011) provides calculations that suggest length and stiffness of the vocal folds, rather than mass, are factors most influential to F0 (see Box 5–1).

Note these surgeries target F0 increase only. Yet it is widely accepted that formant frequencies, determined by vocal tract configuration, make important contributions to feminine-sounding voices. Thomas and MacMillian (2013) describe a surgical procedure to shorten the vocal tract length by removing some superior thyroid cartilage, then very closely suspending it from the hyoid bone. This procedure was done, along with removing anterior segments of thyroid cartilage and true and false vocal folds and creating a new anterior commissure and overall smaller larynx, for 54 patients. Their

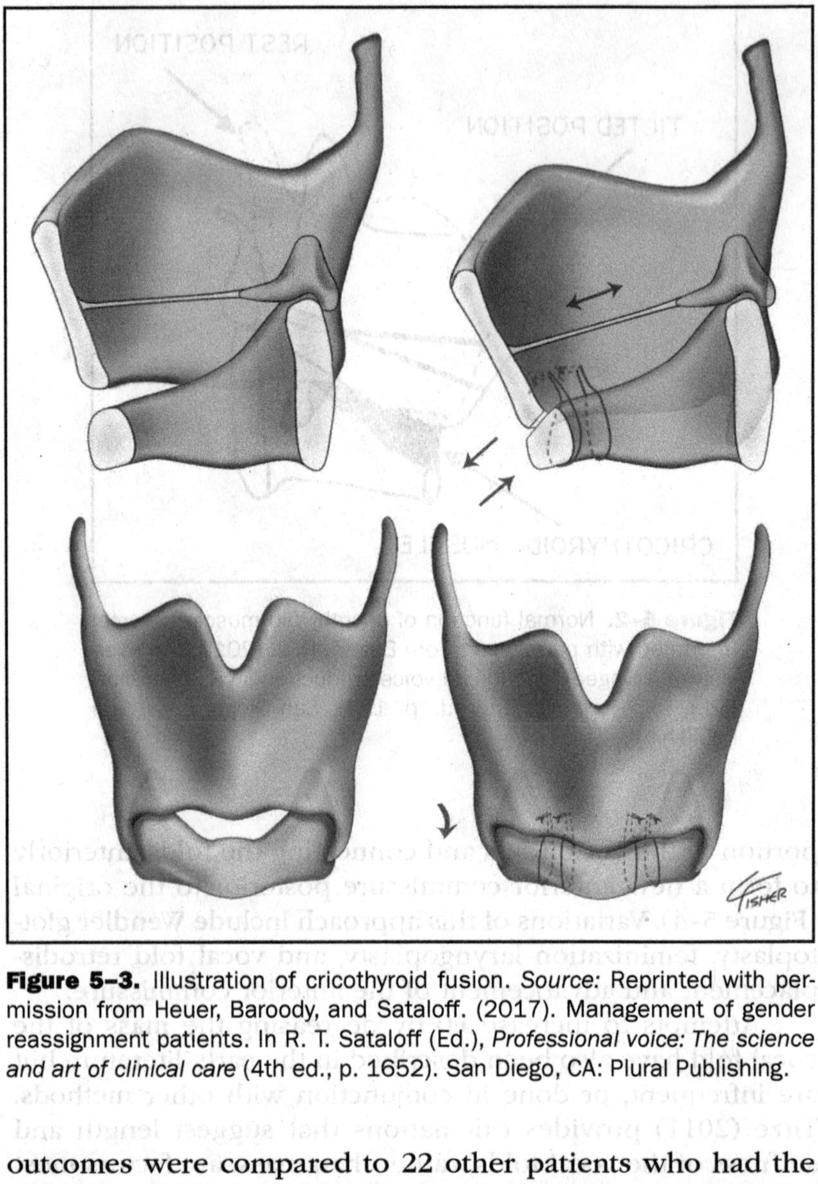

Figure 5–3. Illustration of cricothyroid fusion. *Source:* Reprinted with permission from Heuer, Baroody, and Sataloff. (2017). Management of gender reassignment patients. In R. T. Sataloff (Ed.), *Professional voice: The science and art of clinical care* (4th ed., p. 1652). San Diego, CA: Plural Publishing.

outcomes were compared to 22 other patients who had the anterior modification but not the thyrohyoid approximation procedure (Thomas & MacMillan, 2013). Both groups experienced significant increase in mean F0 (average of 5.5 and 6 ST), and decrease in F0 range (overall average of 10 ST), but no measures of formants or perceptual ratings were collected. Effectiveness of surgical approach to anything besides increase of F0 remains unknown but could be explored as it does not appear to affect an outcome of primary concern: resonance.

In a meta-analysis of 13 studies (six classified as CTA, six as shortening glottoplasty and one as reduction glottoplasty),

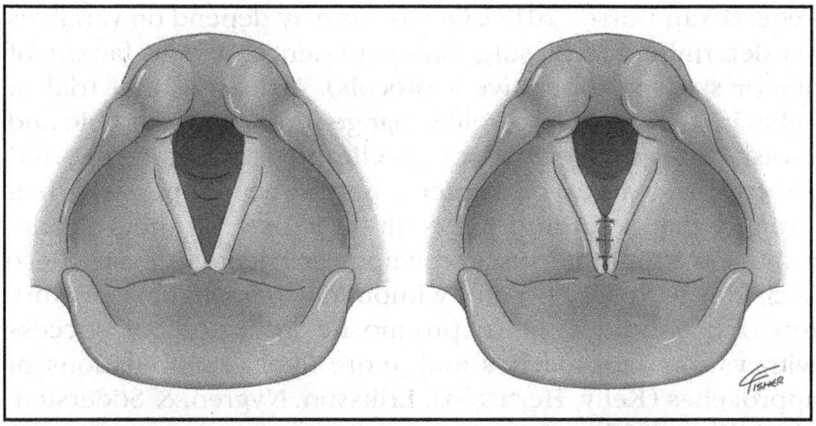

Figure 5–4. Illustration of vocal folds of normal and shortened length. Source: Reprinted with permission from Heuer, R. J., Baroody, M., and Sataloff, R. T. (2017). Management of gender reassignment patients. In R. T. Sataloff (Ed.), *Professional voice: The science and art of clinical care* (4th ed., p. 1654). San Diego, CA: Plural Publishing.

the shortening technique resulted in the greatest F0 increase, but also the greatest heterogeneity of outcomes (Song & Jiang, 2017). In this meta-analysis, the shortening glottoplasty was most successful for F0, but unique complications included scar tissue or dehiscense of the new web, whereas the CTA did not have these complications but more commonly did not raise F0 and did not maintain F0 over time. In a direct comparison of long-term outcomes for CTA and glottoplasty procedures, outcomes for CTA were so relatively poor that the procedure is no longer performed at that institution (Kelly, Hertegård, Eriksson, Nygren, & Södersten, 2018). Specifically, mean F0 increased and was maintained after both types of surgery, but F0 range decrease was significantly greater for the CTA group (14.5 ST) than the glottoplasty group (4.4 ST), both primarily from the upper end of their total frequency range. Additionally, more patients in the CTA group reported dysphonia, and satisfaction measures were better in the glottoplasty group. It is of note that all patients in this longitudinal study increased F0 to a gender-neutral range with voice modification services with a speech therapist before deciding to have surgery.

One meta-analysis of pitch-raising surgeries acknowledged the overall positive outcomes of F0 and patient satisfaction reported in the research literature, but ultimately concluded that existing evidence for effectiveness of surgical procedures was insufficient because of low-quality research designs and analyses (Van Damme, Cosyns, Deman, Van den

Eede, & Van Borsel, 2017). Outcomes may depend on variables yet determined (e.g., surgeon's experience, patient factors of age or size, postoperative protocols). At least a brief trial of behavioral approach to voice change prior to irreversible and invasive surgery seems worthwhile no matter the reported effectiveness rates of surgery, but some people will feel strongly that a surgical intervention is best for them. Again, providers should inform and empower clients to make these decisions with support and without our personal bias. Future research should explore prognostic indicators of success with various approaches and, more likely, combinations of approaches (Kelly, Hertegård, Eriksson, Nygren, & Södersten, 2018; Kim, 2017).

Behavioral Approach

Empirical evidence for behavioral interventions for trans women wishing to have a more feminine-sounding voice is presented in Table 5–1. As with investigations of surgical approaches, there are no randomized control trials (RCTs) but quasiexperimental, observational-analytical, and observational-descriptive studies have consistently showed marked progress. Treatments generally target increasing pitch and more anterior resonance—often via precise articulation—with attention to respiratory-phonatory support and pitch variation (i.e., intonation). Often service delivery involves weekly sessions for several months at a university clinic. Outcome measures tend to be limited to acoustic with some indication of speaker satisfaction. Perceptual ratings by naive listeners in a few studies were not significantly influenced, although those same studies were of short intervention periods and also had fewer acoustic changes than other studies (Gelfer & Tice, 2013; Gelfer & Van Dong, 2013).

When selecting targets and discussing the general sequence of indirect and prepatory work followed by direct voice work, a chart similar to Figure 5–5 may be helpful. Some targets will take longer than others to develop—for trans women, resonance often takes the longest—and targets will be developed and integrated before being mastered. This may seem obvious to a practitioner familiar with voice, but clients should be educated about the need to address the speech system as a whole, as opposed to changing pitch only, for example. We find this tends to be particularly enlightening for clients who have explored the internet for videos and tutorials about voice change.

Table 5–1. Empirical Studies of Voice Treatment for Trans People

	Participants	Intervention	Outcome	Additional notes
Quasiexperimental (Level 2)				
Meszaros et al., 2005	Three MtF (two untreated MtF) Vocally healthy, taking estrogen	One session per week (8 to 19 months) incorporating auditory discrimination and audiovisual feedback using the voice range profile to target "high-pitch vocalization by using the first articulation zone, a costoabdominal breathing technique to lengthen the time of expiration, to decrease laryngeal muscle tension, and to increase head resonance as compared to chest resonance. Careful attention was paid to the formation of soft tones, precise articulation, and the attainment of a female intonation [and] increasing the intensity."	For trained group only: • Habitual pitch shifted into female levels. • Pitch range shifted upward on the scale, sometimes diminishing due to greater elevation of the lower limit than the upper limit. • Improved or maintained healthy levels for: intensity range, maximum phonation time, self-rating of communicative impairment, and Friedrich's dysphonia index. One untrained person worsened on ratings of voice quality, MPT, and Friedrich's dysphonia index.	Trans women on estrogen but without voice training do not improve, and may develop dysphonia.

continues

Table 5–1. *continued*

	Participants	Intervention	Outcome	Additional notes
Gelfer & Tice, 2013	Five trans women (comparison: five cis men and five cis women matched by age and height) at an American university's speech clinic	8 weeks of two 1-hour group sessions per week (groups were either two or three people) incorporating immediate audiovisual feedback about voice frequency and quality using pitch trace software. Each session began with /m/-vowel syllable on target SFF with good oral resonance and progressed to words beginning with nasal and liquid phonemes. Then, at phrase level, "intonation and natural-sounding speech" was added to the focus. This progressed through complete sentences, increasing first by length and complexity then by emotional content, and finally picture descriptions, role-playing, or open-ended questions.	**Perceptual:** Percentage of voice samples (pooled across five speakers) judged by listeners to sound "female" went from 2% pre- to 51% immediately post-treatment (individual percentages ranged from 10 to 92%), and from 8% pre- to 33% 15 months post-treatment (range 12 to 96%). These results are mirrored in interval-scale ratings of femininity and masculinity. **Acoustic:** Statistically significant change from pre- to immediate-post and 15-month post-treatment for SFF in spontaneous speech, reading, and vowels, as well as SFF upper and lower limit of semispontaneous answers to questions, and first formant frequency of sustained /i/.	• On average, SFF during even spontaneous speech changed significantly, and was somewhat maintained more than a year later. • Although every person moved toward their goals, large perceptual outcome variability across the five participants limited statistical significance. Why some people make large gains and others don't remains unclear in this study.
Gelfer & Van Dong, 2013	Three trans women (comparison: three cis men and three cis women matched by age and height) at an American university's speech clinic	6 weeks of two 1-hour group sessions per week (groups were either two or three people) and Stemple's VFE two times each, twice per day at home, for the entire 6-week period.	**Perceptual:** Immediately following training, the three participants' speech samples were judged to sound female at rates of 15%, 7%, and 0%.	• Participants reported VFE was a positive experience but insufficient without the voice training.

	Participants	Intervention	Outcome	Additional notes
Gelfer & Van Dong, 2013 *continued*		Two additional sessions provided training and follow-up on the VFEs. Group sessions used symptomatic therapy protocol as described above for Gelfer and Tice, 2013.	However, they all gained in listener ratings of femininity, to various degrees.	• Addition of VFE did not appear to contribute to measured outcomes.
Observational-Analytical (Level 3)				
Carew, Dacakis, & Oates, 2007	10 "male-to-female transsexuals" aged 25 to 64 years, six of whom were living full-time in female roles and receiving care at an Australian university's speech clinic in 2002	Five 45-minute weekly sessions to increase use of lip spreading and forward tongue carriage during speech. These were targeted separately until both were mastered in complete sentences. Instructional techniques included clinician models and clients' positive and negative practice in vowels, syllables, words, phrases, sentences, and conversation. Clients were asked to complete at least 15 minutes of daily home practice with reading.	• Gains in group mean and median F1 were significant for /a/ and /u/, for F2 only for /a/, and for F3 /i/, /a/, and /u/. • Post-treatment gains in F0 were significant, but the group mean only went from 119 Hz to 133 Hz. • Listener's ratings of speaker femininity increased for seven participants, decreased for two and was stable for one. • Participant's self-ratings of satisfaction and femininity of voice improved significantly, both ratings changed from a mean of 3.4 to 5.6 on a 10-cm horizontal line scale.	• Large individual variation • Average gains were statistically significant, but post-treatment measures still appear to be in the range of cisgender male norms. • Possible more gains would be made with this approach if more sessions.

continues

Table 5–1. *continued*

	Participants	Intervention	Outcome	Additional notes
Dacakis, 2000	10 "male-to-female" transsexuals aged 32 to 58 years receiving care at an Australian university's speech clinic	Received training for between 1 and 8.9 years (mean = 4.3 years) prior to this follow-up assessment. The techniques are only described as "focused primarily on increasing mean fundamental frequency."	Comparison of SFF during monologue at initial session, discharge, and follow-up revealed some, but not all, gains were maintained. At follow up, six people were within 3 Hz of discharge level and four others lost 20 to 30 Hz but not all the way to initial levels. Satisfaction ratings were high (mean = 78/100 at discharge)	More sessions were significantly correlated to maintenance of SFF gains.
Hancock & Garabedian, 2013	Retrospective review of 25 "male-to-female" clients receiving care at an American university's speech clinic from 2006 to 2010	Weekly 1-hour sessions during semester schedule with home practice assigned for semester breaks. Average of 22 sessions (range 2 to 77) typically targeting increase in F0 by 5 Hz increments as well as forward oral resonance beginning with bilabial and semi-vowel phonemes, and progressing through hierarchy of linguistic complexity. Relaxation, reducing phonotraumatic behaviors, and breath control were common goal targets. Vocal variety and upward intonation were also addressed by a majority of clients. Less than half of the clients targeted pragmatics, language, and nonverbal language.	Average gains of 6 semitones for vowel and 5 semitones in reading and monologue were statistically significant, with large effect sizes. No significant changes in intensity or MPFR.	F0 gains were correlated with greater number of sessions, but not with age, percent of time presenting as female, or initial acoustic measures of F0, SFF, MPFR, or intensity.

	Participants	Intervention	Outcome	Additional notes
Soderpalm et al., 2004	22 "male-to-female" and three "female-to-male" transsexuals referred to voice clinic in Sweden between 1991 and 2002.	21 trans women received treatment: Vocal hygiene exercises (relaxation, balance of expiratory and laryngeal/muscular effort) and pitch raising exercises of gradual climbing/gliding, exactness of articulation, and encouraging more anterior articulation. Built on "accent method but broadened and individualized." Three of these trans women were referred for phonosurgery.	F0 significantly increased for trans women. Vocal fatigue was reduced.	• More than half showed supraglottal constriction during phonation. • Degree of satisfaction with post-treatment voice was not correlated with number of sessions.

Note. Levels according to Joanna Briggs Institute (2011), http://joannabriggs.org/

Treatment Periods	1	2	3	4	5	6	7	8	9	10
Postural alignment	D	I	I	M	M	M	M	M	M	M
Relaxation	D	I	I	I	M	M	M	M	M	M
Breathing	D	I	I	I	I	M	M	M	M	M
Pitch	E	D	D	D	D	D	I	I	M	M
Resonance	E	D	D	D	D	D	D	I	I	M
Prosody	E	E	D	D	D	I	I	M	M	M
Pragmatics, etc.	E	E	E	E	D	D	I	M	M	M

E = May be emerging skill, occasional feedback but not a focus

D = Developing, primary focus of session

I = Integrating use with other skills and more contexts

M = Mastered, independent with occasional feedback

Figure 5–5. General progression of skill development.

PROCESS PERSPECTIVE

Unfortunately, no amount of research or expertise can provide a magic potion. The idea that perfection is possible, required, or even desired in training needs to be debunked. Vocal training takes time and requires intentional and active daily practice, dedication, discipline, patience, and progressive skill. "Getting ready" can be a time when assumptions and fears clients may hold are realized and adjusted. It will be important to be comfortable with the idea that this training is essentially a process of exploring the voice.

Focusing on a final outcome too much can distract them from the process. Sometimes clients express resistance or frustration, saying things like, "But that doesn't sound like me," or "I feel ridiculous using this voice." This may seem like a "vocal adolescence" stage, in which the voice is not what it was and feels awkward and far away from what it could be, is inevitable in the vocal transformation process. Accepting and working through this leads to the final stage of growth and achieving vocal goals. If a client fixates too much on where they are not and where they should be vocally, the process will get stuck. The example of a client, Karen, in Box 5–2 illustrates one way this obstacle can be uncovered and addressed.

Box 5–2. Case Example: Developing a Process Perspective

Karen had been training for a more feminine-sounding voice for five months. She attended sessions regularly and was receptive to home practice but was developing slowly. She expressed frustration with herself often. When we explored this together, she shared that she approached voice training with the idea that her voice needed to sound a certain way now. Because of this, she was resistant to the evolving voice. Her inner reaction was that "this voice is not what I want". She often became quite depressed at the end of a session, and from week to week there was little allowance for process, only for outcome. Once we discussed it openly, she revealed that she believes that "if I feel dissatisfied until I get what I want, this will help me get what I want." This simply does not work in any facet of life.

With the help of counseling support in the session, she was able to allow greater acceptance of her voice from session to session. Learning a new skill is similar to a child learning to stand, then walk, then run. They develop balance, then apply balance in function, and finally use balance at higher levels of function. We make allowances in evolving function, and deeply enjoy witnessing the independence develop—and they do too! Vocal feminization work is not that different, it is just that we have to learn how to focus on what we can do versus what we are not doing.

To help Karen move forward with a process perspective, she was guided to write a couple of sentences in her journal at the end of each day to train her brain to look at what worked, what helped, and what she liked about her "practice" voice. She then brought her journal to our sessions and we discussed it together. Occasionally we look would back over time to notice the ebb and flow of a natural process of progress. Learning to accept and be in the process keeps one more present, aligned with the needs of the moment, and more open and relaxed mentally, emotionally, and physically.

It helps clients to know that progress is not usually a straight line upward. Seeing an image such as the one in Figure 5–6 can be helpful for clients to understand that growth is inconsistent from session to session as the brain rewires, personal resistances are explored and integrated, and life circumstances arise and pass. In Figure 5–6, the lower left corner represents the starting point in training and the right upper most corner the end of training where clients goals have been met. The solid line shows a constant upward progression, while the dotted line indicates the ups and downs along the way. Knowing that they both meet at the upper right corner of the graph can be illuminating. See the companion website for this book for videos of clients at various intervals in their transformation.

While you are educating, counseling, shaping the client's vocal patterns, and guiding the client through the process, the client is the one who will have to apply what they are learning in daily practice. They will change and grow through attending sessions regularly, developing awareness, asking

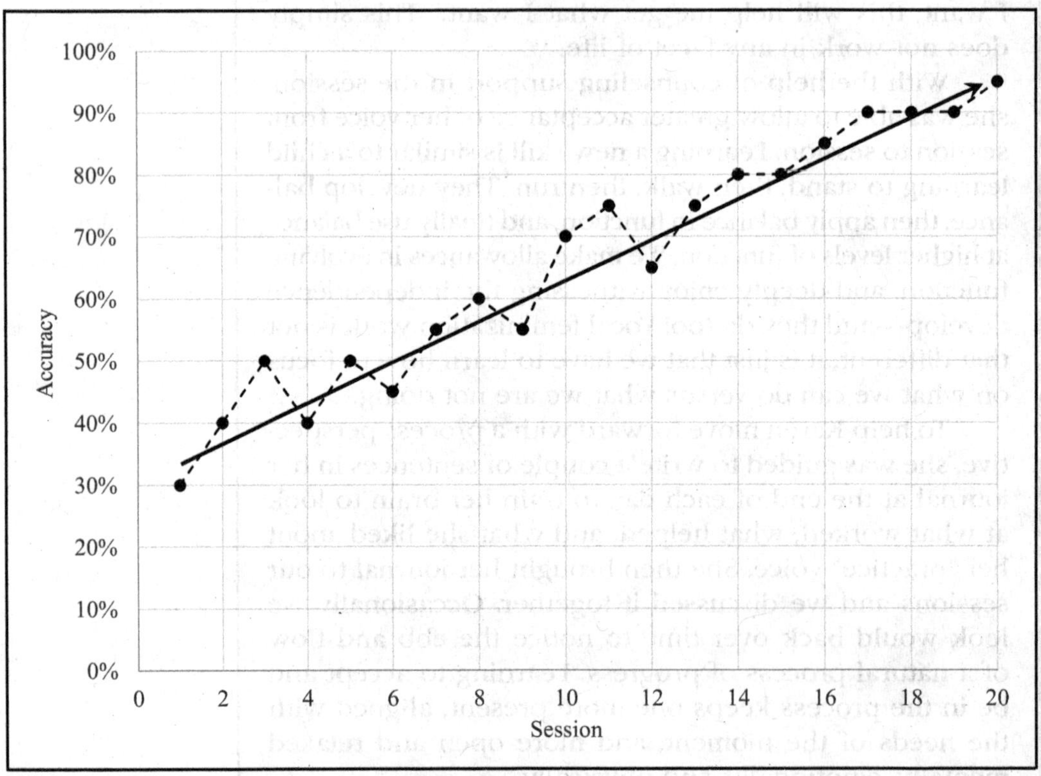

Figure 5–6. Normal variation in progress.

questions, following their home program, expressing personal roadblocks, using apps for accurate levels, and so on. Being independent, consistent, and reliable in their approach creates shorter training time and integration of a new voice more easily into life.

Clients are naturally concerned that they will not be able to achieve a satisfactory voice, even while knowing others that have. For some, making such significant changes to their voice is difficult to imagine. Part of the reason is that voice training is the only part of the physical transition that is not done for them or to them. Consider electrolysis, hair transplantation, taking hormones, or surgeries. While these procedures involve major medical processes, requiring responsibility, healing time, and expense for clients, the process must be entrusted to the hands of the provider. What can be daunting for new voice clients is that now they must rely more on themselves to make changes, and they rarely feel equipped to do so alone.

Training is highly personal and as such, taps into a vulnerable emotional area for all clients. An important understanding appears to be the feedback process itself. It is helpful for clients to know in advance the difference between feedback to shape their production and criticism. Promise an intention, always, to guide clients along the path, with feedback never meant to be a personal judgment. Practitioners must be aware of the sensitive nature of feedback regarding one's voice and learn to guide gently and with care.

CONCLUSION

It should now be clear that a client's mindset to "just raise my pitch to 200 Hz" is a sign of an incomplete and unhelpful understanding of the factors that should be considered in this process. Auditory perception of speaker's gender can be greatly influenced by the speaker's F0 and formant frequencies. We are less certain about the factors of prosody, vocal quality, articulation, and verbal and nonverbal language, but they may be worth considering with some clients. We have growing evidence that speakers can make modifications to their voice and communication, via training, surgery, and/or hormone treatment, and achieve goals regarding how others attribute gender to them. Still, all the speech and language flexibility at the speaker's disposal may not be enough for them to receive desired gender attributions from themselves or from others. This may come as an unpleasant reality to be processed with extreme sensitivity. Thus, attention to coping and navigating occurrences of misgendering should be a priority in the client's care.

As one of many factors in the ASSEMBLE model, the speaker's communication practices are viewed not as a list of features to be habituated, but rather a skilled use of interpersonal communication cues from an expanded repertoire of possibilities. After your assessment and prior to charging ahead with behavioral voice modification is prime time to help the client understand this so they can collaborate with appropriate providers as they move forward. Like the coach with the runner at the beginning of this chapter, it is the practitioner's role to educate the client about the process so they may be an engaged and helpful collaborator in planning the strategy, or "getting ready" before they "get set" and "go!"

REFERENCES

Abitbol, J., Abitbol, P., & Abitbol, B. (1999). Sex hormones and the female voice. *Journal of Voice*, *13*(3), 424–446.

Ahearn, L. M. (2010). Agency and language. In J. Jaspers, J. O. Östman, & J. Verschueren (Eds.), *Society and language use* (pp. 28–48). Amsterdam, The Netherlands: John Benjamins.

Andrews, M., & Schmidt, C. P. (1997). Gender presentation: Perceptual and acoustical analyses of voice. *Journal of Voice*, *11*(3), 307–313.

Avery, J. D., & Liss, J. M. (1996). Acoustic characteristics of less-masculine-sounding male speech. *Journal of the Acoustical Society of America*, *99*(6), 3738–3748.

Azul, D. (2015). Transmasculine people's vocal situations: A critical review of gender-related discourses and empirical data. *International Journal of Language and Communication Disorders*, *50*(1), 31–47.

Azul, D. (2016). Gender-related aspects of transmasculine people's vocal situation: Insights from a qualitative content analysis of interview transcripts. *International Journal of Language and Communication Disorder*, *51*, 672–684.

Azul, D. Nygren, U., Södersten, M., & Neuschaefer-Rube, C. (2017). Transmasculine people's voice function: A review of the currently available evidence. *Journal of Voice*, *31*(2), 261.e9–261.e23.

Bailey, A. H., & Kelly, S. D. (2015). Picture power: Gender versus body language in perceived status. *Journal of Nonverbal Behavior*, *39*, 317–337.

Baken, R. J. (1998). An overview of laryngeal function for voice production.. In R. Sataloff (Ed.), *Vocal health and pedagogy* (pp. 65–84). San Diego, CA: Singular Publishing.

Baken, R. J., & Orlikoff, R. F. (2010). *Clinical measurement of speech and voice* (2nd ed.). Clifton Park, NY: Delmar Cenage Learning.

Berg, M., Fuchs, M., Wirkner, K., Loeffler, M., Engel, C., & Berger, T. (2017). The speaking voice in general population: Normative data and associations to sociodemographic and lifestyle factors. *Journal of Voice, 31*(2), 257.e13–257.e24.

Berry, D. A., Verdolini, K., Montequin, D. W., Hess, M. M., Chan, R. W., & Titze, I. R. (2001). A quantitative output-cost ratio in voice production. *Journal of Speech, Language, and Hearing Research, 44*, 29–37.

Block, C. (2017). Making a case for transmasculine voice and communication training. *Perspectives of the ASHA Special Interest Groups, SIG 3, 2*(1), 33–41.

Boker, S. M. et al. (2011). Something in the way we move: Motion Dynamics, not perceived sex, influence head movements in conversation. *Journal of Experimental Psychology, 37*(3), 874–891.

Booz, J. A. (2017). Perceived gender in clear and conversational speech. *Journal of the Acoustical Society of America, 139.* https://doi.org/10.1121/1.4950261

Bralley, R. C., Bull, G. L., Gore, C. H., & Edgerton, M. T. (1978). Evaluation of vocal pitch in male transsexuals. *Journal of Communication Disorders, 11*, 443–449.

Carew, L., Dacakis, G., & Oates, J. (2007). The effectiveness of oral resonance therapy on the perception of femininity of voice in male-to-female transsexuals. *Journal of Voice, 21*(5), 591–603.

Cargile, A. C., & Bradac, J. J. (2001). Attitudes toward language: A review of speaker-evaluation research and a general process model. In W. B. Gudykunst (Ed.), *Communication yearbook 25* (pp. 347–382). Mahwah, NJ: Erlbaum.

Childers, D. G., & Wu, K. (1991). Gender recognition from speech. Part II: Fine analysis. *Journal of the Acoustical Society of America, 90*(4), 1841–1856.

Clopper, C. G., Levi, S. V., & Pisoni, D. B. (2006). Perceptual similarity of regional dialects of American English. *Journal of the Acoustical Society of America, 119*(1), 566–574.

Coleman, R. O. (1971). Male and female voice quality and its relationship to vowel formant frequencies. *Journal of Speech and Hearing Research, 14*, 565–577.

Cuddy. A. (2012). *Your body language may shape who you are.* TED-Global Talk. Retrieved from https://www.ted.com/talks/amy_cuddy_your_body_language_shapes_who_you_are?language=en

Dacakis, G. (2000). Long-term maintenance of fundamental frequency increases in male-to-female transsexual. *Journal of Voice, 14*(4), 549–556.

Davies, G. (2018). *Gender and body language in Roman art.* Cambridge, UK: Cambridge University Press.

Davies, S., Papp, V., & Antoni, C. (2015). Voice and communication change for gender nonconforming individuals: Giving voice to the person inside. *International Journal of Transgenderism, 16*, 117–159.

De Vries, K. M. (2012). Intersectional identities and conceptions of the self: The experience of transgender people. *Symbolic Interaction, 35*(1), 49–67.

Fitch, J. L., & Holbrook, A. (1970). Modal vocal fundamental frequency of young adults. *Archives of Otolarngology, 92*, 379–382.

Fitzsimons, M., Sheahan, N., & Staunton, H. (2001). Gender and the integration of acoustic dimensions of prosody: Implications for clinical studies. *Brain and Language, 78*(1), 94–108.

Gallena, S. J. K., Stickels, B., & Stickels, E. (2018). Gender perception after raising vowel fundamental and formant frequencies: Considerations for oral resonance research. *Journal of Voice, 32*(5), 592–601.

Gelfer, M. P. (1999). Voice treatment for the male-to-female transgendered client. *American Journal of Speech-Language Pathology, 8*, 201–208.

Gelfer, M., & Bennet, Q. E. (2013). Speaking fundamental frequency and vowel formant frequencies: Effects on perception of gender. *Journal of Voice, 27*(5), 556–566.

Gelfer, M., & Schofield, K. J. (2000). Comparison of acoustic and perceptual measures of voice in male-to-female transsexuals perceived as female versus those perceived as male. *Journal of Voice, 14*(1), 22–33.

Gelfer, M. P., & Tice, R. M. (2013). Perceptual and acoustic outcomes of voice therapy for male-to-female transgender individuals immediately after therapy and 15 months later. *Journal of Voice, 27*(3), 335–347.

Gelfer, M. P., & Van Dong, B. (2013). A preliminary study on the use of vocal function exercises to improve voice in male-to-female transgender clients. *Journal of Voice, 27*(3), 321–334.

Gorham-Rowan, M., & Morris, R. (2006). Aerodynamic analysis of male-to-female transgender voice. *Journal of Voice, 20*, 251–262.

Graddol, D. (1986). Discourse specific pitch behavior. In C. Johns-Lewis (Ed.), *Intonation in discourse* (pp. 221–237). London, UK: Croom Helm.

Gunzberger, D. (1995). Acoustic and perceptual implication of the transsexual voice. *Archives of Sexual Behavior, 24*(3), 339–348.

Hai, D. M., Khairullah, Z. Y., & Coulmas, N. (1982). Sex and the single armrest: Use of personal space during air travel. *Psychological Report, 51*, 743–749.

Hall, J. A., Coats, E. J., & LeBeau, L. S. (2005). Nonverbal behavior and the vertical dimension of social relations: A meta-analysis. *Psychological Bulletin, 131*(16), 898–924.

Hancock, A.B. & Azul, D. (2018). *Theory-guided, person-centered voice and communication support for gender-diverse people.* Presented at the World Professional Association of Transgender Health Conference, Buenos Aires, Argentina.

Hancock, A. B., Childs, K., & Irwig, M. (2017). Trans male voice in the first year of testosterone therapy: Make no assumptions. *Journal of Speech, Language, and Hearing Research*, *60*(9), 2472–2482.

Hancock, A. B., Colton, L., & Douglas, F. (2014). Intonation and gender perception: Applications for transgender speakers. *Journal of Voice*, *28*(2), 203–209.

Hancock, A. B., & Garabedian, L. (2013). Transgender voice and communication treatment: A retrospective chart review of 25 cases. *International Journal of Language and Communication Disorders*, *48*(1), 54–65.

Hancock, A. B., & Gross, H. E. (2015). Acoustic and aerodynamic measures of the voice during pregnancy. *Journal of Voice*, *29*(1), 53–58.

Hancock, A. B., & Helenius, L. (2012). Adolescent male-to-female transgender voice and communication. *Journal of Communication Disorders*, *45*, 313–324.

Hancock, A. B., & Rubin, B. (2015). Influence of communication partner's gender on language. *Journal of Language and Social Psychology*, *34*(1), 46–64.

Hardy, T., Boliek, C. A., Wells, K., Dearden, C., Zalmanowitz, C., & Rieger, J. M. (2016). Pretreatment acoustic predictors of gender, femininity, and naturalness ratings in individuals with male-to-female gender identity. *American Journal of Speech-Language Pathology*, *25*, 125–137.

Henton, C. G. (1989). Fact and fiction in the description of female and male pitch. *Language and Communication*, *9*, 299–311.

Henton, C. G. (1995). Pitch dynamism in female and male speech. *Language and Communication*, *15*(10), 43–61.

Hillenbrand, J. M., & Clark, M. J. (2009). The role of F0 and formant frequencies in distinguishing the voices of men and women. *Attention, Perception, and Psychophysics*, *71*(5), 1150–1166.

Hooper, C. R. (1985). Changing the speech and language of the male to female transsexual client: A case study. *Journal of the Kansas Speech-Language-Hearing Association*, *25*, 6.

Hudson, A. I., & Holbrook, A. (1982). Fundamental frequency characteristics of young black adults: Spontaneous speaking and oral reading. *Journal of Speech and Hearing Research*, *25*, 25–28.

Irwig, M., Childs, K., & Hancock, A. B. (2016). Effects of testosterone on the transgender male voice. *Andrology*, *5*, 107–112.

Kadakia, S., Carlson, D., & Sataloff, R. T. (2013). The effect of hormones on the voice. *Journal of Singing*, *69*(5), 571–574.

Kalra, M. A. (1977). Voice therapy with a transsexual. In R. Gemme & C. Wheeler (Eds.), *International congress on sexology* (pp. 77–84). New York, NY: Plenum Press.

Kaye, J., Bortz, M. A., & Toumi, S. I. (1993). Evaluation of the effectiveness of voice therapy with a male-to-female transsexual subject. *Scandinavian Journal of Logopedic and Phoniatrics*, *18*, 105–109.

Kelly, V., Hertegård, S., Eriksson, J., Nygren, U., & Södersten, M. (2018). Effects of gender-confirming pitch-raising surgery in transgender women: A long-term follow-up study of acoustic and patient-reported data. *Journal of Voice.*

Kim, H. (2017). A new conceptual approach for voice feminization: 12 years of experience. *Laryngoscope, 127*(5), 1102–1108.

Klatt, D. H., & Klatt, L. C. (1990). Analysis, synthesis, and perception of voice quality variations among female and male talkers. *Journal of the Acoustic Society of America, 87*(2), 820–857.

Krumhuber, E., Manstead, A. S. R., & Kappas, A. (2007). Temporal aspects of facial displays in person and expression perception: The effects of smile dynamics, head-tilt, and gender. *Journal of Nonverbal Behavior, 31*(1), 39–56.

LaFrance, M., Hecht, M. A., & Paluck, E. L. (2003). The contingent smile: A meta-analysis of sex differences in smiling. *Psychological Bulletin, 129*(2), 305–334.

Lakoff, R. (1973). Language and women's place. *Language in Society, 2*, 45–80.

Lakoff, R. (1975). *Language and women's place*. New York, NY: Harper & Row.

Leaper, C., & Ayres, M. M. (2007). A meta-analytic review of gender variations in adults' language use: Talkativeness, affiliative speech, and assertive speech. *Personality and Social Psychology Review, 11*(4), 328–363.

Leaper, C., & Robnett, R. D. (2011). Women are more likely than men to use tentative language, aren't they? A meta-analysis testing for gender differences and moderators. *Psychology of Women Quarterly, 35*(1), 129–142.

Leung, Y., Oates, J., & Chan, S. P. (2018). Voice, articulation, and prosody contribute to listener perceptions of speaker gender: A systematic review and meta-analysis. *Journal of Speech, Language, and Hearing Research, 61*, 266–297.

Lutz, K. C., & Mallard, A. R. (1986). Disfluencies and rate of speech in young adult nonstutterers. *Journal of Fluency Disorders, 11*, 307–316.

McDuff, D., Girard, J. M., & Kaliouby, R. (2017). Large-scale observational evidence of cross-cultural differences in facial behavior. *Journal of Nonverbal Behavior, 41*, 1–19.

Mehrabian, A. (1972). *Nonverbal communication*. Chicago, IL: Aldine-Atherton.

Mészáros, K., Vitéz, L., Szabolcs, I., Goth, M., Kovács, L., Görömbei, Z., & Hacki, T. (2005). Efficacy of conservative voice treatment in male-to-female transsexuals. *Foliz Phoniatrica et Logopaedica, 57*, 111–118.

Moore, E., Wisniewski, A., & Dobs, A. (2003). Endocrine treatment of transsexual people: A review of treatment regimens, outcomes, and adverse effects. *Journal of Clinical Endocrinology and Metabolism, 88*(8), 3467–3473.

Mount, M. H., & Salmon, S. J. (1988). Changing the vocal characteristics of a post-operative transsexual patient: a longitudinal study. *Journal of Communication Disorders, 21*, 229–238.

Mulac, A. (2006). The gender-linked language effect: Do language differences really make a difference? In K. Dindia & D. J. Canary (Eds.), *Sex differences and similarities in communication* (2nd ed., pp. 219–239). Mahwah, NJ: Erlbaum.

Mulac, A., Bradac, J. J., & Gibbons, P. (2001). Empirical support for the gender-as-culture hypothesis: An intercultural analysis of male/female language differences. *Human Communication Research*, 27, 121–152.

Mulac, A., Giles, H., Bradac, J. J., & Palomares, N. A. (2013). The gender-linked language effect: An empirical test of gender process model. *Language Science, 38*, 22–31.

Mulac, A., & Lundell, T. L. (1982). An empirical test of the gender-linked language effect in a public speaking setting. *Language and Speech, 25*, 243–256.

Mulac, A., Lundell, T. L., & Bradac, J. J. (1986). Male/female language differences and attributional consequences in a public speaking situation: Toward an explanation of the gender-linked language effect. *Communication Monographs, 53*, 115–129.

Munson, B., McDonald, E., DeBoe, N. L., & White, A. R. (2006). The acoustic and perceptual bases of judgments of women and men's sexual orientation from read speech. *Journal of Phonetics, 34*, 202–240.

Owen, K., & Hancock, A. B. (2010). The role of self- and listener perceptions of femininity in voice therapy. *International Journal of Transgenderism, 12*(4), 272–284.

Palomares, N. A. (2004). Gender schematicity, gender identity salience, and gender-linked language use. *Human Communication Research, 30*(4), 556–568.

Palomares, N. A. (2008). Explaining gender-based language use: Effects of gender identity salience on references to emotion and tentative language in intra- and intergroup contexts. *Human Communication Research*, 34, 263–286.

Palomares, N. A. (2009). Women are sort of more tentative than men, aren't they? How men and women use tentative language differently, similarly, and counter-stereotypically as a function of gender salience. *Communication Research*, 36, 538–560.

Palomares, N. A. (2016). Language and gender. In C. R. Berger & M. E. Roloff (Eds.), *The international encyclopedia of interpersonal communication* (pp. 1–11). Hoboken, NJ: John Wiley & Sons.

Pemberton, C., McCormack, P., & Russell, A. (1998). Have women's voices lowered across time? A cross-sectional study of Australian women's voices. *Journal of Voice, 12*(2), 208–213.

Postmes, T., & Spears, R. (2002). Behavior online: Does anonymous computer communication reduce gender inequality? *Personality and Social Psychology Bulletin, 28*, 1073–1083.

Rendall, D., Vasey, P. L., & McKenzie, J. (2008). The Queen's English: An alternative, biosocial hypothesis for the distinctive features of "gay speech." *Archives of Sexual Behavior*, *37*, 188–204.

Saito, Y., Nakamura, K., Itani, S., & Tsukahara, K. (2018). Type 3 thyroplasty for a patient with female-to-male gender identity disorder. *Care Reports in Otolaryngology*, 1–4.

Shport, I. A. (2018). The roles of vowel fronting, lengthening, and listener variables in the perception of vocal femininity, *Journal of Speech, Language, and Hearing Research*, *61*, 130–144.

Söderpalm, E., Larsson, A., & Almquist, S. (2004). Evaluation of a consecutive group of transsexual individuals referred for vocal intervention in the west of Sweden. *Logopedics Phoniatrics Vocology*, *29*(1), 18–30.

Södersten, M., Hertegård, S., & Hammarberg, B. (1995). Glottal closure, transglottal airflow, and voice quality in healthy middle-aged women. *Journal of Voice*, *9*(2), 182–197.

Södersten, M., & Lindestad, P. (1990). Glottal closure and perceived breathiness during phonation in normally speaking subjects. *Journal of Speech and Hearing Research*, *33*, 601–611.

Song, T. E., & Jiang, N. (2017). Transgender phonosurgery: A systematic review and meta-analysis. *Otolaryngology-Head and Neck Surgery*, *156*(6), 803–808.

Stathopoulos, E. T., Huber, J. E., & Sussman, J. E. (2011). Changes in acoustic characteristics of the voice across the life span: Measures from individuals 4 to 93 years of age. *Journal of Speech, Language, and Hearing Research*, *54*, 1011–1021.

Thomas, J. P., & MacMillan, C. (2013). Feminization laryngoplasty: Assessment of surgical pitch elevation. *European Archives of Otorhinolaryngology*, *270*, 2695–2700.

Titze, I. (2011). Vocal fold mass is not a useful quantity for describing F0 in vocalization. *Journal of Speech, Language, and Hearing Research*, 520–522.

Trimboli, A., & Walker, M. (1987). Nonverbal dominance in the communication of affect: A myth? *Journal of Nonverbal Behavior*, *11*(3), 180–190.

Tsao, Y. C., & Weismer, G. (1997). Interspeaker variation in habitual speaking rate: Evidence for a neuromuscular component. *Journal of Speech, Language, and Hearing Research*, *40*(4), 858–866.

Van Borsel, J., De Cuypere, G., & Van den Berghe, H. (2001). Physical appearance and voice in male-to-female transsexuals. *Journal of Voice*, *15*(4), 570–575.

Van Borsel, J., & De Maesschalck, D. (2008). Speech rate in males, females, and male-to-female transsexuals. *Clinical Linguistics and Phonetics*, *22*(9), 679–685.

Van Borsel, J., de Pot, K., & De Cuypere, G. (2009). Voice and physical appearance in female-to-male transsexuals. *Journal of Voice*, *23*(4), 494–497.

Van Borsel, J., Janssens, J., & De Bodt, M. (2009). Breathiness as a feminine voice characteristic: A perceptual approach. *Journal of Voice*, *23*(3), 291–294.

Van Damme, S., Cosyns, M., Deman, S., Van den Eede, Z., & Van Borsel, J. (2017). The effectiveness of pitch-raising surgery in male-to-female transsexuals: A systematic review. *Journal of Voice*, *31*(2), 244.e1–244.e5.

Wingate, V. S., & Palomares, N. A. (2017). Gender issues in intergroup communication. In *Oxford research encyclopedia of communication*. UK: Oxford University Press.

Wolfe, V. I., Ratusink, D. L., Smith, F. H., & Northrop, G. E. (1990). Intonation and fundamental frequency in male-to-female transsexuals. *Journal of Speech, Language, and Hearing Disorders*, *55*, 43–50.

Zemlin, W. R. (1998). *Speech and hearing science* (4th ed.). Boston, MA: Allyn and Bacon.

Ziegler, A., Henke, T., Wiedrick, J., & Helou, L. B. (2018). Effectiveness of testosterone therapy for masculinizing voice in transgender patients: A meta-analytic review. *International Journal of Transgenderism*, *19*(1), 25–45.

Zraick, R. I., Gentry, M. A., Smith-Olinde, L., & Gregg, B. A. (2006). The effect of speaking context on elicitation of habitual pitch. *Journal of Voice*, *20*(4), 545–554.

Zraick, R. I., Kempster, G. B., Connor, N. P., Thibeault, S., Klaben, B. K., Bursac, Z., . . . Glaze, L. E. (2011). Establishing validity of the CAPE-V. *American Journal of Speech-Language Pathology*, *20*, 14–22.

6

Intervention Phase 2: Get Set . . .

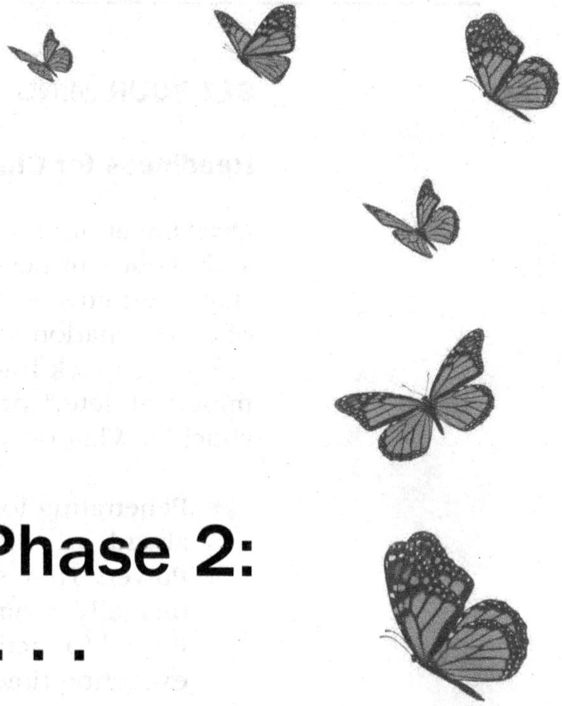

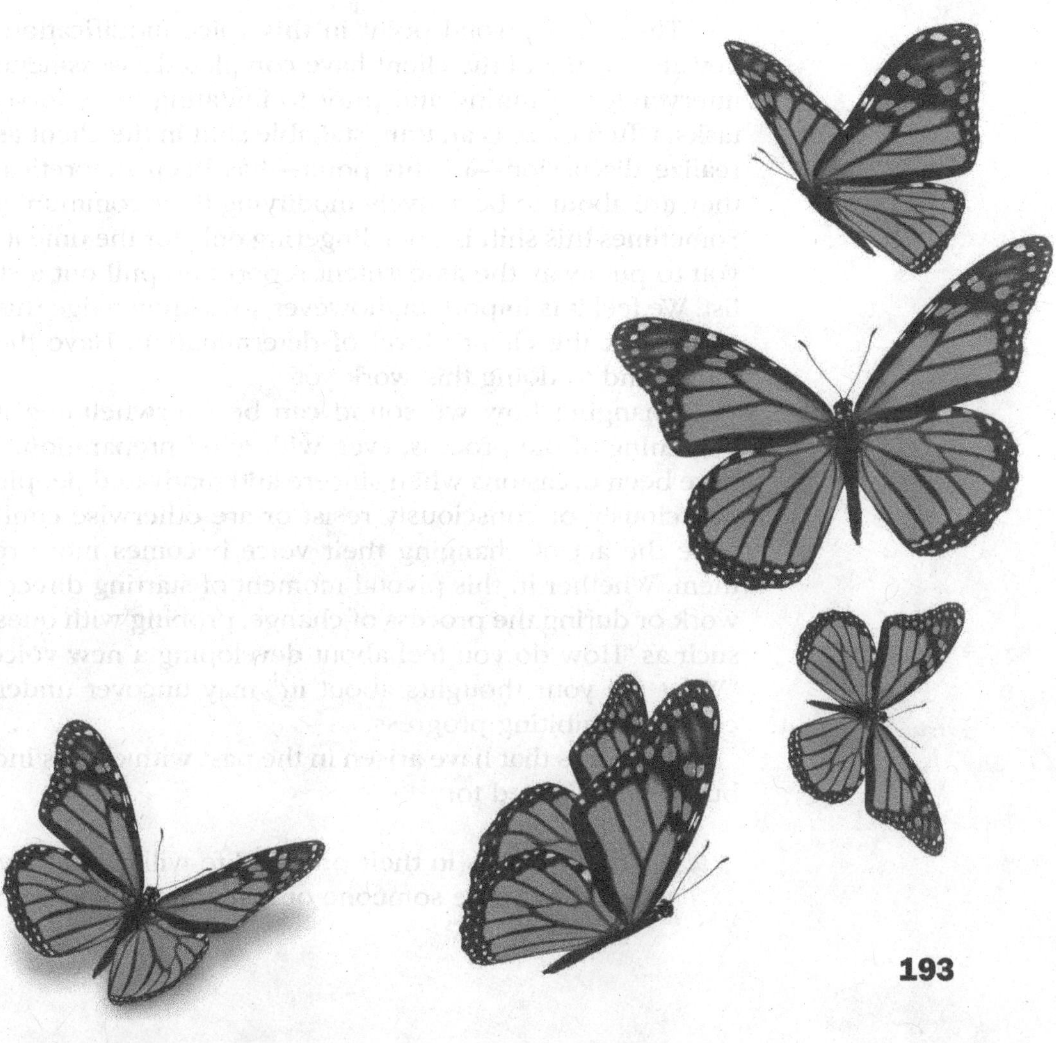

SET YOUR MIND TO IT

Readiness for Change

Determination is required. It is also rewarded. The provider and client will need to be determined and help one another stay determined in moments of uncertainty or fear. The rewards of determination are innumerable and invaluable.

Do a quick Internet search for "determined look," "determined athlete," or even "determined baby" if you want a chuckle. What do you notice?

- Penetrating focus: Eyes are steady, looking straight ahead.
- Power: They seem physically, emotionally, and mentally strong (even the babies!).
- Poised for action: Preparation time is over; plan execution time is imminent.

There is a pivotal point in this voice modification journey after you and the client have completed assessments and intervention planning and prior to initiating the intervention tasks. Often there is an unmistakable shift in the client as they realize discussion—to this point—has been theoretical, but they are about to be actively modifying their communication. Sometimes this shift is brief, lingering only for the time it takes you to put away the assessment report and pull out a stimuli list. We feel it is important, however, to acknowledge this shift and check the client's level of determination. Have they set their mind to doing this work yet?

Changing how we sound can be overwhelming at the beginning of the process, even with good preparation. There have been occasions when sincere and motivated people subconsciously or consciously resist or are otherwise conflicted once the act of changing their voice becomes more real to them. Whether in this pivotal moment of starting direct voice work or during the process of change, probing with questions such as "How do you feel about developing a new voice?" or "What are your thoughts about it?" may uncover underlying conflict, inhibiting progress.

Concerns that have arisen in the past with clients include, but are not limited to:

- Fear that others in their present life will think they are pretending to be someone or something they are not.

- Unexpected sounds: "Doesn't sound real," "doesn't sound like me," "doesn't sound feminine."
- Reluctance because a significant family member has not accepted their transition.
- Feeling disoriented or disconnected from the new voice, as if not their own.
- Arising conflict related to gender positioning, presentation, and attributions.

These responses do not necessarily mean they haven't set their mind to the work, or that they will not or should not proceed with intervention. The responses may, however, uncover the need for further education and counseling about the somewhat awkward beginning phases of vocal transition or perhaps lead to further psychological support. Asking your client about their readiness is a large part of compassionate and competent health care. A mismatch between readiness and intervention, known in the literature as *strategy-to-stage mismatch*, is an unfortunate cause for program failure but can be avoided by using client-centered communication, such as active listening and motivational interviewing techniques (Behrman, 2006; Van Leer, Hapner, & Connor, 2007).

When the client has largely set their mind to continue, make use of the moment (in so far as it can be restricted to a single moment) of transition from a preparation to an action phase of change to honor and reward the client for a significant accomplishment, acknowledging it was made possible by their determination (Prochaska & DiClemente, 1982). Client self-efficacy is improved with each success and with verbal encouragement (Van Leer, Hapner, & Connor, 2007). Even a brief exercise, such as the one scripted below, is an investment in the client's self-efficacy and a good introduction to the "get set" practices described in this chapter.

> ***Not yet, but when I tell you in a moment, you're going to take a very slow inhale, hold the breath, then a very slow exhale. As you do each of these three phases of a breath, I will be comparing it to the process or journey we are on. Think of "ready, set, go." We've been getting ready, we're getting set now, and we're about to go. Part of that middle "get set" is to pivot from preparation mode to action mode, sort of like pivoting from an inhale to an exhale. This exercise can help us mark this pivotal session. Shall we do it?***

As you slowly inhale, recall finding out about voice, sharing personal information, doing voice assessment, making intervention decisions, so much you've done!

Now, while you hold your breath, know we are ready. We are looking ahead. Feel brave and strong. Set your mind to it.

As you exhale, feel the relief of letting go.

Keep breathing gently and congratulate yourself for being right where you are. You have taken important steps. You are committed to the steps in front of you, exploring them, even stumbling and overcoming them if needed.

When you are ready and before we move forward, please share how you are thinking or feeling.

Mindfulness

A growing body of empirical evidence supports using mindfulness-based practices involving "full, direct, and active awareness of experienced phenomena" in health care, education, and workplace environments (Van Gordon, Shonin, Zangeneh, & Griffiths, 2014, p. 130). In addition to mental health domains, cognitive function and task performance improves after mindfulness-based interventions (Chiesa et al., 2011; Sedlmeier et al., 2012). Mindfulness is the term we use to demonstrate the process of using a meditation practice at the start of each session. As described in Chapter 1, the benefits of even a brief 5-minute mindful meditation includes greater calm, clarity, and concentration and a general sense of greater well-being (Walsh & Shapiro, 2006). Beginning a session with a clearer, calmer mind and body can enhance learning.

With regard to vocal training, the greater the physical tension carried by the client, the greater the potential imbalance in systems that impact vocal function. Identifying poor posture, breath-holding, and abdominal, shoulder, back, cervical, laryngeal, jaw, lingual, and facial tension may be a clue to underlying muscular tension. Therefore, including general relaxation prior to direct voice work can be essential.

The specific benefits to clients may include:

- relaxing the systems related to vocal function;
- heightening awareness of their physical body, essential for voice training and personal growth;

- exposure, perhaps for the first time, to the total health benefits of mindfulness; and
- taking an active and powerful role in their own vocal transition process.

Guiding clients to develop a "feeling" sense is important. The more they are in tune with their bodies, the more they can feel alignment in the body, feel air flow through the vocal tract, feel laryngeal structures release, feel resonance focus in the oral cavity, and so on. These sensations can range from openness, ease, and flow at one end of the continuum to restriction, effort, holding, and detachment at the other end. It is important that we gauge our clients' awareness, as it will be necessary for voice training. Only what one is aware of can be volitionally changed toward a desired result. Finally, emotional release may also occur as clients become more in touch with themselves during this process.

SET THE ENVIRONMENT

Equipment

- A good chair allows one to sit upright easily while leaning back on the backrest. Usually a straight-backed, stationary chair is effective.
- A pillow may come in handy for clients that cannot feel comfortable and relax in the chair.
- A visual feedback tool such as mirror, video, or photo from a phone or other electronic device.
- A treatment table or yoga mat or large towel.

Materials

Scripts for the deep breathing and body scan approaches below are available in Appendix 6–A. Direct provider guidance allows you to escort the client live, interjecting personal language and directing focus that may best benefit the client. Playing prerecorded audio recordings, such as the one available on the companion website for this book, allow the provider to participate with the client. Not only is this helpful for us personally, but participating together in this exercise can also increase rapport with your client.

SET THE MIND AND BODY

The approaches suggested below can gently guide participants to bring their attention to the sensations in the body, thereby relaxing the body and freeing the mind from the day's activities or struggles. There are numerous other methods available on the Internet should you want to explore visualization, progressive relaxation, the relaxation response, or another approach. Most of our clients look forward to participating in the mindfulness practice at the start of the session. It is an opportunity for them to let go of the stresses of the day and increase readiness for upcoming voice training. Some clients rarely allow this time for themselves.

Describe the process ahead of time so clients know what to expect. The following points make it a safe and approachable experience for most new clients:

- You will be guided in a relaxation exercise for about 3 to 5 minutes.
- You will be completely aware and in control at all times.
- You can close your eyes or lower them.

The techniques are described below.

Deep Breathing

The deep breathing relaxation approach can be effective as a 3- to 5-minute process. Ask the client to approach this process gently and with curiosity rather than as something to accomplish. When the client is ready to begin:

1. Guide them to take in a breath as slowly as they can until they comfortably reach the top of the breath.
2. Ask them to pause at the top of the breath briefly, noticing the pause.
3. Then, just as slowly, release the breath, letting all the air out.
4. Direct their awareness to how it feels to be at the bottom of the breath.
5. Have the client repeat the whole cycle very slowly. It is often helpful to talk them through to keep a slow pace.
6. Pause frequently between instructions to allow the client to feel what is happening as an observational

practice without judgment (e.g., "notice what you feel or sense," "simply observe without judging it as good or bad"). There is no good or bad way; there is only their unique way. Have them notice everything about their body as it shifts from inhalation to exhalation:

- The movement of the body as the air goes deeply in and then out again.
- The airflow itself as it passes through the body.
- Feel the air as it flows through the nostrils. The sensation and intensity may vary from the left side to the right side. Notice if there is a difference.
- Observe. Investigate. Feel. Explore.
- Notice any thoughts or feeling that arise, simply observing them as they arise and pass.
- Awareness of the breath, body, emotions, and thoughts is a necessary part of the process and is accepted without judgment.

Body Scan

This process is similar to Vipassana meditation and will also feel familiar as a part of mindfulness-based stress reduction (MBSR) process to those with some experience with the program. MBSR was created in 1979 by Jon Kabat-Zinn, the founding executive director of the Center of Mindfulness at the University of Massachusetts medical school. This is a gentle approach of focusing on the sensation of various parts of the body without judgement.

Introduce the approach as a body scan, suggesting that the client will feel the sensations in each part of the body with your guidance, starting from the top of the head, scanning downward slowly part by part to the feet. For some clients, starting at the feet and moving up toward the head could work better—feel free to explore these options with each client. Here, we are interested in sensing the body versus thinking about the body. If thoughts or judgments arise, which is an automatic and habitual response, simply acknowledge that thought and then gently move back to sensing into the body. Over time, the practice of returning attention to the body will become easier and needed less often.

Feel each part of the body for whatever that sensation is. There will be some parts that you may not feel, and that is perfectly fine. Simply note, "How interesting, I cannot really feel my left eyebrow right now" and continue down through the rest of the body without any judgment that it is good or bad, right or wrong. Returning to the observation of it, the watching of it, and the awareness of it allows it to be an experience. Then continue with your body scan.

There may also be sensations in the body related to physical discomfort or emotions such as fear, anger, or sadness. By observing them compassionately, clients allow these reactions to arise and dissipate. This takes practice and understanding. Until we slow down, it is hard to see how our mental, emotional, and physical patterns influence our day. Meditation allows us to begin the process of intentionally developing present-moment awareness within a controlled setting. Mindfully incorporating this into daily life continues the process of mindfulness practices.

Both the body scan and deep breathing meditation scripts have been adapted to meet the needs of the 1-hour training session. It may be helpful to know that both were originally much longer and include much greater detail when utilized for longer periods of time. Feel free to adjust the length of time and level of detail to suit the needs of the client and your session. Sometimes clients meditate in the waiting room before the session, giving us more time for direct voice work within the session. Conversely, if a client is having a difficult day, allowing more meditation time may serve the needs of the client and the overall effectiveness of the session.

SET POSTURAL ALIGNMENT

Aim and Purpose

Posture is not one position and should not appear rigid. Posture is fluid, mobile, adjustable, and appropriate to position, emotion, and communication. When the weight of the body shifts as we move and change positions, it is natural for the body to rebalance itself as is appropriate. We all have an optimal posture that is unique to our bodies and—adjusts automatically and subconsciously as the need arises. The human body functions best when it is aligned. In this state, the musculoskeletal system is the most efficient and functions with ease, power, and flexibility whether standing or sitting.

Given the proximity of the cervical spine to the larynx and the influence of vocal tract shape on voice, it is not a surprise that neck and head position influences the sound of the voice. For example, tilting or turning the head left or right can change the sound of the voice. For some clients, if they are working on oral resonance or projection skills with the cervical spine even slightly out of alignment, they will not be able to fully achieve the target, even with the best support and technique.

The causes of postural misalignment are varied and multifactorial, including but not limited to: habituated patterns learned early in life, years of being hunched over a computer, medical/spinal conditions, aging, or long-term stress throughout stages of life. A forward head position and rounded spine and shoulders (e.g., slouched posture) can directly restrict rib-lung expansion and optimal function of the diaphragm during inhalation, contributing to a shallow breathing pattern (Albarrati, Zafar, Alghadir, & Shahnwaz, 2018). While the laryngeal muscles automatically compensate for the restricted breath, habituation of compensatory patterns over time can lead to higher vocal and respiratory efforts, strain, and early vocal fatigue while training (Lewandowski & Gillespie, 2016). Alignment of the body prepares clients for optimal vocal training by:

- increasing general relaxation of the body,
- increasing freedom of the breath,
- increasing flexibility of the larynx,
- allowing an open vocal tract, and
- enhancing control, flexibility, and power of the voice.

On the psychological level, body positions can induce desirable states of being. For example, open and expansive postures (e.g., arms wide out to side, hands behind neck with elbows out) reduce stress hormones, boost confidence, and positively influence thinking and decision making (Briñol, Petty, & Wagner, 2009; Eerland, Guadalupe, & Zwaan, 2011). Research participants standing in an open and more expansive body posture were 45% more likely to take risks compared to those with a closed, rounded, and restricted posture (Peper & Lin, 2012). Aligned posture and open body positions are foundational to the client's physical and psychological readiness for the session, and greater well-being in general.

Unique Considerations

There are unique considerations when addressing mind-body connection with clients who struggle with body dysphoria or self-consciousness. Clients may attempt to conceal or contort their body to alleviate their distress. For example, a client may consciously or subconsciously conceal their shape by presenting with a rounded forward posture with their arms crossed over the lap and their legs crossed at ankles or knees.

Another example relates to a client who came to sessions in very high heels and short dresses. Understandably, the only comfortable position for her was to cross her legs, angling them to one side. Because her posture restricted her breath and affected head position, she had to address it directly. It caused her great anxiety to align her torso even while keeping her legs crossed. To serve the voice and the client, both client and provider agreed that wearing short skirts to voice therapy did not serve her, so she would plan her wardrobe so her garments would afford her greater comfort and flexibility in the session. Later, when her voice was more stable, she would have greater control and be less vulnerable to the effects of varied body positioning.

Misalignments are revealed during the assessment. Stimulability testing will demonstrate the influence posture has over their voice by simply exposing the change in the client's voice once realignment has been established. Consider the misaligned postures presented in Figure 6–1 A–D—notice that a variety of adjustments may be necessary to find the alignment that will facilitate desired vocal quality (i.e., Figure 6–1E). In addition, making these adjustments may uncover the client's level of resistance to modifying this pattern and the level of tender care, education, and shaping that may be needed to achieve the desired result.

Client education relating to posture's important influence over voice production as well as to the client's emotional state will be helpful. Since postural alignment may feel unfamiliar, it is normal and expected for there to be an adjustment period. Posture affects how we feel and how we see ourselves. Describe the upcoming process, letting them know that many clients report that using a new posture feels different at first. Your goal is to encourage relaxed alignment without struggle, working with clients to find the shape that produces optimal voice and is acceptable and comfortable for them.

Techniques for Posture Modification

Below are many options that can be used to guide clients to attain optimal alignment. Choose the one that is most effective

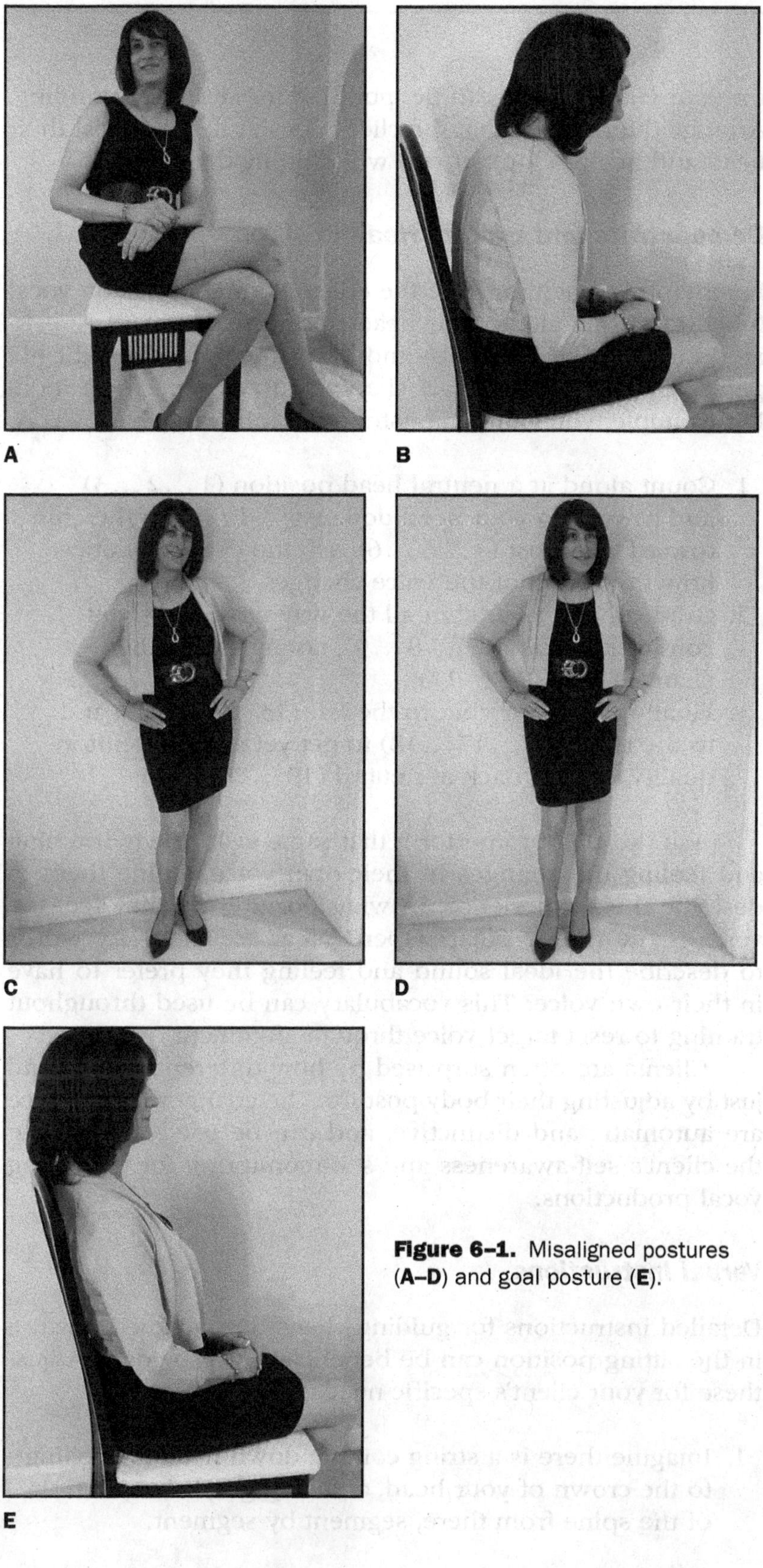

Figure 6–1. Misaligned postures (**A–D**) and goal posture (**E**).

for your client. These can be modified for sitting or standing. Arrange the room so that the client doesn't have to twist their head and neck to look at you while phonating.

Demonstrate and Explore Head Position

It is helpful to demonstrate the effect alignment has on vocal function. If one alters their head position as they are speaking, shifts in vocal quality and resonance are dramatically perceived as the vocal tract shape adjusts for each position. For example, you can demonstrate the following:

1. Count aloud at a neutral head position (1 . . . 2 . . . 3) and as you tip your head downward, bringing the chin toward the chest (4 . . . 5 . . . 6), ask the client to notice how the sound of the voice changes.
2. Gradually tip your chin all the way upward as you continue to count (7 . . . 8 . . . 9), noting the further changes (10 . . . 11 . . . 12).
3. Finally, turn your chin to the left (13 . . . 14 . . . 15) and to the right (16 . . . 17 . . . 18) to get yet another shift in quality, ending back at neutral (19 . . . 20 . . . 21).

Ask the client to perform that same task slowly listening and feeling the changes in their own voice. Guide them to describe their experience. In what position do they feel the voice is the freest? Clear? Open? What are their key words to describe the ideal sound and feeling they prefer to have in their own voice? This vocabulary can be used throughout training to reset target voice through alignment.

Clients are often surprised by how different they sound just by adjusting their body posture. The changes to the voice are automatic and distinctive, and can be used to cultivate the client's self-awareness and self-monitoring for upcoming vocal productions.

Verbal Instructions

Detailed instructions for guiding clients into aligned posture in the sitting position can be beneficial for providers. Adjust these for your client's specific needs:

1. Imagine there is a string coming down from the ceiling to the crown of your head, allowing gentle suspension of the spine from there, segment by segment.

2. While you are imagining your spine is suspended, put both feet flat on the floor.
3. The "sitz bones," (ischial tuberosity) rather than the lower back (the sacrum), should have contact with the seat of the chair. It may help to lean forward and shift the hips back as far as they can go in the chair to set the position more easily, and then sit upright.
4. Align the body so the shoulders float above the hips and the ears float over the shoulders. The chest is lifted gently as if a light were shining upward from the center.
5. Relax the spine and abdomen within this alignment. (Using language such as "make them soft" or to "imagine the inside of your body is liquid" is often effective in releasing more of the body before you give further instructions. This alone will allow a shift toward more optimal alignment.)
6. Broaden the shoulder blades and soften them back and down. (The distance between the shoulders and the ears will broaden simply by releasing elevated shoulders.)
7. Head position should be level, guiding the crown of the head to the highest point as it reaches toward the ceiling. The spine is gently suspended from the base of the skull.
8. The chin is level: neither up or down nor left or right.

Use the above as a guide only. The body functions optimally when there is a flow or "liquidity" at all times in place of a static or fixed position. It helps clients to release any residual head position tension by gently nodding a few times as in "yes" and then shaking head left to right as in "no" to find the balance around the midline without tension.

Imagery

For those clients who try too hard, or where verbal instructions appear to make the client more tense, tapping into the right brain more can be highly effective. Instructions to the client are as follows:

1. Imagine a scene (past experience or desired) where you experience a positive feeling such as confidence, strength, love, prosperity, generosity, or any other desirable feeling.
2. Nod your head when you feel it.

3. Good, now take a moment to enjoy this feeling. Note all the support around you, scents, tastes, colors, sounds, etc. Whatever is there is perfect.
4. Envision or imagine how your body feels and the body language expressed.
5. Now, allow your body's shape to reflect that experience or inner feeling.
6. Open your eyes when your body is ready for some final adjustments.

At this point, the provider gently cues the client for maximum postural potential. Some clients spontaneously began using diaphragmatic breathing once the alignment has been set. For others, resonance becomes more oral and vocal quality improves. After 2 or 3 minutes in this new pattern, clients have begun to smile for no apparent reason and reported a vague feeling of well-being they could not put words to.

Whichever approach your client benefitted from, the focus throughout the rest of the session is on allowing the body to remain soft as they move through the training segments from here into laryngeal massage, breathing, and direct voice work.

SET THE MUSCULATURE

Once the client is relaxed and aligned, we flow into the next component, which is relaxing related muscular groups. Move and speak slowly, gently taking advantage of the client's relaxed state as we move forward. See Box 6–1 for tips when working on these goals. Once you train your client, these exercises can also be completed as part of the home program prior to vocal practice (see Appendix 6–B).

Aim and Purpose

The degree of laryngeal repositioning and repatterning required during vocal adjustments may trigger maladaptive patterns such as lifting the head or restricting the jaw or lingual position instead of contracting of the laryngeal elevators with optimal respiratory support. Therefore, relaxing the musculature surrounding and supporting the larynx may be necessary before optimum phonation for vocal transition can occur, especially if associated with posture and associated stress or anxiety. Being aware of related musculature and how it impacts

Box 6–1. Relaxation and Massage Tips

- Clients should use aligned and relaxed posture unless specified throughout all activities.
- There should be constant flow of the breath for all activities. If you, as the provider, are breathing and relaxed, your client will be more likely to do the same.
- **Do not continue if there is pain.** Clients may be forcing into a stretch, have mechanical issues beyond the scope of this work, or have an unresolved injury or condition that needs to be evaluated. For discomfort during laryngeal massage, talk to the client, follow the guidance provided, and use your own clinical intuition and insight into the issue.
- Stay aware and attuned to your client during all of this work. Gentle, patient, and slow motions as muscles release during a stretch or massage enhance effectiveness.
- Clients can learn to do exercises independently, safely, and accurately as part of a home program once they have been trained in the session. It is important that clients are following instructions and performing the massage and all stretches consciously. If clients do too much, they may experience physical discomfort, lack of vocal control, or other unnecessary difficulties.
- Use visual feedback where appropriate.

vocal function is important. Please seek more detailed anatomy and physiology as needed from other sources designed to provide this information. We provide guidance to relax five related areas, starting with the largest muscles: shoulders, neck, jaw, tongue, and extrinsic laryngeal muscles.

Beginning with the shoulders will indirectly optimize postural alignment and provide early warming and release of the smaller related muscles such as the neck and larynx. You will not have to do every exercise to be effective in vocal training. Instead, use the exercises as appropriate for your particular client. As you go through these with your client, identify effectiveness by asking your client to notice if there is greater flexibility, ease, and comfort. These are very common exercises for release of certain problematic muscular holding patterns, but please always be cautious and aware of client needs and tolerance level. Refer to the photos in this chapter and a video of laryngeal massage on the companion website for this book. Watching the process and effectiveness with a client can improve another client's self-efficacy and, therefore, the effectiveness of this technique.

Before you begin any practice, make sure that the client does not have pain, and has not had a surgery or injury to the areas addressed. Always get a doctor's approval before you make any recommendations to a client with medical, surgical, or pain issues.

Releasing Shoulder Tension

Clients with one or more of the following can benefit from shoulder release activities:

- unilateral or bilateral shoulder elevation;
- rolled forward position of the shoulders;
- rigidity and tension in the shoulders, upper torso, neck, and jaw; and
- client report of tension in the area.

Shoulder Shrugs

Gently have them elevate their shoulders all the way up, holding them up for approximately 5 seconds (but use what feels best to the client), and then letting them fall back downward to a relaxed position. It is important to keep the neck relaxed. Repeat 3 to 5 times.

Shoulder Rolls

While your clients' hands are resting open on their lap, have them slowly and gently rotate one shoulder in a circle rotation forward, upward, back, and down. Repeat five to 10 times, and then change direction (i.e., rotate backward). Repeat for the opposite shoulder.

Clients who are very stiff and have limited range of motion may find success by fully bending the elbow and making a circle in the air with the elbow. It will feel like the elbow is leading the way going around in a circle one way and then the other way.

Releasing Neck Tension

The neck is an important and delicate area. Never force or push the neck into any position. Clients with one or more of the following may benefit from neck stretches:

- forward head posture,
- visible or functional neck and/or shoulder tension or rigidity,
- postural asymmetries,
- complaints of neck tension, and
- dysphonia.

Neck Rotation

Guide the client to gently and slowly turn the head to look over the right shoulder to a comfortable range until they feel a stretch on the left side of the neck. Hold for about 5 seconds, then return to starting position. Repeat, this time over the left shoulder (Figure 6–2A). Repeat the set three times.

Side Tilts

Ask your client to slowly and consciously tilt their head so the right ear drops toward their right shoulder until they feel a stretch on the left side of the neck. Encourage the client to allow the weight of the head to enhance the stretch without pushing into it (Figure 6–2B). Guide them to consciously keep the shoulders relaxed and posture aligned. Allow the release to continue for approximately 10 seconds then return to starting position. Repeat on the left so the left ear is tilting toward the left shoulder, stretching the right side of the neck. Repeat three times.

Chin Tucks

Have your client slowly tuck their chin and look down toward the floor in front of them until they feel a stretch in the back of the neck, but without any discomfort. It should be a passive stretch, which allows the weight of the head to enhance the stretch without pushing into it. Hold for 10 seconds, then return to starting position (Figure 6–2C). Repeat three times. The opposing stretch is neck extension, which is lifting the head upward as they look at the ceiling and feel a stretch in

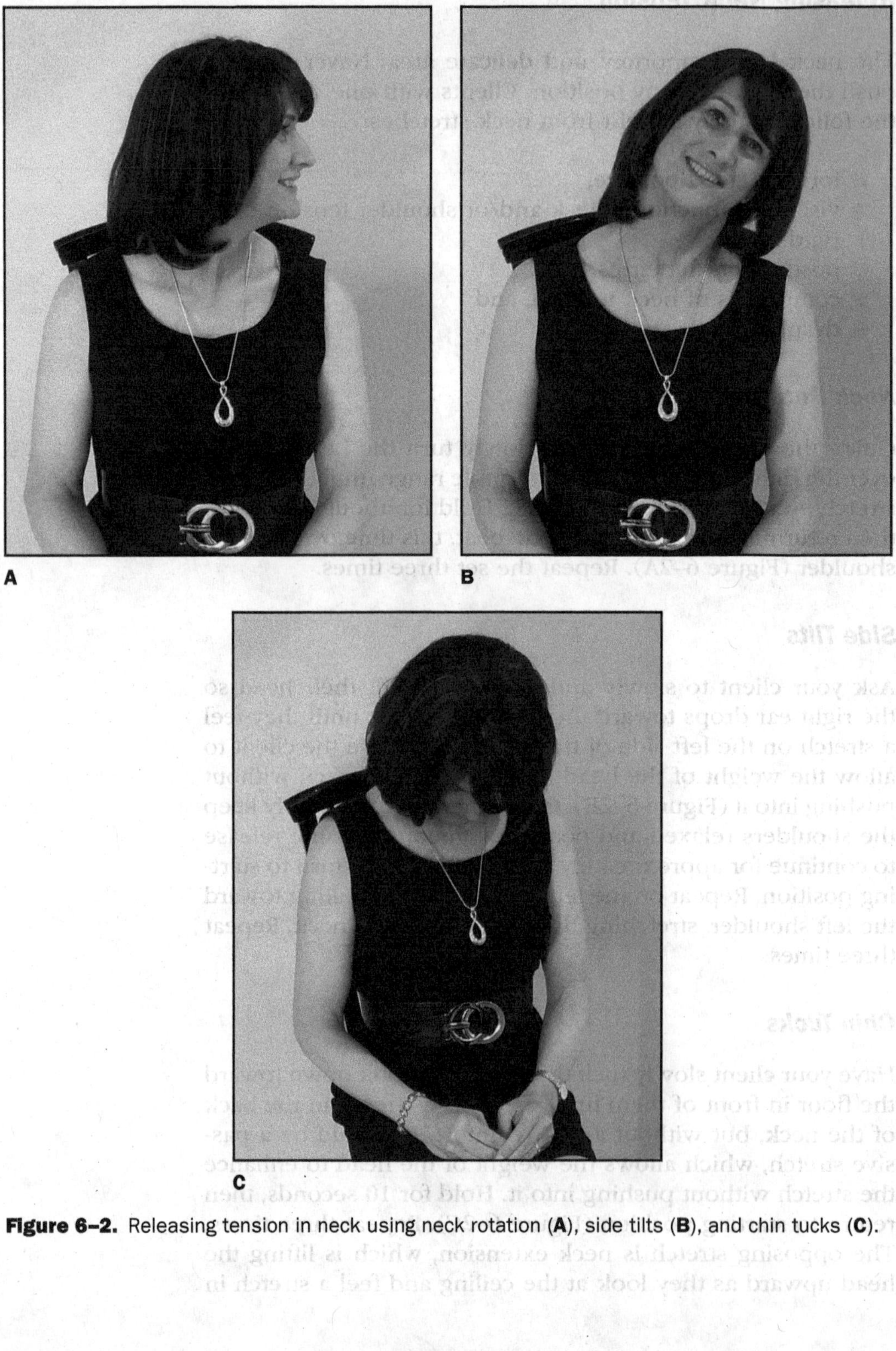

Figure 6–2. Releasing tension in neck using neck rotation (**A**), side tilts (**B**), and chin tucks (**C**).

the front of the neck. Do not perform this stretch without physician approval because of clients' tendency to overdo and the risk of neck injury.

Releasing Jaw Tension

Ask the client if they have ever had temporomandibular joint (TMJ) issues. It is recommended that you avoid jaw work with any client who has been treated in the past for TMJ issues without approval from their physician or physical therapist. Clients perform the following exercises with a provider model and guidance. Those with one or more of the following may benefit from jaw releases and stretches:

- mandibular restriction,
- lingual tension, and
- visible masseter contraction or jaw clenching.

Phase one: Tell your client to press the mid portion of the tongue upward firmly against the hard palate with their lips together. The jaw will open slightly. Encourage your client to consciously let this happen naturally. Hold for about 10 seconds, then release the tongue. Have them notice how their jaw muscle feels for another few seconds to memorize what relaxation here feels like.

Phase two: Encourage your client to allow the jaw to remain slightly open. Have them place their fingertips in the center of the masseter muscle between the mandible and maxilla. Have them gently, slowly, and gradually add light pressure and wait for some release (Figure 6–3A). It is very important that the client stays aware of the feeling in the muscle and follow the release by observing that there is a softening of the muscle under their fingertips. Discourage pushing too hard without waiting for the muscle to release first, then follow the depth from the release, versus forcing depth before the muscle has softened. Hold for 20 to 30 seconds. The jaw opening will increase naturally. Adjust the pressure gradually if you feel it will enhance the effect. If it doesn't, stop. Do not overdo.

Phase three: Finally, have your client open their hand as if about to salute, with the palm face down, place the inner edge of the open hand comfortably between the chin and lower lip. Press downward, opening the jaw, and allow the jaw to release upward (it will close reflexively), consciously allowing the motion of the jaw to be passive (Figure 6–3B).

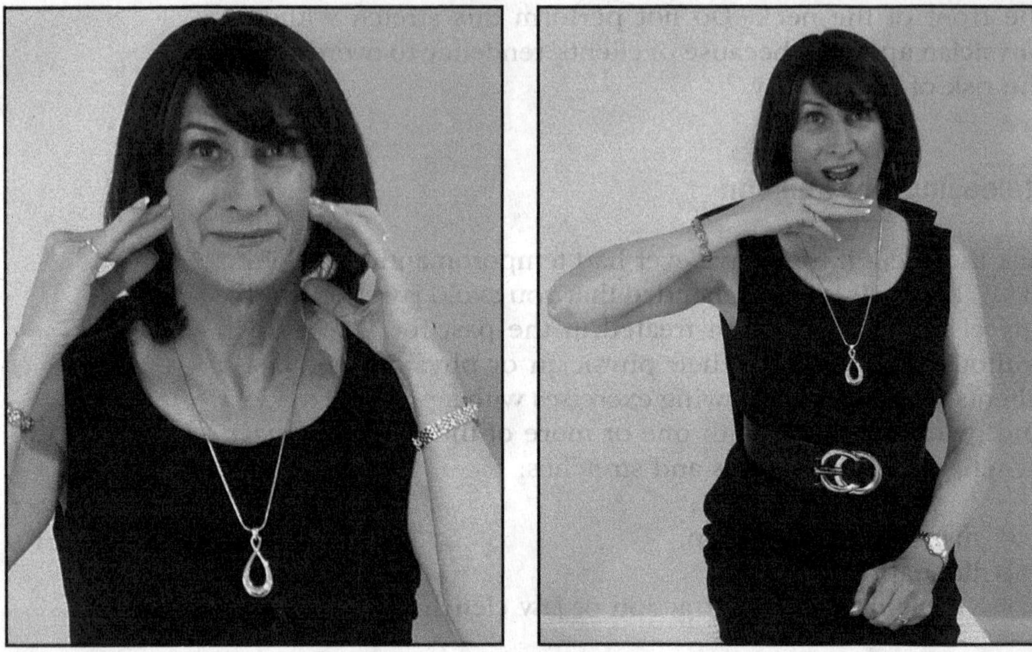

A B

Figure 6–3. Releasing tension in face using pressure (**A**) and stretch (**B**). Note (**A**) demonstrates finger placement, but mouth will be open when applying pressure.

Letting go of control can be challenging for clients. Do this repeatedly for about 10 seconds. With time, increase passive motion of the jaw.

Releasing Tongue Tension

Tongue stretches can improve vocal function, voice quality, and resonance. Because of the intensity of vocal training and its potential for hyperfunction, it is important to release any identified buildup of tension. When the tongue muscles (e.g., genioglossus and hyoglossus) are tense, the tongue bulks, the larynx is pulled upward, and overall the vocal tract is smaller (Figure 6–4). Following the release of tongue musculature, many clients express a feeling of openness and freedom—the sense of "more space" in the throat. We offer two approaches to release tongue muscle tension.

Tongue Stretch

The first approach is the simplest. Have the client open their mouth all the way and protrude their tongue downward and

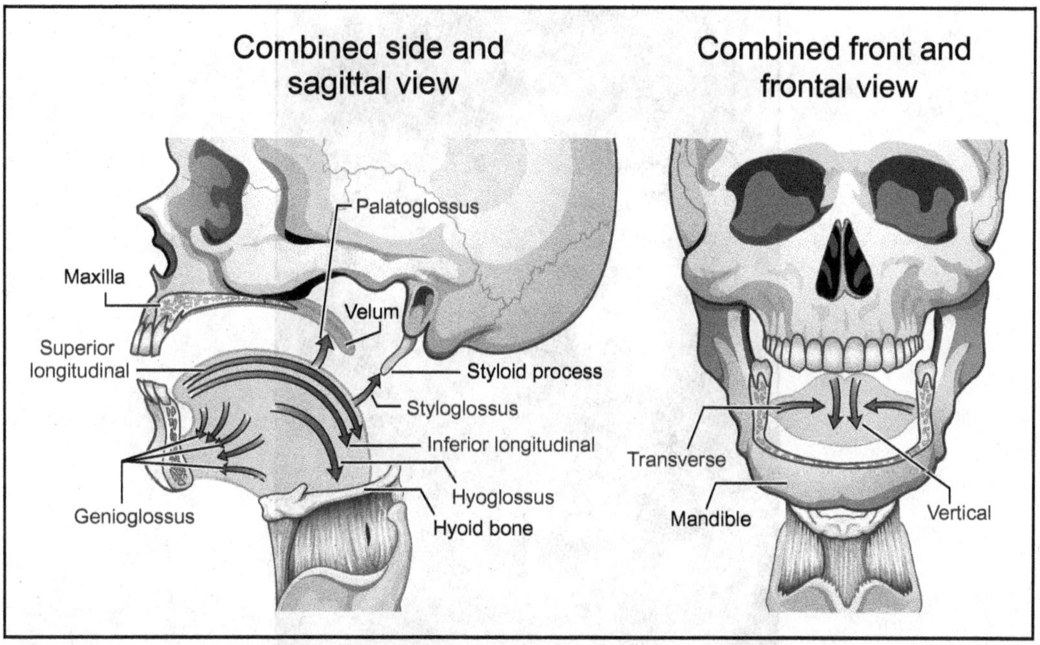

Figure 6–4. Tongue muscles shown from side and front views with major actions of each muscle shown. *Source:* Reprinted with permission from Hixon, Weismer, and Hoit (2020). *Preclinical speech science: Anatomy, physiology, acoustics, and perception* (3rd ed.). San Diego, CA: Plural Publishing.

hold for 20 to 30 seconds as they focus on stretching the back of their tongue (Figure 6–5A). Repeat three times. This often results in greater laryngeal and jaw mobility, providing a sense of greater vocal freedom.

Tongue Pull

If you sense that the client can benefit from a more intense approach, we suggest a tongue-pull technique. Tell the client in advance exactly what to expect (likening it to a doctor or dentist visit can be helpful) and how long it will take. The whole process should not take much more than 60 to 75 seconds. It should not be painful *at all*. If it is, stop and examine factors such as technique or unknown medical or psychological issues. When a tongue pull is paired with laryngeal massage, it can be a powerful vocal release. Before you begin, give your client a tissue for saliva that collects in the corners of their mouth during the procedure.

1. Ask the client to maximally protrude their tongue. Wearing gloves, wrap gauze around the client's tongue and then grip the tongue, holding it in protrusion. Ask

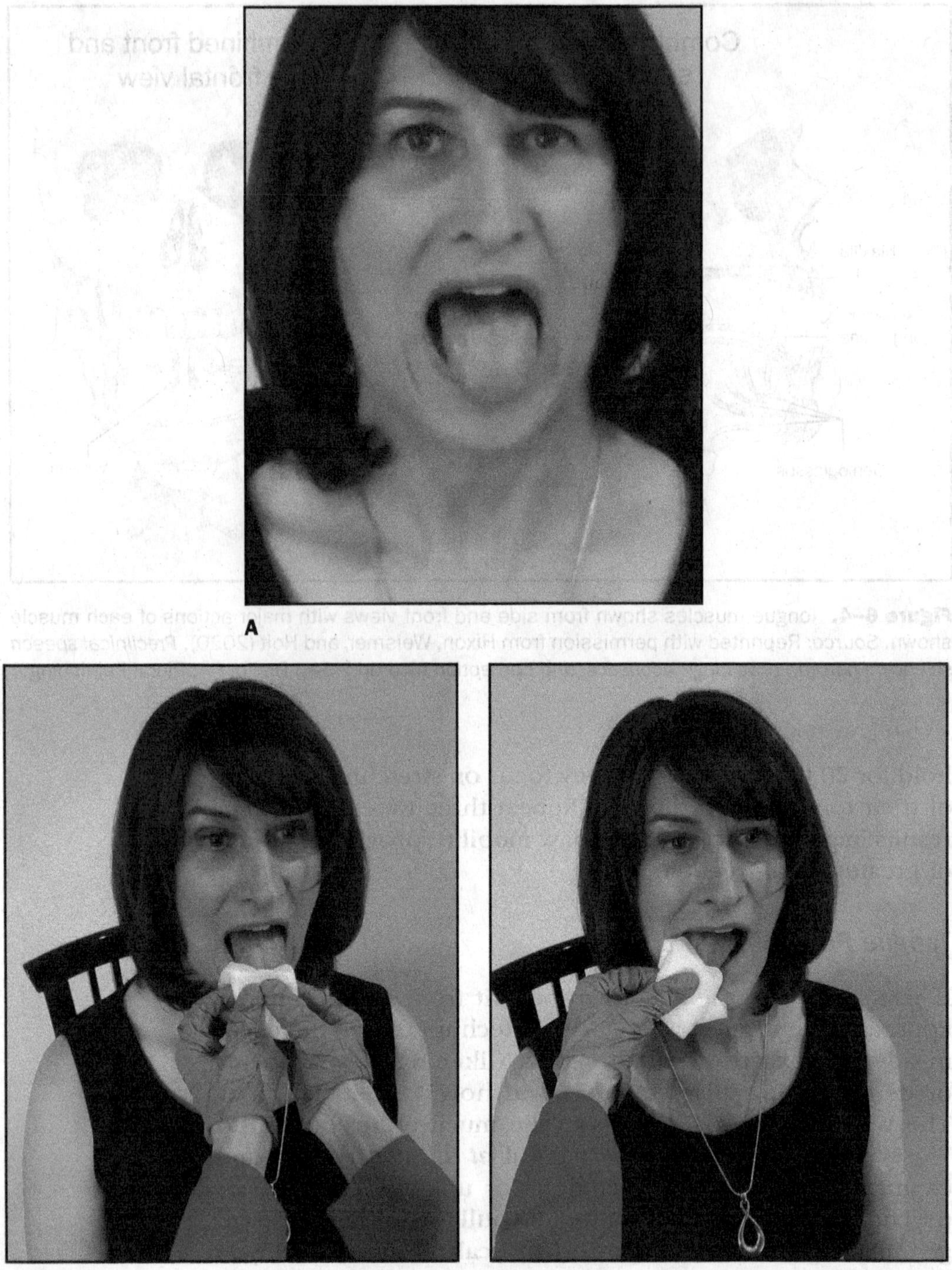

A

B C

Figure 6–5. A–C. Releasing tension in tongue using stretch.

them to release it completely, allowing you to hold their tongue in position. Encourage the client to let you do all the work.

2. Gently hold the tongue predominantly downward to its passive limit (never pull past that limit) and hold it in place waiting to release. Telling them that it will be in this position for about 30 to 40 seconds helps them to relax and participate more fully.
3. Wait for 20 to 30 seconds, and the tongue will release. When it does, it will slacken slightly, allowing you to stretch it slightly further and hold for another release (Figure 6–5B).
4. Gently stretch the tongue to one side to its limit. Feel and wait for about 10 to 15 seconds for its release. Do the same to the opposite side (Figure 6–5C).
5. Return to the center and gradually let go of the pull to avoid spasm. Encourage the client to keep their tongue as relaxed as possible until you let go of their tongue.

Ask the client to describe the difference following this procedure. Note changes in quality of voice, resonance, pitch, and client sensation of spaciousness and freedom in both vocal function and the swallow. If either of the tongue releases are highly effective, teach the client to perform the most effective independently at home between training sessions. It may be especially helpful before and after home vocal practice.

Extrinsic Laryngeal Muscle Massage

Aim and Purpose

Massage of the extrinsic and supplementary laryngeal muscles is important because of their direct influence on voice production. They are responsible for laryngeal elevation and depression, anterior and posterior motion and fixing the larynx into one position in the neck. For example, the infrahyoid (i.e., below the hyoid bone) muscles pull the larynx downward so when they are tense it is difficult to elevate the larynx (Figure 6–6). Freedom in laryngeal movement improves the speaker's ability to manipulate pitch and resonance of the voice.

The underlying anatomy and physiology of easy voice production is why we integrate massage into each session. Teaching the clients to do self-massage between sessions can

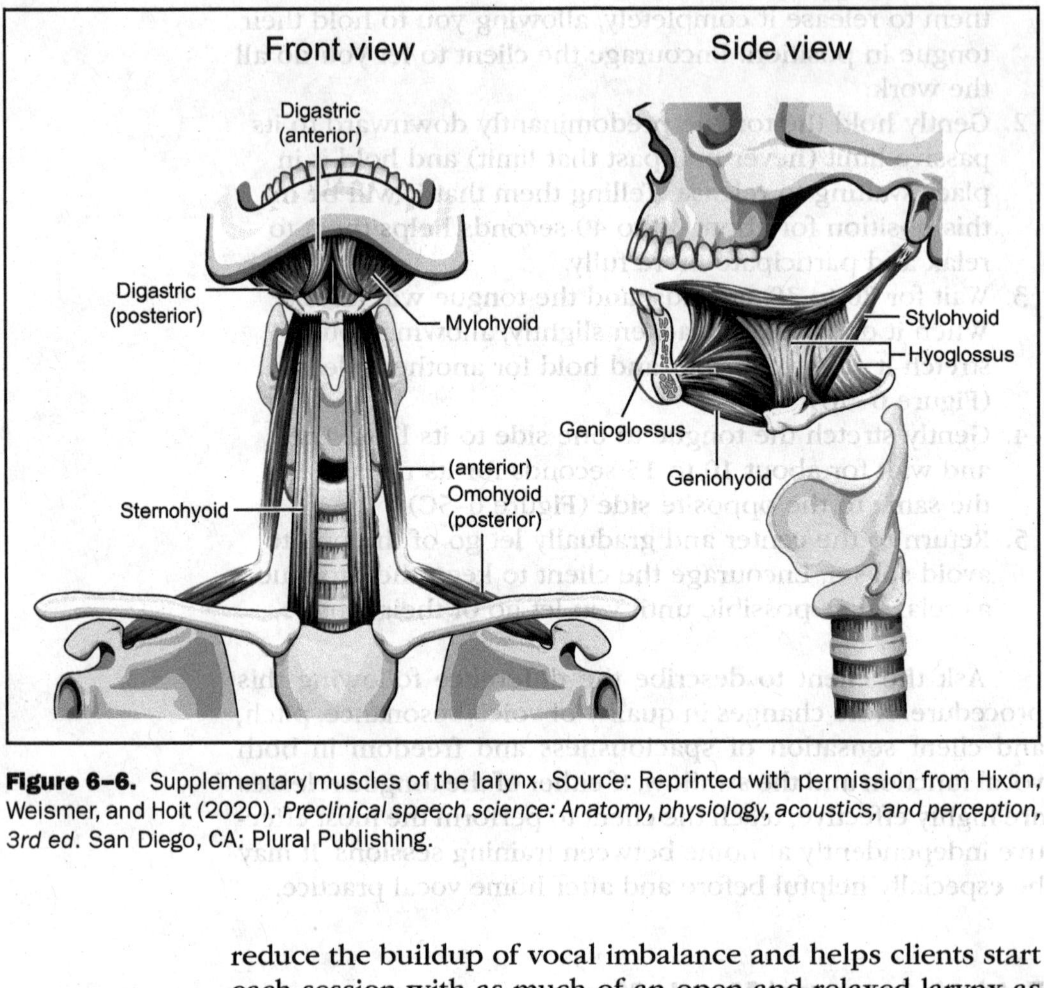

Figure 6–6. Supplementary muscles of the larynx. Source: Reprinted with permission from Hixon, Weismer, and Hoit (2020). *Preclinical speech science: Anatomy, physiology, acoustics, and perception, 3rd ed*. San Diego, CA: Plural Publishing.

reduce the buildup of vocal imbalance and helps clients start each session with as much of an open and relaxed larynx as possible.

The goals for massage of the laryngeal muscles are:

1. To heighten the client's awareness of their own level of laryngeal tension so they can monitor it outside of the session independently.
2. To establish a baseline rating for yourself and the client. Ultimately, we want the client's and provider's awareness and experience to eventually be heightened enough so that the ratings are similar.
3. To release laryngeal structures of tension thereby enhancing vocal function and ease of production.

Before you begin, it is very important to obtain your client's permission to touch them. Explain in advance what you want to do, how it will benefit them and how it will feel. Some clients with previous trauma are sensitive to being touched. One client who was attacked would get highly anxious when she was approached. Since she was uncomfortable talking about it, she could not bring the subject up on her own and agreed to the massage. When the provider sensed the client's anxiety and asked the client about it, they were able to discuss it and find a solution. In this case, self-massage was possible and effective to release tension as long as the provider was continuously talking aloud explaining each step of the process to her.

Measure Baseline Suprahyoid and Infrahyoid Tension

You want to be able to assess the level of tension before and after the massage. Once the massage is complete, examine the effect of the massage to determine that there is appropriate laryngeal freedom before you begin voice training.

To assess the degree of suprahyoid (e.g., geniohyoid, mylohyoid) tension, start by having your client reset their posture. Stand beside them so that your dominant side is toward the front of them. Ask them to drop their head slightly down (about a couple of inches). This will slacken the structures enough for you to achieve greater depth during palpation. Support the client's head with the nondominant hand to keep it from drifting up. Using the dominant hand, place your thumb against your client's chin and your index finger underneath in the center of the *V* of the mandible to palpate the suprahyoid muscles. Use deep circular strokes beginning in the middle portion (geniohyoid), then right of center and left (mylohyoid) to assess the degree of tension and rate it (see Figure 6–6).

A 1-to-10 tension scale can be used to rate your impressions for comparison later. A rating of "1" is the most relaxed, and your fingertips will tell you the tissue is soft, flexible, and deeply palpable without resistance. A rating of "10" is the highest degree of tension and can be identified by significant rigidity and firmness. Clients may report tenderness to the touch, but not always.

To assess infrahyoid (i.e., sternohyoid, omohyoid) tension, ask your client to sit aligned and relaxed with head position downward about 2 inches. Stand behind the client and use two hands, one on either side of the larynx. Using the thyroid notch as a landmark, place your fingertips on either side of the notch and gently slide them posteriorly over the sternohyoid and omohyoid (see Figure 6–6). Stay anterior to the bulky sternocleidomastoid. Stay aware! If you feel a pulsing under your fingertips, you are too far back; you want to be anterior to the carotid artery.

Use your fingertips to palpate the musculature for rigidly or flexibility in the tissues throughout the structure from the hyoid bone to the base of the larynx, as well as anteriorly to posteriorly. Start with very light pressure and learn what level of pressure the client responds to. In general, the pressure directly over the laryngeal cartilage will not be forceful. Then, with open fingers, manually rock the larynx laterally, left to right and right to left, to assess flexibility. The flexible and responsive larynx has a lot of lateral range and a rigid larynx has resistance to the motion.

It is not at all unusual to identify left to right asymmetries. We find it easier to assess asymmetries, mobility, and muscular patterns in the two-handed position, when there is symmetrical digital placement, pressure and manipulation on both sides. Some providers prefer to sit in front or beside their client and use one hand to assess and massage. Both approaches are highly effective and it is completely determined by the comfort and experience of the provider. Again, a 1-to-10 scale to subjectively assess tension is helpful for later comparisons. A "1" rating indicates that the larynx glides easily without resistance, is soft to the touch, and is relaxed. A "10" is significant tension, and can be identified by its rigidity, as it is fixed into one position and is firm to the touch. A client at more severe levels may complain of tenderness to the touch.

Client Self-Assessment

Obtain your client's self-assessment for general laryngeal tension before the massage to get a baseline and then after the massage to assess its effectiveness. Have them listen and feel as they count aloud to five to assess the sound and feeling of vocal function (i.e., ease and relaxed vs. effortful and tense), and then feel the swallow. Have them self-rate using the same subjective rating scale that you use, and then discuss the results. The purpose of the client self-rating is to heighten client awareness of sensation of laryngeal tension and associated changes in voice quality, pitch, and resonance. Some clients cannot sense laryngeal release from counting at all, but feel it dramatically in the swallow. Others may have the opposite experience. Eventually their perceptions will increase in accuracy and more closely match provider pre-

and post-assessment. Their feedback is extremely important in how we proceed with our work, and we want to train them to become self-reliant monitors of their own laryngeal tension and vocal function.

Administer Massage

Because of the direct relationship to vocal function, we almost always provide a massage to our clients. Some clients, however, simply do not carry tension there on a regular basis and while we examine the musculature each time, we can move forward without a massage if it is appropriate. Use your judgement and involve the client in this process as much as possible.

To provide timing for this procedure, massage for approximately 1 or 2 minutes for each area, then retest and move forward from there. Do more where it is needed. It is important not to overdo, but do enough to assure optimal results. Continue to attune to the client as you touch them while identifying the physical response of each client's musculature, which is highly individual. Please see the video demonstration of this massage on the book's accompanying companion website for greater understanding and ease in learning this massage.

If your baseline assessment tells you that one area is significantly tighter, it may be beneficial to start where there is the least amount of tension. This way we can start to release tension indirectly, making it more comfortable for the client and easier to massage directly later. For example, if there is significant tension in the infrahyoid musculature, starting indirectly in the suprahyoid musculature typically reduces some infrahyoid tension allowing for deeper direct laryngeal work that will follow.

Suprahyoid Massage. In general, if there is suprahyoid tension, we massage it directly. For severe tension, however, it can be helpful to release above and below the structure first to free some of the tension and make it more comfortable for the client when you address it directly afterwards. Specifically, performing a tongue pull from above described earlier in this chapter, and an infrahyoid massage from below can be an effective strategy for reducing significant tension. Even with this preparation, clients who prefer not to be touched at such severe levels may do better with self-massage at first to free up surface tension. With time you will be able to take over and go deeper without much, if any, discomfort.

If tension is noted anywhere in the extrinsic laryngeal muscles, we perform a suprahyoid massage because of the impact that it has on the entire mechanism, even if it feels that there is minimal tension in those muscles.

To begin the massage:

1. Think of the suprahyoid musculature in thirds: the middle section, the left of the middle, and the right. Start in the middle, soft, fleshy portion of the mylohyoid using the index finger with the thumb against the chin for leverage. Be aware that you are not too anterior (against the mandible) or too posterior (into the larynx). Then move to the left and right of center to make sure to release the tissue there.
2. Use circular, deep motions of the index finger. You can go quite deep with most clients and have it be comfortable for them. Always ask the client for feedback, "Is this enough pressure? Too much pressure?" It will be more work if the client is tight, and less if they are open and free there. You should have the sense after about 15 seconds that it is starting to release and it will become easier to massage more deeply. As there is greater freedom, go deeper into the tissue. For most clients this feels really good. It is not unusual for a client to express initial mild discomfort if there is significant tension, but this releases gradually during massage. Most clients really look forward to their massage.
3. Teach the client self-massage for between sessions to reduce the accumulation of daily tension:
   a. The client sits with aligned posture.
   b. Their head is slightly down from level by about 2 inches.
   c. The client grounds their hand by putting the outer edge of the index finger against the tip of the chin and uses the tip of the thumb to massage deeply into the musculature for about 1 minute.
   d. It is critical that they learn how to feel what they are doing and how it makes them feel. It is recommended that you limit it to about a minute since some clients will believe that more is better. Eventually they will become more aware and sensitive to the needs of their larynx and can sense when to do more and when to do less.

Infrahyoid Massage. Clients with more severe tension will benefit from the massage starting indirectly, such as beginning with the suprahyoid muscles before the infrahyoid massage. This will safely free up some of the tighter musculature, making it easier to move in more directly afterward.

Note if there is clicking, restriction, or rigidity on one side more than the other. The clicking is related to tension and will be reduced or eliminated following an effective massage. While a video demonstration is available on this book's companion website, it is also helpful that you have a mentor and practice on many volunteers before you work with a client. Practice on several different people (e.g., all sizes of larynges and necks) because the landmarks feel quite different at first.

1. Standing behind the client, place your index fingers on the posterior horn of the hyoid bone bilaterally. The middle and ring fingers can line up just below. As you encircle the major horns of the hyoid bone with the index fingers anteriorly, you can simultaneously massage the posterior borders of the thyroid cartilage with the lower fingers. It is more effective if you use the finger tips versus the pads of the fingers. Focus on the feeling under your fingers.
2. Using light pressure, alternate the hands in a "locomotive" pattern, with your right hand rotating forward and down while the left rotates around toward the back, and vice versa. You can move them simultaneously if it feels appropriate. Notice what is needed. Slowly allow the fingers to massage anteriorly rotation by rotation toward the thyroid notch, and back again. Finally, come downward in the same manner, about one-half to 1 inch with your whole hand, and find any remaining tension. Come back up to the starting position. You should have greater lateral range when the massage is completed.
3. Always ask the client for feedback for the amount of pressure and comfort level. This should feel comfortable for most clients unless there is a significant amount of tension. For clients with severe tension, work indirectly first and start with the suprahyoid structures, then move more directly into the infrahyoid musculature.
4. Clients who express the sensation of being choked are telling you that you are pressing too hard into the structure with your fingers. Simply trust your fingertips to

sense into the muscles and gently rotate the surface tissue. There is no need to squeeze.

5. This whole process can take about 1 minute for mild tension to more time for significant tension. You are aiming for the tissue under your fingers to get softer allowing fingers to go slightly deeper and the range of motion to increase, indicating greater relaxation and flexibility of the musculature. Your fingers will be able to feel releases and increased freedom as you practice and trust yourself more and more. Clicking will dissipate and usually completely disappears.
6. Once complete, we recommend you go back to the suprahyoid musculature briefly to release any new tension that has occurred.

Reassess the Level of Tension

Using the same methods as before the massage, client and provider reassess the level of tension after the massage and compare the results. The provider and client should find similar degrees of change over time as the client becomes more aware. It is important to perform the massage at the start of the session but also throughout the session if dysphonia or altered resonance occurs during training. Most clients benefit from laryngeal massage and are often shocked at the difference in how they feel afterwards. Many become aware that having an open and relaxed larynx is a new experience. While they are trained in self-massage for home practice, most just enjoy turning it over to us during the session and appreciate the difference when completed. Now the client is prepared, relaxed, and aligned, and the foundation is set for them to begin diaphragmatic breathing training and direct voice work.

SET BREATHING FOR SPEECH

Aim and Purpose

The breath supports vocal production in all contexts of voice use whether we are working with clients with voice difficulties and disorders, singers, professional speakers, or actors. Proper breath support is particularly important for trans people because they are in a sense creating an entirely new physiological vocal program for their anatomical structures.

Proper diaphragmatic breathing, depth of inhalation, ease of function, and coordination of the breath with the newly developing voice are critical. Not only do these support significantly altered frequencies, resonance, and intonation patterns, but they also discourage maladaptive compensatory habits from creating strain and tension potentially interfering with target productions.

In preparation for phonation, the diaphragm and external intercostals contract, enlarging the thoracic cavity and creating a negative pressure, which brings environmental air into inflating lungs. We can perceive the abdomen and lower ribs visibly expand in response to this change in pressure (Figure 6–7). If more air is required for the desired task, or if there is restricted contraction of the diaphragm, other muscles can become involved, such as the sternocleidomastoid and scalenes, creating greater expansion of the thorax.

During phonation, the diaphragm and associated musculature release in a gradual and controlled manner; the abdomen supports the flow of air from the lungs through the trachea and into the larynx, inciting the vocal folds into motion. This

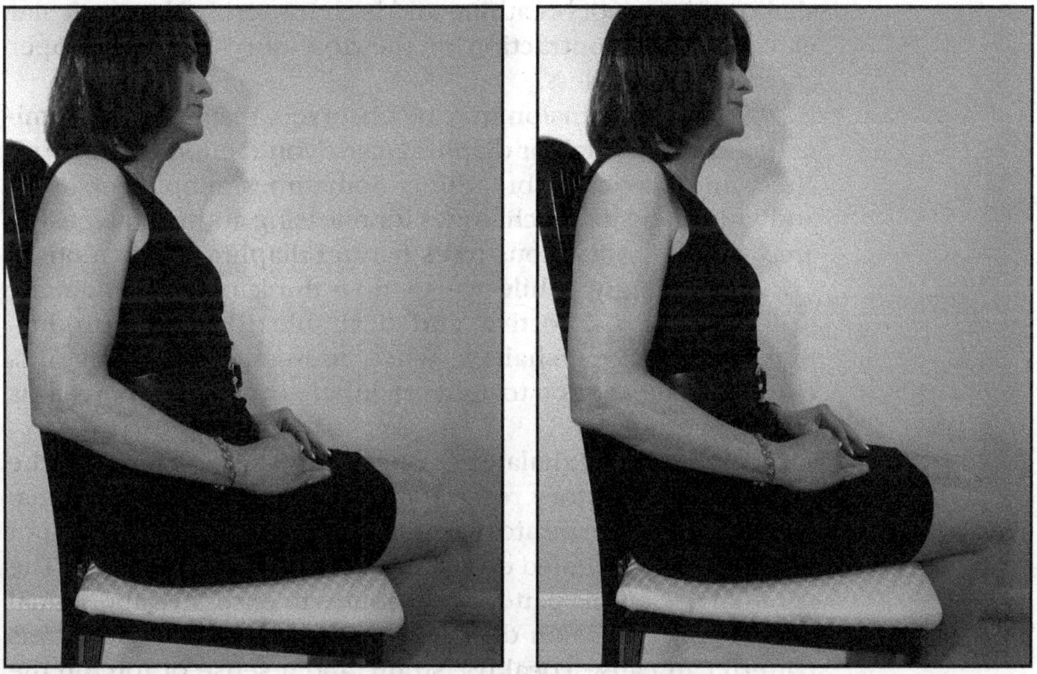

A B

Figure 6–7. Side view of diaphragmatic breathing inhale (**A**) and exhale (**B**).

vibrated air is acoustic energy that flows through the vocal tract, and is shaped during the resonatory and articulatory phases of sound production to give us our unique voice.

Additionally, intentionally relaxing the mind and body prior to the direct breath work is important because the respiratory system is exquisitely sensitive to cognition and emotions (Grassman, Vlemincx, Leupoldt, Mittelstadt, & Van den Bergh, 2016; Von Leupoldt, Vovk, Bradley, Keil, Lang, & Davenport, 2013). It reacts to daily stress by tensing and restricting inspiratory excursion and inhibiting essential voice support as a result. Therefore, having a good working knowledge of the many manifestations of maladaptive breathing patterns as they relate to vocal function is essential. It is important that we identify the unique pattern manifested in each client in the context of voice production.

Maladaptive inspiratory patterns occur when inspiration is shallow, forcing both inspiratory and expiratory muscles to compensate and resulting in high-effort phonation. When the diaphragm is not fully utilized, the chest expands to compensate and supplement inspiration. This may or may not accompany abdominal breathing, and can be commonly associated with clavicular breathing. Clavicular breathing is the shallowest type of breathing and is characterized by clavicular elevation and contraction of the accessory muscles, upper chest, and shoulders.

Abdominal tension may be observed, restricting or eliminating the potential for diaphragmatic contraction during both chest and clavicular breathing. Sometimes simply releasing abdominal tension (techniques for releasing abdominal tension are below) spontaneous frees natural diaphragmatic motion.

Interestingly, while we tend to think of diaphragmatic breathing as supportive and desirable for voice production, it can also be shallow. When addressing breathing, it is extremely important to look at inhalatory depth as well as proper musculature.

In addition, exhalatory issues such as speaking into the end of the expiratory reserve habitually can prevent optimal phonation. The expiratory reserve is the additional amount of air that can be exhaled effortfully after normal expiration. The habitual use of this pattern contributes to excessive abdominal and laryngeal tension during phonation. Habitual use of this pattern can cause vocal fry, strain, and a sense of forcing the voice at the ends of utterances before replenishing the breath. This is such a stable pattern for some clients that it may be initially difficult to release the abdomen.

Unique Considerations

Due to the dramatic changes in laryngeal positioning and function necessary to accommodate the newly developing voice, it is not uncommon for compensatory patterns to take the place of optimal respiratory support. Patients with abdominal fixation or restriction during phonation may develop secondary to high efforts during the vocal modification process, or self-consciousness because of their physical shape or binding their abdomen over a long period of time. Symptoms of poor respiratory support for voicing may include impaired projection ability, vocal fatigue, strain, or harsh or rough voice quality (Azul, Nygren, Södersten, & Neuschaefer-Rube, 2017). For transgender clients AMAB, other characteristics may include laryngeal resonance, low pitch, and restricted intonation. It is important to identify these undesirable patterns early in the process. It is even more important that clients work with us to develop healthy breathing habits. Therefore, helping them understand the relevance of breath support in voice production is a good next step.

Educate About Breathing

No matter how we describe the instructions, conscious breathing will initially feel quite awkward to new clients. They will be relieved to learn that this will become automatic once again with practice. It is important that clients understand breath support in a practical way as it relates specifically to upcoming voice development. For example, there is a connection between the breath coming out and the vocal production. Additionally, the fact that it is so critical in supporting pitch elevation and intonation targets can motivate a client to become more aware of their breath and engage more consistent breath support when using their voice.

Voice quality as a result of shallow breath support may be strained, rough, and effortful. A deeper inhalation often solves the problem and can be stabilized and generalized to all voice work. Anchor the experience by asking the client to demonstrate what feels like too much and too little support for them. Clients with histories of prolonged stress with high verbal output, high general anxiety, forcing the voice into an inappropriate pitch or volume level, asthma or other respiratory or medical difficulty, or complications with reflux often need retraining.

Before you start breath work, encourage clients to prepare the environment first. The environment for the breath is the aligned and relaxed body. If they are binding their abdomen, gently discuss comfortable approaches for them to be able to develop enough expansion of the diaphragm and abdominal region to support their voice goals. Loosening or perhaps removing binds during the practice may be an option with time. For many, once this method's value is recognized, exploring other options is more approachable.

Experiment with the techniques below as they suit your clinical style as well as client effectiveness. Once diaphragmatic breathing has been established in any of the following, generalize the target breathing pattern to higher and more functional levels, eventually merging breathing goals with other voice modification goals.

Techniques for Freeing the Diaphragm

Explore the approaches below that are appropriate for your client. Focusing on abdominal release alone can spontaneously free up diaphragmatic breathing and improve voice quality. If abdominal release occurs during any of the following approaches, immediately heighten client awareness of the new and natural motion of the diaphragm. Have the client intentionally gently increase depth as appropriate. Stabilize the newly developing pattern and generalize gradually to complex levels of speech. Box 6–2 illustrates a client who needed multiple approaches before finally identifying the appropriate technique to release her abdominal tension.

Heighten Client Awareness

Bring client's attention to the fact that they are sitting with tense abdominals and ask the client to release abdominal tension volitionally. Many clients have no idea that they are holding. If your client has difficulty after a few attempts using verbal instructions and modelling, move on to other options below.

Forward Fold

From the sitting position, have the client lean forward placing their elbows on their knees. The abdomen and upper legs will touch in this position. During inhalation, with the help of gravity, there is often a release of the abdomen, increasing the pressure of the abdomen against the legs (Figure 6–8).

Box 6–2. Case Example: Fixed Abdomen

One of our clients AMAB progressively developed difficulties reaching previously attainable pitch goals accompanied by mildly strained quality.

Further investigation revealed that her abdomen was so fixed (in contraction), she could not release it enough for the diaphragm to fully engage. It was not until we looked at her respiratory function habitually that we realized that modification approaches had to focus primarily on abdominal release before we could move forward with direct voice goals.

She initially could not perceive the tension in her abdomen and therefore even with guidance could not release what she could not feel. We tried modeling with visual and tactile feedback, verbal instructions, and "hand over hand," among other techniques. Finally, we applied abdominal pulsing to manually release abdominal tension followed by "cat-cow" positioning to influence natural patterns to emerge. Only then was it easy for the client to feel the change and identify what it was like to have diaphragmatic freedom and expansion.

The improvement in the ease and quality of her voice was surprising to her and she was now able to understand the relationship between relaxed and flowing breath and ease in vocal function. It was critical for this client to anchor this new awareness and change in breathing behavior. Working with negative practice gave her confidence in how to come out of any future tension patterns that may redevelop.

Once she became more consistent with her breathing and vocal pattern, we asked her why she thought the issue developed. She reported that she felt she was trying too hard in the modification process during home practice. She forced her abdominals to squeeze to push out the voice versus releasing the breath, naturally guiding it to connect to and support the voice. We were able to reinforce the value of ease in her new clinical and functional voice goals by having her journal her new awareness for future practice, video record herself using her phone so she could objectively see the difference in her new breathing pattern to practice at home, and audio record her new vocal quality that occurred as a means of reinforcement.

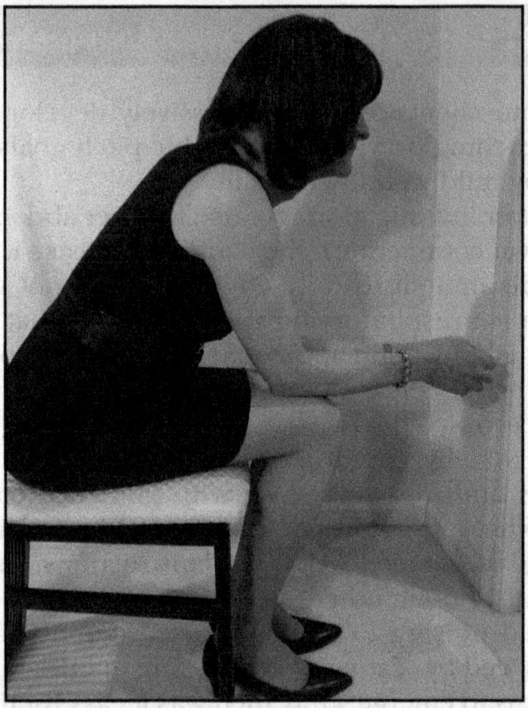

Figure 6–8. Side view of forward fold.

This heightens client awareness of motion in the abdomen for perhaps the first time in a very long time. Encourage the client to mindfully follow the motion of their new breathing pattern until it becomes more consistent. Then when the client feels they can, have them continue with this pattern as they slowly sit up, generalizing diaphragmatic breathing to the sitting position.

Abdominal Pull-In and Push-Out

1. Pull in: Have the client pull in the abdomen as tightly as they can, hold for the count of five, and release completely. Have the client note the release of the abdomen and the spontaneous rush of air into the body. Ask the client to focus on the feeling of the release and allow that freedom to continue.
2. Push Out: Ask the client to push the belly out consciously to make it really big and round, hold for the count of five and release dramatically. Have the client feel the release and allow that freedom to continue.

Cat-Cow

This is a common yoga posture that is done while on hands and knees on a yoga mat, but it is highly effective for our purposes in the seated modification. Clear this with your client before you begin in case there are contraindicated medical or structural issues, particularly when overarching the back. We are going to do the cat-cow stretch in the seated position for ease in the clinical setting, but feel free to apply it on a yoga mat or treatment table if you feel it is more effective for your client to be in the hands and knees position.

In this technique, the rounding of the back takes place during exhalation and is representative of the cat and arching of the back takes place during inhalation and is representative of the cow. This technique can naturally stimulate diaphragmatic breathing, without the client focusing on it specifically.

To begin, have client sit in a chair with both feet on the floor (Figure 6–9A).

1. With their hands resting gently on their lap, ask them to inhale while lifting the chest up and forward, rolling the shoulders back and down into an arched position (Figure 6–9B).
2. Have them look up comfortably.
3. Then, with the palms still resting on their lap, release the breath while rounding the back, pulling the navel inward toward the spine (Figure 6–9C).
4. Look downward.

You may have to repeat the above several times until the provider identifies its effectiveness. This can stimulate the diaphragm organically for many clients which is what makes it quite effective. When diaphragmatic breathing is identified, the client is made aware and asked to consciously follow the natural motion of the breath. When they feel they can duplicate the same motion without the cat-cow in a stable sitting position, ask them to slowly release the cat-cow motion and continue with the breathing.

For all of the above techniques, once abdominal tension is released, often the diaphragm begins to function with greater freedom and depth with very little effort. If there is still excessive upper thoracic activity, try the techniques below for volitional control and optimal coordination. If the client needs more breath support, try the techniques for increasing depth of inhalation.

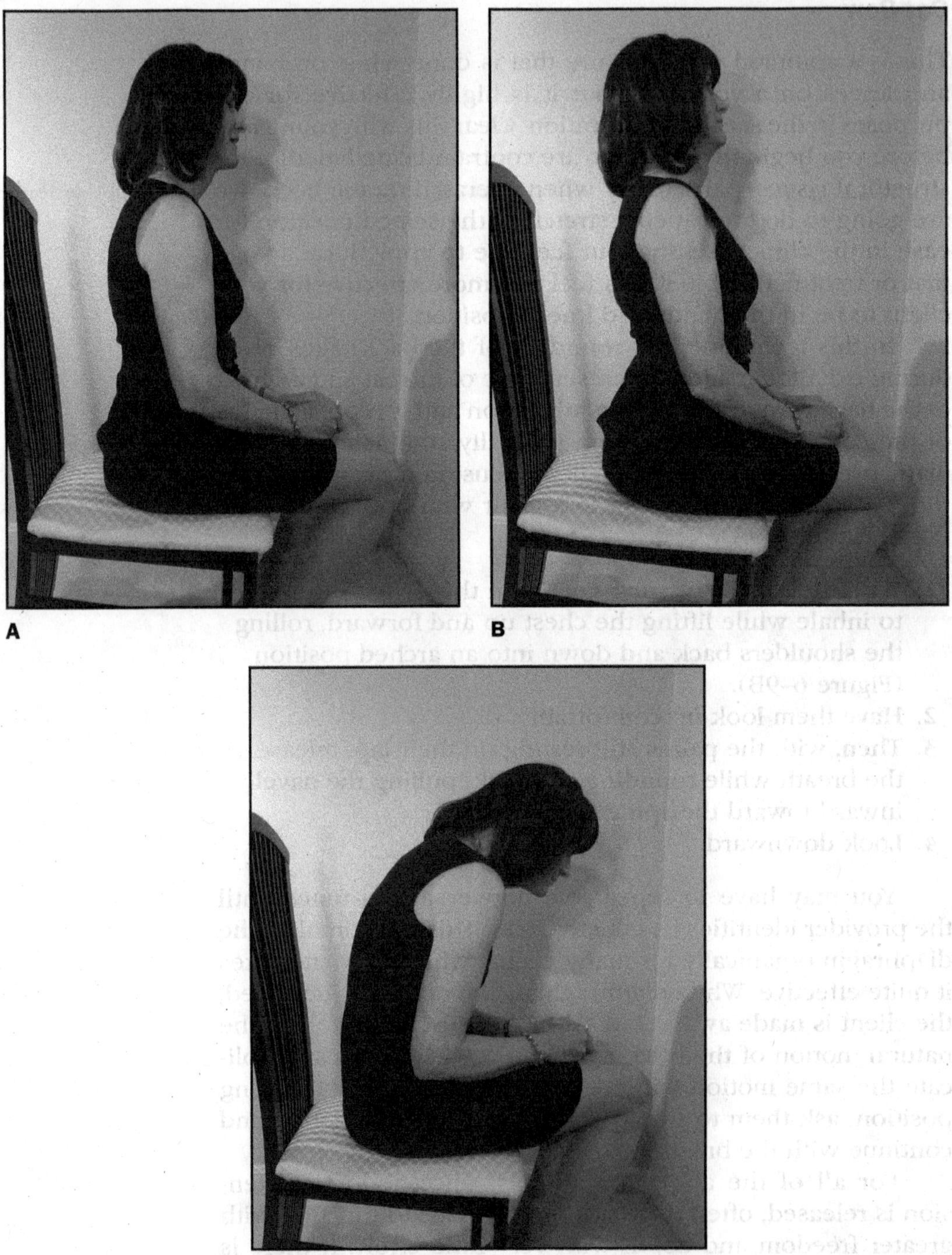

A B C

Figure 6–9. Cat-cow in a seated position. Baseline (**A**), cow (**B**), cat (**C**).

It is important that our clients realize that breath work is the foundation of their upcoming pitch work. We can take it a step further in the diaphragmatic breathing component of the session by helping them make the connection between the inhalation they are working on with the diaphragm, and the use of that breath for vocal production for feminization on the exhalation. Please read about one client who benefited from this approach in Box 6–3.

Box 6–3. Case Example: Diaphragmatic Breathing

Our new client was a 64-year-old transgender woman. She had fully transitioned with the exception of her masculine-sounding voice. She was a musician and played the clarinet as a part of a local symphony orchestra. When we introduced diaphragmatic breathing, she had difficulty expanding her diaphragm and releasing it freely during phonation. We started by heightening her awareness of the new pattern in contrast to her current breathing pattern. We used the verbal description and clinician model, the hand over hand approach, and the abdominal pull in and push out method with little result on a consistent basis. She became very discouraged and lost confidence in her ability to learn how to breathe correctly.

She reported that she could not feel what we were describing as the target. We shifted focus and introduced the forward fold approach. She immediately responded to the sensation of the inhalatory pressure of her belly against her lap for feedback and excitedly said, "I can feel it!"

She now realized the contrast of the free and released abdomen through the changes she felt in pressure. Once she was consistent with the diaphragmatic pattern in the forward fold, we guided her to sit upright while maintaining the pattern. Although she became consistent, she had difficulty understanding that the breath is what moves the vocal folds and drives the sound.

As she was an instrumentalist, we compared it to any reed instrument: "Your own voice operates in the same way as your clarinet, by taking in a diaphragmatic breath and then release it from your lungs through your voice box (the reed) and out of your mouth (the bell of the instrument) you can make your unique sound. Feel the connection of the breath coming in and then being used on the outbreath to make sound. Once you inhale the breath, release it while feeling the connection of the breath to the voice as you make some sighing sounds with it, like this.

Now try it. Take a breath in and then breathe it out connecting it to your voice as you breathe out, saying "aaaaaaahhhh." Feel the breath go all the way up connecting to the sound of your voice and go out. Now say prolonged 'one.' Good, now allow that breath to lift your voice without forcing it happen, allow it to just flow up and out."

After two or three times, she lifted her head and with great surprise said, "Oh my gosh, that sounds like me!"

From here the process became more effective as she developed confidence. By the end of the session she shared that she could imagine applying this in her daily practice with greater consistency over time.

Techniques for Volitional Control and Coordination of the Diaphragm

The following techniques can stimulate the diaphragm and discourage chest and clavicular patterns. They are in no particular order. Helpful inhalatory verbal cues include:

- "Soft body,"
- "No effort,"
- "Breath down,"
- "Think down,"
- "Direct the air through the seat of the chair and floor,"
- "When you feel the chest start to rise, stop,"
- "Let your body take over," and
- "Don't overthink."

Abdominal Pressure

Before using this approach, make sure that the client does not have abdominal pain, new surgical sites or other restrictive issues.

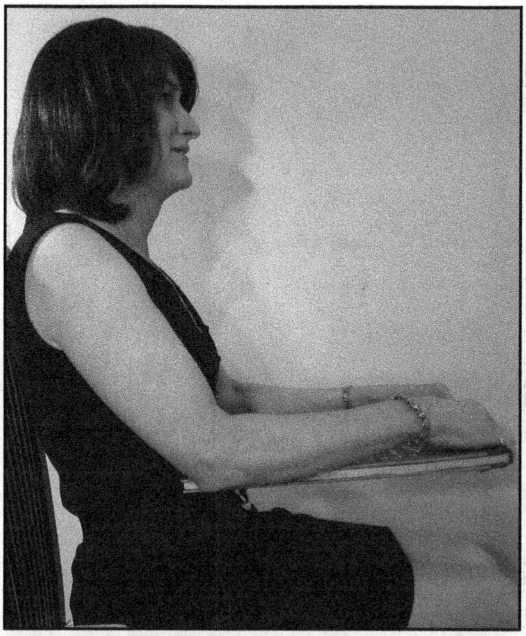

Figure 6–10. External feedback via abdominal pressure.

1. Place the edge of a book or the bottom of a full water bottle against the diaphragm/abdomen as they hold the opposite edge with both hands and relax their arms (Figure 6–10). The prominence of these items allows for sensory and visual feedback.
2. Ask the client to inhale allowing the breath to move the book outward. Be aware that some clients will "muscle it," forcing the abdomen outward. Support the client to allow that the motion be powered by the breath instead of the muscles.
3. Encourage inhalation to the point just before the chest wants to lift. Then release gently.
4. Repeat several times until the client tells you they can do it independently, then remove the feedback tool and have them duplicate the same diaphragmatic inhalation with 5 to 10 passive breaths, progressing to automatic sequences and up the continuum.

Hand Over Hand

1. Direct the client to place one hand over the abdomen and the other over the chest (Figure 6–11).

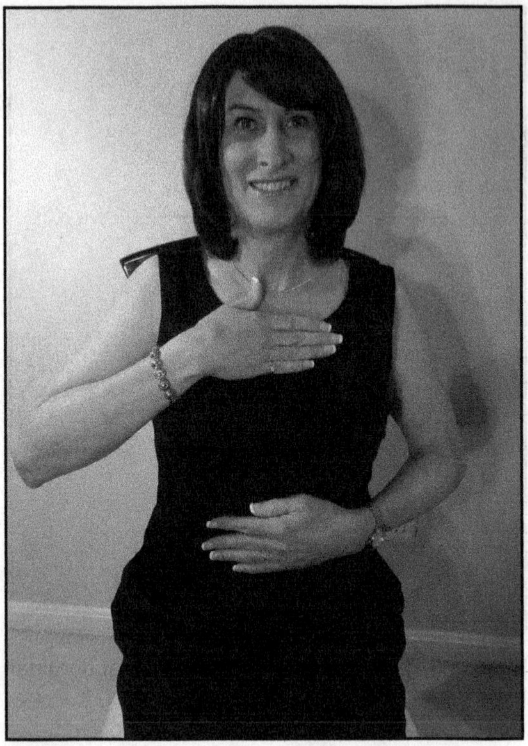

Figure 6–11. External feedback via hand-over-hand posture.

2. During a comfortable inhalation, encourage the client to allow the lower hand to rise in response to abdominal expansion. The upper hand should remain stable during this time.
3. During exhalation, guide the client to release the abdomen with ease. The motion should be smooth and fluid without effort or gripping.
4. Repeat as needed. Ask the client to tell you when the motion can continue without feedback from the hands. Then ask the client to remove the hands and continue the same motion from passive breaths to vocalization during automatic sequences and then up the continuum as appropriate.

If sitting upright was not effective in eliciting the target, the next step is to apply the instructions above while the client leans way back on a chair, or lies on their back on a treatment table or a yoga mat on the floor. This may allow the process to occur with greater ease as the body responds differently with the benefit of gravity.

Techniques to Increase Depth of Inhalation

Discuss how appropriate depth of inhalation is relevant to the health and balance of the speaking voice. While they may be using the correct musculature, it may not be enough to support functional voice and communication with ease.

1. Compare the target inhalatory depth, which produces the best vocal quality with the least effort, with the client's habitual pattern. Ask the client to discriminate between the two productions and describe the difference in how it feels and sounds. Add negative practice to anchor the new learning if needed.
2. Ask them to duplicate the target inhalation progressing from automatic sequences to more challenging levels.
3. Teach clients that strain or roughness can be a symptom that they need to replenish the breath, and to stop to inhale.

Some clients are underconditioned and have difficulty increasing depth of inhalation. With doctor approval, they can build up their core respiratory strength through exercise. Box 6–4 gives an example of a client with poor physical conditioning that appeared to affect vocal transformation.

Box 6–4. Case Example: Physical Activity

H. P. is a 64-year-old retired transgender woman with the desire for a more feminine-sounding voice. She lives alone, volunteers two days a week, and is inactive most of the rest of the week. She presented with a breathy, strained, and gravelly voice with significant roughness at the ends of phrases. The client complained of vocal fatigue and poor projection ability. She felt it began several years ago. She did not remember situations that made it better or worse. She had no known history of a voice disorder. There was no tremor, weakness, swallowing issue, speech difficulty, or reason to suspect neurological involvement at that time. She had no history of smoking, asthma, or emphysema. She did recall having bronchitis for a long period of time about 5 years ago. The client was referred to an Ear, Nose and Throat physician for a direct examination. She was diagnosed with presbyphonia and referred back to us for voice therapy.

Traditional diaphragmatic breathing exercises and methods of voice modification such as vocal function exercises, establishing the best pitch for optimal vocal production, and increasing oral resonance using various approaches including semioccluded vocal tract were effective for improving vocal quality but could not be generalized functionally over time. It was observed by clinicians and confirmed by the client that there was generally poor physical conditioning, she walked quite slowly, alignment was rounded, cues to align her posture produced short-lived change, and her breathing was shallow, limited, and insufficient to support healthy phonation for any length of time.

Objective measures were as follows:

- Speaking fundamental frequency: 140 Hz
- Maximum phonation frequency range: 111 to 280 Hz (16 ST)
- Frequency range during conversation: 124 to 160 Hz (4.5 ST)
- Maximum intensity: 62 dB
- Maximum phonation time: 6 seconds

With the hopes of improving breath support through general conditioning, the client was asked to see her primary care doctor to rule out neurological and other influences on respiratory and vocal function, and to get medical clearance for a progressive walking program 30 minutes daily. She was referred to neurology and pulmonology and cleared for neurological and respiratory disease. Within 8 weeks, breath support and vocal quality improved and we were able to progress more intensively with vocal feminization modification. Maximum phonation time increased from 6 to 12 seconds, and max intensity increased to 68 dB. Pitch at the top of her total range increased by 2 semitones (ST).

The client generally was more energized and appeared to enjoy this newer vocal result. There was hope that this would lead to further progress, but unfortunately the client did not maintain her walking routine consistently and returned to her pretreatment state. H. P. was not interested in pursuing the viability of medical or surgical approaches to improve her voice quality overall or for pitch elevation. She was encouraged to find a walking partner and ways to stay active throughout the week and to let us know if she felt ready to resume vocal modification.

Coordinate Posture and Breathing with Phonation

Automatic Sequences and Memorized Productions

Automatic sequences are a good bridge from establishing the initial target to higher levels. Counting to 10 provides stimuli of one to two syllables, days two to three syllables, and months progress to four syllables. Since these sequences are "automatic," they allow the client to focus on the breath as they go up in syllable length, without having to sacrifice much attentional energy to the utterance. Once the client has learned the skill enough, generalize to phrases such as a memorized poem.

Reading Simple Sentences

Here are some examples of simple sentences to have your client practice reading:

1. Listen to me.
2. Let me know.
3. Trust yourself.
4. Send me a text.
5. Create a vision.
6. A piece of pizza.
7. Tug at your heart.
8. Let's get together.
9. Watch that movie.
10. Drink your coffee
11. Answer the phone.
12. You are masterful.
13. Conscious control.
14. Wait for an answer.
15. Believe in yourself.
16. We're having lunch.
17. Mint ice cream cone.
18. A piece of chocolate.
19. Expand your horizon.
20. Use your imagination.

Reading Sentences of Progressive Length for Breathing, About Breathing

Have your client practice reading longer sentences such as these:

1. Align your spine now.
2. Keep energy in the breath.
3. Always keep the spine soft.
4. Keep freedom in the breath.
5. Keep movement in the breath.
6. Feel your abdomen go in and out.
7. The chest and shoulders are quiet.
8. Always keep the shoulders relaxed.
9. Release the breath easily and freely.
10. The diaphragm moves the breath in.
11. Inhale while expanding the abdomen.
12. Let the air flow out easily as you speak.
13. Make sure that you are taking enough air.
14. Keep the chest and shoulders relaxed and calm.
15. The air comes in and the air goes out as you speak.
16. Always keep the breathing muscles calm when you speak.
17. Use supportive breath support while reading these sentences.
18. The longer the sentence, the deeper the inhalation to support it.
19. You may notice that there is plenty of air to finish this sentence.
20. Once you have gone through all the sentences, consider yourself a success!

Generated Sentences

Name items around the room in a short sentence.

1. I see a picture.
2. I see ___.
3. I see ___ and ____.
4. I see a ____ next to a ____.

State Personal Information

1. My name is ___.
2. I live in ___.
3. My phone number is ___.
4. I am __feet, __inches tall.
5. My eyes are ______.
6. My favorite color is _____.
7. I enjoy eating at _____ restaurant.
8. My favorite beverage is ______.

9. My favorite food is ______.
10. It took me ____ minutes to get here today.

See Appendix 6–C for additional stimuli and tips for making stimuli personally meaningful. Ask the client to verbally identify changes in pitch, resonance, quality, and tension as is appropriate to reinforce the effectiveness of proper postural alignment, relaxation of voice and related muscles and proper breath support on the vocal production.

Gaining Independence

Initially, setting the ideal vocal environment will take more time in the session. Once the client is able to discriminate tension from relaxation, misaligned body position from aligned, and a relaxed and supportive breath from a constrained pattern, the client will be more able to independently incorporate a more relaxed physical and mental state throughout the session. Encourage clients to complete their own mindfulness practice just prior to the start of their session.

READY, SET . . .

Exhale. The next phase of intervention, "Go," will probably be the most highly anticipated and longest. But don't rush to it. Time spent learning about the client, making informed plans collaboratively, and setting the mind and body for intense changes is an investment. If the client is not fully ready or set when pitch elevation work is started, for example, they will end up backtracking when the pitch isn't changing and stabilizing well. Just as exhaling without a good inhale results in strain and pressure, so does voice work without a good plan and preparation.

REFERENCES

Albarrati, A., Zafar H., Alghadir, A., & Shahnwaz, A. (2018). Effect of upright and slouched sitting postures on the respiratory muscle strength in healthy young males. *BioMed Research International*, 1–5. doi:10.1155/2018/3058970

Azul, D., Nygren, U., Södersten, M., & Neuschaefer-Rube C. (2017). Transmasculine people's voice function: A review of the currently available evidence. *Journal of Voice*, *31*(2), 261.e9–261.e23.

Behrman, A. (2006). Facilitating behavioral change in voice therapy: The relevance of motivational interviewing. *American Journal of Speech-Language Pathology*, *15*, 215–225.

Briñol, P., Petty, R. E., & Wagner, B. (2009). Body posture effects on self-evaluation: A self-validation approach. *European Journal of Social Psychology*, *39*(6), 1053–1064.

Chiesa, A., Calati, R., & Serretti, A. (2011). Does mindfulness training improve cognitive abilities? A systematic review of neuropsychological findings. *Clinical Psychology Review*, *31*(3), 449–464.

Eerland, A., Guadalupe, T. M., & Zwaan, R. A. (2011). Leaning to the left makes the Eiffel tower seem smaller: Posture-modulated estimation. *Psychological Science*, *22*(12), 1511–1514.

Grassmann, M.,Vlemincx, E., von Leupoldt, A., Mittelstadt, J. M., & Van den Bergh, O. (2016). Respiratory changes in response to cognitive load: A systematic review. *Neural Plasticity*, 1–16.

Lewandowski, A., & Gillespie, A. (2016). The relationship between voice and breathing in the assessment and treatment of voice disorders. *Perspectives of the ASHA Special Interest Groups*, *1*(3), 94–104.

Peper, E., & Lin, I. (2012). Increase or decrease depression: How body postures influence your energy level. *Biofeedback*, *40*(3), 125–130.

Prochaska, J. O., & DiClemente, C. C. (1982). Transtheoretical therapy: Toward a more integrative model of change. *Psychotherapy Theory, Research and Practice*, *19*, 276–288.

Sedlmeier, P., Eberth, J., Schwartz, M., Zimmerman, D., Haarig, F., Jaeger, S., & Kunze, S. (2012). The psychological effects of meditation: A meta-analysis. *Psychological Bulletin*, *138*(6), 1139–1171.

Van Gordon, Shonin, Zangeneh, & Griffiths (2014). Work-related mental health and job performance: Can mindfulness help? *International Journal of Mental Health Addiction*, *12*, 129–137.

Van Leer, E., Hapner, E., & Connor, N. (2007). Transtheoretical model of health behaviour change applied to voice therapy. *Journal of Voice*, *22*(6), 688–698.

Von Leupoldt, A., Vovk, A., Bradley, M. M., Keil, A., Lang, P. J., & Davenport, P. W. (2010). The impact of emotion on respiratory-related evoked potentials. *Psychophysiology*, *47*(3), 579–586.

Walsh, R., & Shapiro, S. L. (2006). The meeting of meditative disciplines and Western psychology: A mutually enriching dialogue. *American Psychologist*, *61*, 227–239.

APPENDIX 6–A
Relaxation Scripts

MEDITATION SCRIPTS

Deep Breathing Script

"Let's begin.

Feel the weight of your body as you relax in the chair.

[Pause]

That's it . . . good . . . really allow the chair to hold you up as you relax into it . . .

[Pause]

Now, as slowly as you can, inhale as deeply as you comfortably can, as if in slow motion, pausing at the top of the breath consciously . . . being aware of that pause . . .

And then even . . . more . . . slowly, exhale . . . to the end of the breath.

That's it, yes . . . I am going to have you do this as . . . slowly . . . as . . . you . . . can . . . three times.

Go ahead and slowly repeat this now . . . as you put all your attention on how your body moves as you breathe . . . the belly . . . the chest . . .

[Pause and watch them. See if they need to go slower or deeper, and coach them on the next one to "go even deeper and slower on this next one . . . "]

Noticing there is air passing through your nose or mouth . . . feeeeeel it . . . sense into it, allowing it to be exactly as it is . . . there is no wrong way to do this . . . there is just your way.

[Pause for a few seconds.]

Any thoughts that arise are perfectly natural . . .

Simply observing them . . . allowing them to pass . . .

Observing feelings . . .

Gently allowing yourself to go back to the breath . . .

[Pause for a few seconds.]

Yes . . . nice . . . and as you [depends where they are, if they are on the exhalation say, "as you slowly let go of the breath . . . "] notice the body . . . feel how it moves to the motion of the breath."

[Pause for a few seconds.]

Keep track of the time as well as the state of the client to know how you want to proceed. If you want them to do one more breath, for example, say something like, "and as you approach your last breath, make it the slowest and deepest of all the breaths . . . focusing on the sensations in the body, the motions in the body, the feelings in the body."

If they are following your cues, affirm them: "Yes, good . . . "

If the client needs more time, it is fine to continue.

When you want to prepare them to end the meditation, you can guide them by the tone of finality in your voice and by saying something like:

"Finally, letting go of any last thoughts . . . focusing on the sound of my voice . . . feeling your body in the chair . . . your feet on the floor . . . the air in the room touching your skin . . .

. . . when you are ready . . . you can slowly . . . open your eyes."

When completed, continue using a gentle voice, slow pace for a few minutes so as to maintain the level of relaxation as you go into laryngeal massage.

General Relaxation Script for the Body Scan Meditation

"OK, shall we begin?

Allow yourself to sit aligned and relaxed . . .

Gently focus your attention on the top of your head . . . the back and sides of your head . . . your ears . . .

You may notice different sensations there . . . such as tingling . . . or maybe warmth or coolness . . . heaviness . . . or lightness . . .

[Pause for a few seconds.]

There is no limit to the sensations that you may feel . . .

And there is no wrong way to perceive this . . .

There may be no sensation at all, and this is perfect . . .

You are aware of all experiences you have as you put your attention there.

[Pause]

If your mind starts to wander . . . just observe it and allow it to pass . . . it is all good.

This is just an observation exercise and we are noticing what is there . . .

[Pause for a few seconds.]

Notice the hair on your head . . . and the scalp . . . going deeper beneath the scalp . . . good.

Put your attention lightly on your face . . . perhaps feeling the air touching the surface of your skin . . . going deeper into the muscles in the mask of the face . . .

[Pause]

Now let's go lower to the neck and torso . . .

[Pause]

Feel all the sensations in the muscles in the front, sides, and back of the neck.

[Pause]

Gently . . . go deeper into the center of the neck and throat, feeling the air flowing through . . .

Notice any sensations.

[Pause]

Go down to the shoulders now . . . releasing them even more . . . as you feel the sensations of the fabric of your clothing against your skin . . . going deeper into the muscles . . . tendons . . . joints . . . yes . . . good.

[Pause]

Feel the sensations of the upper arms . . . and the lower arms . . . notice the sensation in the hands, fingers . . .

[Pause]

Go lower now into the torso . . . feeling all the space between your chest and upper back . . . your abdomen and lower back . . . your spine . . .

[Pause . . . and give them time to notice.]

Feel the motion in your body as your body breathes you . . . good . . .

[Pause]

Become mindful of your hips, and feel their connection against the seat of the chair.

[Pause]

Coming down and noticing the upper legs . . . lower legs . . . connecting to the feet.

[Pause]

And feeling their connection to the floor . . .

[Pause]

As you sit there and listen to my words, let go of all points of attention . . . let your attention go . . .

[Pause about 20 seconds, let the client savor this.]

Bring your attention back to all the sounds in the room . . . my voice . . .

[Pause]

The feeling of sitting in the chair . . .

[Pause]

And take three conscious natural breaths . . .

And when you are ready . . .

[Pause]

You can open your eyes."

APPENDIX 6–B
Home Program Worksheets

SHOULDER STRETCHES

Client Name:	**Date Prescribed:**
Home Program: Shoulder Stretches	
Before you begin, remember the following:	
■ Use aligned posture throughout these activities. Be aware that the head position is aligned and level throughout if possible. ■ Relax your body. Using a brief body scan is helpful; feel the body as it softens. ■ Maintain natural motion of the breath. Avoid holding your breath. ■ At no point should there be pain. If there is, please stop and talk to your provider about it. ■ Reset alignment and the softening of the neck and shoulders as needed. ■ As muscles release during the stretch, stretch them a bit more. ■ Do not do any of the activities more than is helpful or feels good. More is not always better. The result may be physical discomfort and lack of vocal control. ■ Use a mirror for feedback where appropriate.	
Exercises:	
A. Shoulder Shrugs: ____ time/s each day/week	
1. Raise your shoulders all the way up to your ears, 2. Hold them there for a few seconds, and then let them fall to a relaxed position. It is important to keep the head and neck relaxed. Repeat 3 to 5 times.	
B. Shoulder Rolls: ____ time/s each day/week	
1. Rest your hands in your lap. 2. Doing one shoulder at a time, slowly and gently rotate the first shoulder in a circle rotation forward, upward, back, and down. 3. Repeat 5 to 10 times, and then change direction and rotate backward. 4. Repeat Steps 2 and 3 for the opposite shoulder.	
Tip: *If you are very stiff and unable to produce the optimal position, you may find success rotating the arm with a bend at the elbow. It will feel like the elbow is leading the way going around in a circle.*	

NECK STRETCHES

Client Name: **Date Prescribed:**

Home Program: Neck Stretches

Before you begin, remember the following:

- Use aligned posture. Be aware that the head position is aligned and level throughout if possible.
- Relax your body. Using a brief body scan is helpful; feel the body as it softens.
- Maintain natural motion of the breath. Avoid holding your breath.
- At no point should there be pain. If there is, please stop and talk to your provider about it.
- Reset alignment and the softening of the neck and shoulders as needed.
- As muscles release during the stretch, stretch them a bit more.
- Do not do any of the activities more than is helpful or feels good. More is not always better. The result may be physical discomfort and lack of vocal control.
- Use a mirror for feedback where appropriate.

Exercises:

1. Neck Flexion (Chin Tucks): ____ time/s each day/week

As you exhale, slowly tuck your chin, dropping your head slowly down until you can look down at your toes while feeling a stretch in the back of the neck. There should be no discomfort. Allow the weight of the head to enhance the stretch without pushing into it.

2. Neck Rotation: ____ time/s each day/week

Keeping the shoulders relaxed, slowly turn your head to look over your right shoulder as you exhale, until a stretch is felt on the left side of the neck. Repeat on the other side.

3. Side Flexion (Side Tilts): ____ time/s each day/week

Slowly tilt your right ear toward the right shoulder as you exhale, until a stretch is felt on the left side of the neck. Again, allow the weight of the head to enhance the stretch without pushing into it. Consciously keep the shoulders relaxed. Repeat on the other side.

- *Hold each for a count of 10, then come up to the starting position.*

- *Repeat each set 3 times.*

Client Name:	**Date Prescribed:**
Home Program: Instructions for Reducing Jaw Tension	
Before you begin, remember the following:	
■ Use aligned posture throughout these activities. Be aware that the head position is aligned and level throughout if possible. ■ Relax your body. Using a brief body scan is helpful; feel the body as it softens. ■ Maintain natural motion of the breath. Avoid holding your breath. ■ At no point should there be pain. If there is, please stop and talk to your provider about it. ■ Reset alignment and the softening of the neck and shoulders as needed. ■ As muscles release during the stretch, stretch them a bit more. ■ Do not do any of the activities more than is helpful or feels good. More is not always better. The result may be physical discomfort and lack of vocal control. ■ Use a mirror for feedback where appropriate. ■ Avoid holding your breath during the exercises.	
Reducing Jaw Tension: ___ time/s each day/week	
Phase One:	
With the lips together, press the mid portion of the tongue upward firmly against the hard palate. The jaw will open slightly. Consciously let this happen. Hold for about 10 seconds, then release the tongue. Notice how the jaw muscles feel for another few seconds to memorize what relaxation here feels like.	
Phase Two:	
Allowing the jaw to remain slightly open, place your fingertips in the center of the masseter muscle between the mandible and maxilla. Take a relaxed breath and—starting on the exhalation—gently, slowly, and gradually add light pressure and wait for some release. Follow the release, going deeper as it allows, by observing that there is a softening of the muscle below your fingers and allowing it to continue. Hold for 20 to 30 seconds. The jaw opening will increase naturally. Apply more pressure gradually if you feel it will enhance the effect. If it doesn't continue to release tension, ease the pressure or stop.	
Phase Three:	
Finally, open the hand as if about to salute, with the palm face down, place the inner edge of the open hand comfortably between the chin and lower lip. Press downward (opening the jaw) and allow the jaw to release upward (it will close reflexively), consciously allowing the hand to passively open the jaw. This can be challenging for clients to let go of control. Relax the jaw enough so that only the hand is opening and closing the jaw. Do this repeatedly for about 10 seconds.	

REDUCE TONGUE TENSION

Client Name: **Date Prescribed:**

Home Program: Instructions for Reducing Tongue Tension

Before you begin, remember the following:

- Use aligned posture throughout these activities. Be aware that the head position is aligned and level throughout if possible.
- Relax your body. Using a brief body scan is helpful; feel the body as it softens.
- Maintain natural motion of the breath. Avoid holding your breath.
- At no point should there be pain. If there is, please stop and talk to your provider about it.
- Reset alignment and the softening of the neck and shoulders as needed.
- As muscles release during the stretch, stretch them a bit more.
- Do not do any of the activities more than is helpful or feels good. More is not always better. The result may be physical discomfort and lack of vocal control.
- Use a mirror for feedback where appropriate.

Release Lingual Tension: ____ time/s each day/week

A. Tongue Stretch

1. Open your mouth all the way.
2. As you exhale, protrude your tongue downward and hold for 20 to 30 seconds focusing on stretching the back of their tongue.
3. Gently relax and release the tongue. Repeat three times.

B. Tongue Pull

1. Protrude your tongue and wrap gauze around it. Relax it as much as possible.
2. Gently pull the tongue downward to its first limit as you exhale (never pull past that limit) and hold it in place.
3. Wait for 20 to 30 seconds, and the tongue will release. When it does, it will slacken slightly, allowing you to stretch it slightly further and hold for another release.
4. Then, gently stretch the tongue to one side, to its limit. Feel for its release, which is usually about 10 to 15 seconds.
5. Repeat on the opposite side.
6. Return to the center and gradually let go of the pull.

In both exercises, notice if there are improvements in quality of voice, resonance, pitch, and the sensation of spaciousness and freedom in your throat.

Client Name:	**Date Prescribed:**

Home Program: Massage the Muscles Under the Chin (Suprahyoid Muscles)

Only Do This Massage with Direct Training From Your Provider

Before you begin, remember the following:

- Use aligned posture throughout these activities. Be aware that your head position is aligned and level before you start.
- Relax your body, maintaining natural motion of the breath. There should be constant flow of the breath throughout all activities below.
- At no point should there be pain. If there is, please stop and talk to your provider about it.
- As muscles release during the stretch, go into the stretch a little deeper.
- Do not overdo any of the activities recommended. The result may be physical discomfort and lack of vocal control.
- Use a mirror for feedback where appropriate.
- Do this massage daily before and after home practice, and when you feel you need it; however, do not do more than 5 or 6 times each day.

Steps to Follow:

1. Sit with aligned posture.
2. Lower the head slightly by about 2 inches.
3. Place the tip of your thumb under your chin, feeling the space just behind the jaw bone and in front of the Adam's apple. Rest your index finger against the chin and use the tip of the thumb to massage in deep small circles into the muscles in the soft space under the chin.
4. Massage for approximately 1 minute.

Avoid pushing into the Adam's apple/voice box at all times.
Do not overdo. More is not necessarily better.

LARYNGEAL MASSAGE

Client Name:	**Date Prescribed:**
Home Program: Massage the Muscles of the Voice Box	
Only Do This Massage with Direct Training From Your Provider	
Before you begin, remember the following:	
■ Use aligned posture throughout these activities. Be aware that your head position is aligned and level before you start. ■ Relax your body, maintaining natural motion of the breath. There should be constant flow of the breath throughout all activities below. ■ At no point should there be pain. If there is, please stop and talk to your provider about it. ■ Do not overdo any of the activities recommended. The result may be physical discomfort and lack of vocal control. ■ Use a mirror for feedback where appropriate. ■ Do this massage daily before and after home practice, and when you feel you need it; however, do not do more than 5 or 6 times each day	
Steps to follow: review this carefully with your provider	
1. Lower the head slightly by about 2 inches. 2. Using a thumb and index finger, touch the Adam's apple (a swallow will make it move up) and then slide them back slowly, staying on the smooth muscles under each digit. 3. Just before you reach the bulky neck muscle, slowly and gently massage in small circles. Rotate toward the back, then down, forward, and up, and repeat for about 1 minute. 4. Your hand can also come forward, and then also down slightly (perhaps ½ to 1 inch) and then up again, and back again, as long as it feels comfortable. 5. Your fingers should be able to feel softening and increased motion of the voice box through this process. 6. Massage for approximately 1 minute. More is not necessarily better.	

SAMPLE HOME PROGRAM

<table>
<tr><td>Daily Practice</td><td>Date of Session:</td></tr>
<tr><td colspan="2">Instructions:</td></tr>
<tr><td colspan="2">1. Use soft and aligned posture
2. Self-massage: Before and after practice for 1 to 2 minutes
3. Diaphragmatic breathing practice: 5 minutes using attached worksheet and instructions</td></tr>
<tr><td>4. Practice oral resonance at the target pitch of 170 Hz (match to Pitch Perfect app) for attached homework</td><td>Practice in a quiet space for 10 minutes 3 to 5 times daily: Take a supportive breath before you begin each response. Use your app to monitor frequency level during the following:
1. Warm-up glides and stabilizing activity
2. Use oral resonance at the target frequency for the practice provided on the attached worksheets.

Explore practice in daily life: Remember to lift forward as often as possible when communication opportunities arise. Focus on your breathing and oral resonance at the target pitch.

Take advantage of going to the market, bank, etc. . . . Just trying it is a success! Accuracy increases with time.

The following was your choice for generalizing during the week:
■ Meet with your practice partner for coffee one time.
■ Plan three phone calls with known or unknown persons.
■ One-on-one communication with your daughter, remembering to lift pitch 3 to 5 times each day.
■ Take advantage of one unexpected opportunity to use this new level.

Journal vocal experiences for discussions in the session. Focus on situation/emotion/experience/ success for next time

Continue writing your gratitudes each day. You were interested in listing three gratitudes per day this week. We will check in on this and see how this is working for you.</td></tr>
<tr><td>Next Session</td><td>Greet provider at the target levels.</td></tr>
</table>

APPENDIX 6-C

Speech Stimuli

STIMULI FOR VOCAL PRODUCTION

Stimuli can be created or modified for any production level, goal area, and communicative context. In general, stimuli will progress from impersonal to personal, short to long, and simple to complex to gradually increase the cognitive-linguistic load. Emotionally loaded topics are initially avoided to give clients a gentle start, making it possible for them to focus more on vocal function. None of us can maintain our best voice when faced with stressful content in a conversational context. Start at levels of production that are realistic for the client's success.

Generic lists are provided in this appendix, but we invite you to create personalized stimuli. Personalized information integrated throughout voice modification will help the client be engaged and help transfer skills into their daily life. Between the structured work we integrate unstructured spontaneous practice in our conversation to help with stabilizing and generalization.

To develop personally meaningful stimuli, discuss with clients their communication situations and the people who are in their lives. You can ask them for a "common vocabulary" list, though most clients need to be guided to collect many examples of verbalizations from daily experiences. Offering a list of questions, such as the one below, can help with this process. You may instruct them to complete the questions at their leisure for homework between sessions, or gradually work on it together over a few sessions as you build rapport.

1. What are the first names of (5 to 10) ___ people that are in your life on a regular basis?
2. What are the names of countries, cities, or towns that you have lived in or visited?
3. List your pets, their names and what you say when you talk to them.
4. What do you say when you answer the phone at home/work?

5. What are some comments and questions that you routinely say relating to:
   a. Home: house/yard/garden/family members/responsibilities/etc.
   b. Work: job/professional responsibilities/personal and phone greetings
   c. Community: post office/bank/supermarket/mall/town center activities
   d. Personal: frustrations/joys/worship
6. Provide information about the following that we can create questions and activities around:
   a. Weekend: getaways/catching up at home/other
   b. Commuter: car/metro/bus/fly/waiting/late/breakdown/station/etc.
   c. Social: bar/party/get-together/reading club/dinner party/drop by/etc.
   d. Exercise: health club/yoga/weights/cardio/bootcamp/tired/sweat/swim/other
   e. Hobbies: outdoor/indoor
   f. Vacation: weekend/local/travel
   g. Mealtime: restaurant/cooking
   h. Meetings: club/professional/meet-ups
7. Daily Phrases: hello, goodbye, please, thank you, you're welcome, yes, no, excuse me [client adds their own]
8. Client suggestions:

When you know enough about the client, you (or the client) can tailor stimuli to facilitate generalization to beyond the training session.

Here are some other stimuli you can use, or inspire you to create your own.

RESPONDING YES AND NO

1. Is your name ________?
2. Do you live in ____________?
3. Do you have a pet?
4. Do you have a hobby?
5. Did you drive to the session today?
6. Do you like to exercise?
7. Are you going away this weekend?

8. Is today Sunday?
9. Will you go out to dinner this evening?
10. Is your birthday this month?

GENERATE PHRASES OR SENTENCES USING THE WORD:

1. Museum
2. Balloon
3. Nails
4. Color
5. Spring
6. Wine
7. Breath
8. Leader
9. Dinner
10. Rose

GENERATE SHORT RESPONSE

1. What day is today?
2. What is your name?
3. Where do you live?
4. Where to you work (go to school)?
5. What do you do for work (what is your major in school)?
6. What do you say when you answer your personal phone/work phone?
7. What form of transportation did you use to get to the session today?
8. What kind of exercise do you do?
9. Where was your last vacation?
10. What is one thing you like to do in your free time?
11. Where do you like to go out to eat and why?
12. What is your favorite meal to cook/eat?
13. Do you have a pet and if so what kind?
14. Who lives in your household?
15. How did you meet your partner/roommate/friend?
16. What are your children/coworkers/friends like?
17. What were you like as a child?
18. What do you like about your friend's/child's/coworker's personality?
19. What would you like to do on your next vacation?
20. What are your professional or personal aspirations?

GENERATE PROGRESSIVELY LONGER RESPONSES

The following list of tasks and contexts can guide you toward creating specific stimuli.

1. Simple greetings that are repetitive and familiar ("Hi, how are you?")
2. Greetings in unfamiliar environments and situations
3. Create a short sentence answering "Who is ___ (famous or familiar people)?" questions.
4. Create a short, simple sentence relating to certain words (e.g., pizza, coffee, computer...).
5. Describe the items in the room, or a room in their home/workplace.
6. Describe the function of the items in the basket, or have them bring an item to describe.
7. Answer "why" questions ("Why do you have to set your alarm in the morning?").
8. Problem solving (e.g., "If you forgot your wallet at home, what would you do?")
9. Metaphor task: What does this metaphor mean to you?
10. Metaphor task: How would you use it in a sentence?
11. Describe steps to the various activities ("Give me directions to getting to my office today").
12. Describe your opinion about ___ (e.g., smoking in public places).
13. Describe your job, or dream job.
14. Describe what in this catalog (e.g., clothing or furniture catalog) appeals to you and why.
15. Monologue related to topics of personal relevance and importance (e.g., family, hobbies).
16. Conversation with familiar and unfamiliar people
17. Conversation in familiar and unfamiliar environments
18. Practice an upcoming speech with an audience they know.
19. Practice an upcoming talk with an unfamiliar audience.
20. Convince me of something.

READING: SHORT SENTENCES

1. I need my coffee!
2. What's new with you?
3. I'll see you tomorrow.
4. Where have you been?

5. Do it your way for now.
6. I'm in the office by nine.
7. I could eat pizza every day!
8. I'd love to lose some weight.
9. Tuesday is my night out with the girls.
10. Can you believe that it's raining again?

READING: 3 TO 8 SYLLABLES PER BREATH GROUP

How Flowers Can Affect Your Mood

1. Being among flowers
2. Can be a way to relax,
3. Simply by looking at them.
4. The variety is amazing.
5. The colors are enticing
6. Whether vivid or subtle.
7. The shapes are unlimited.
8. The sizes have a full range.
9. And combinations are unending.
10. A common daisy
11. Has the power
12. To free the mind.
13. A coneflower's bud
14. Leaves one amazed
15. And in awe of its beauty.
16. It also makes you feel calm
17. When you are upset.
18. In the garden,
19. Plants can change your mood,
20. When you want to renew!
21. Even when nothing
22. Has changed on the outside,
23. Being among plants
24. Can make you feel
25. Changed on the inside.
26. When I do not quite feel right
27. I know that stepping out
28. To my garden
29. Can make all the difference.
30. And I know it will for you!

READING: 5 TO 11 SYLLABLES PER BREATH GROUP

Gardening Can Soothe and Relax You

1. Have you ever had to work in a garden?
2. It turns out that gardening is a surprise!
3. I never thought it could make me feel
4. So deliciously relaxed and happy.
5. It is true, it is hard work, don't let me kid you . . .
6. It is just that when I dig around in the dirt
7. I get so involved in what I am doing,
8. And it brings me such wonderful peace,
9. That I do not notice the work for very long.
10. If you feel low in energy, go out to your yard.
11. Pull a few weeds, then plant a petunia,
12. For beauty and ease of upkeep you would not believe!
13. When you return the next season,
14. You'll find you will be gifted with "free" flowers.
15. Your first petunia will leave seeds in the soil
16. To bloom again, once the sun is high and warm,
17. Without any effort on your part.
18. And that is our gift from the previous generation of flowers.
19. For tending, and digging, and weeding, and bending . . .
20. And for that, we are grateful.

READING IDEAS

1. Text messages
2. Emails
3. Blogs
4. Newspapers
5. Magazines

CHAPTER 7

Intervention Phase 3: Go!

The goal is marked. The mind and body are set. Let's go!

Direct voice work described in this chapter will constitute most of the intervention. This chapter includes multiple approaches and facilitating techniques. Although by no means exhaustive, the variety is intended to equip you for many of the needs that will arise. Some exercises will be familiar to providers already working with voice and speech. Education and experience with voice modification for any reason—gender-related or not—will be helpful.

Each transformation unfolds uniquely, so stay attuned to the process and avoid developing a rut. Assess subjective and objective outcome targets regularly. Continue to collaborate with the client to adjust the strategy as needed as you . . . Go!

PITCH AND RESONANCE

Aim and Purpose

Fundamental and formant frequencies of the voice, perceived as pitch and resonance, respectively, are crucial ingredients in gender attributions. The balance of resonance and pitch at any level produces optimal vocal ease, control, clarity, projection ability, and endurance. While pitch elevation is a dominant feature of vocal feminization in particular, its effectiveness in this process is only realized with the accompaniment of oral resonance. Producing a feminine-sounding voice may involve resonance in a smaller oral cavity (e.g., as when saying "eee"), whereas a masculine-sounding voice involves a larger, open oral cavity (e.g., "ahh"). Either way, free the resonance from the larynx. If we try to modify pitch without attending to oral resonance, there will be poor balance of the voice that can lead to:

- undesirable vocal characteristics, such as monotone falsetto,
- vocal hyperfunction with associated vocal strain or damage, and
- poor efficiency of the system, leading to vocal fatigue.

Therefore, the general approach to pitch modification is to couple the target frequency with oral resonance from the start. In other words, we do not target a pitch level. We target a balanced vocal production at a target pitch level.

Equipment

Recording samples throughout the session can be useful to provide auditory feedback for clients as well as to save, send, and compare samples. If you are using recordings to identify and document change over time, adhere to the recording protocols and equipment standards outlined in Chapter 4. Otherwise, it is reasonable and convenient to use your client's smartphone or personal recording device. This is an invaluable tool for use both in and out of the session. A program that can visually display the target frequency in real time, during the client's production, is also needed for feedback. Many programs can be downloaded to a smartphone, device or computer. At the time of this writing, most of the following are free or inexpensive. This list is not exhaustive.

Praat

Free computer software package for recording and analysis of voice and speech. http://www.fon.hum.uva.nl/praat/

Smart Phone Pitch Apps

Pitch Perfect. This is like a piano keyboard. Tap a button to produce an identified pitch. This app is good for pitch matching and ear training. It displays hertz and the musical note.

https://play.google.com/store/apps/details?id=depollsoft.pitchperfect&hl=en

Voice Analyst. Analyzes fundamental frequency and sound pressure level, and can send and save lives.

https://itunes.apple.com/us/app/voice-analyst-pitch-volume/id732245213?mt=8*Pitch*

Voice Pitch Analyzer. Analyzes average, maximum, and minimum hertz, and saves files for comparison.
https://alternativeto.net/software/voice-pitch-analyzer/

Sonneta Voice Monitor. Analyzes fundamental frequency and sound pressure level (SPL).

https://itunes.apple.com/us/app/sonneta-voice-monitor/id670854671?mt=8

Pitch Lab Pro. Measures frequency, and displays the hertz and musical note.

https://www.amazon.com/PitchLabApp-PitchLab-Pro/dp/B00LOETW3W

Warm-Up

Guided Resonance

Have the client sit in an aligned and soft posture. Following a comfortable breath, have the client say a prolonged "mmm," focusing on the sensation. The use of the nasal "mmm" stimulates "forward focus" that is perceived as a buzzing sensation on the lips and anywhere in the mask of the face (Verdolini, 2000). For transmasculine voices, a more open oral cavity may facilitate an oral resonance with a heavier tone (e.g., "uuuh," "uuum"). The client's lips should be relaxed and the production light and gentle. Note that the pitch will have to change from their habitual voice to achieve this. The ideal fundamental frequency will likely be somewhere in the gender-neutral range unless the client's pitch is already changed from surgery or testosterone. While the client attends to resonance, you should monitor pitch and vocal quality to guard against developing muscle tension patterns.

It is important that the client approach all voice work with the provider in an exploratory manner as opposed to searching for a finite outcome. For example, ask them to describe where they feel vibrations (e.g., "this feels more forward," "I feel it in my throat at this level") as they learn about producing resonance in their body, as well as how each relates to vocal clarity and ease. This awareness is highly valuable, and each small success helps to build skill and self-efficacy (Van Leer, Hapner, & Conner, 2008).

We ask that the client only focus on resonance at this early stage simply because it can be overwhelming to try to focus on more than one new skill at a time. While the client focuses on the sensation of oral resonance, the clinician monitors the frequency to intercede if it becomes too high (i.e., strained and effortful or falsetto phonation) or low (i.e., laryngeal resonance).

Once an agreed upon target production has been achieved, begin to extend the duration of the production. Elicit the prolonged word "mee" in the same way so that the "mmm" is now followed by the forward vowel "eee." The spreading of the lips and elevation of the hyoid bone and larynx required for the "eee" vowel essentially shorten the vocal tract in comparison to other vowels such as "uuu" or "o." This has the effect of subtly raising formant frequencies and having a lighter tone quality (Behrman, 2007), which contributes to a more feminine-sounding voice.

We generalize the acoustic nature of the "eee" to all other vowels in what is commonly called forward focus. This is similar to what is described in most treatment studies for voice feminization (Carew, Dacakis, & Oates, 2007). Another term for this process, coined by Hirsch and Gelfer (2012), is "/i/-ification" (pronounced "eee-i-fi-ka-shun").

As the client prolongs "meeean," draw their attention to the flattened lips and subtle smile of the "eee" vowel and the distinct sound and feel. Then transfer the acoustic nature of the vowel into the following prolonged words: "men," "man," "mun."

Throughout this process, continue to monitor the mean F0 of the production and keep it at an appropriate level. There will come a time when you will be able to target pitch more directly, but the purpose of this warm-up is simply to produce a resonant sound, even if it requires much help from the provider at this point. When your client can produce the above with oral resonance, they will be more likely to apply it to upcoming pitch modification work and therefore more able to approach it safely.

Pitch Glides

After resonance in sustained vowel is established, overlay the skill of varying F0. The client is instructed to prolong the resonant "mee" at a comfortable pitch level, and then slowly glide toward and past the target pitch. Have the client replenish the breath at the highest and lowest pitch levels. Repeat the pitch glide at least three times. This exercise is depicted in Figure 7–1 for people increasing their F0 (i.e., more feminine sound).

The range used in this exercise is usually 8 to 12 semitones (ST) but varies greatly depending upon the client. The whole glide is to be produced in a range where oral resonance is effortless. Gradually shape the range so that the client is aware of starting and ending the glide with oral resonance. Guide the client to be aware of the resonance shifting as the pitch glides up and down. If there is falsetto at the highest

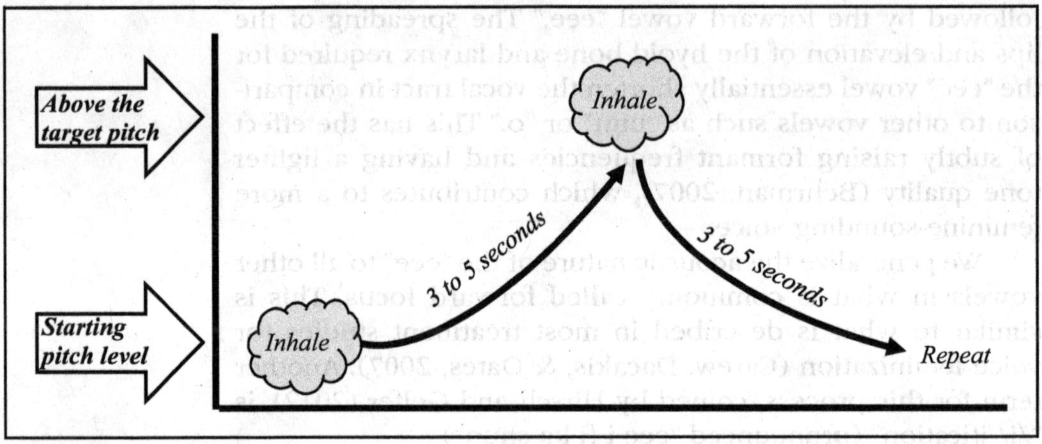

Figure 7–1. Pitch glide.

point, either the pitch is too high or there is not enough oral resonance.

Explore other vowels (e.g., "moo" and "moh"), reinforcing generalization of the "eee" vowel coloring. Again, there should be clear, easy, and pleasant oral resonance throughout each pitch glide.

Pitfalls to Avoid

Throughout this process, help the client vocally explore and search for that sweet spot of vocal balance. Clients should think about what they want to feel and hear. When they focus on what is desired, they are more easily drawn to the target. You as the provider, on the other hand, should be on the lookout for pitfalls. Box 7–1 provides an example of exploring several techniques in response to the client's physical and emotional obstacles. Below is a list of the more common snags clients have encountered, and suggested responses.

Excessive Vocal Intensity

It is important to work at average intensity levels during voice training. Loudness, produced with high subglottal pressure and tight adduction of the vocal folds, will hinder the flexibility required for ease in the vocal modification process. Improvements in pitch and quality can be quite dramatic for some clients when they bring down the volume.

Box 7–1. Case Example: Target Block

This client was a 46-year-old trans female just beginning their vocal transition. During the oral resonance portion of the session, the provider had difficulty establishing a target that was fully forward. The client moved to contrasting the prolonged word "mean" with flattened lips for the vowel against the same word with rounded lips to anchor the target production. The provider felt that the client appeared to be approaching it with tension and that adjusting pitch could enhance vocal clarity and ease. They were guided to elevate pitch using the same word in small steps evaluating the productions along the way. The client had significant difficulty controlling pitch as guided and was getting frustrated.

The provider offered the client a completely new technique using a pitch glide, reasoning that it may be easier to control and hoping to encourage greater optimism and openness in the client's approach. Sure enough, there was greater ease while gliding upward, and with the provider's cues, greater clarity and forward focus emerged. Once the target level was identified, it was repeated after the provider, independently sustained, and then carried into the sentence "My voice feels fine" at the same frequency.

After a few guided trials, the client's face lit up and they said, "Oh, that feels different, I feel it right here" as they pointed to the space above the upper lip. The provider silently noted the frequency to be at 165 Hz while continuing to have the client focus on resonance. The client was more motivated now, saying, "Let me try to go up another time." The provider notes that the level appears free of effort and agrees that going up a little more may be interesting. Because of the difficulty manipulating pitch directly at the start of the session, the client was guided to feel, imagine, or visualize the sensation of resonance a little higher than the lips, such as between the eyes. As hoped, the client's pitch came up slightly and the resonance, vocal quality, and ease were monitored.

Pitch was now up to 178 Hz. The client reported that it felt too hard to maintain and wanted to come down a bit to the level of ease they noticed before. It was determined that based on vocal clarity and ease, their first target level would be established at 165 Hz. The client was completely delighted at their new sound and felt more confident that they could approach pitch and resonance with the same ease during home practice.

Dysphonia

Occasionally the pitch and resonance modification processes reduce dysphonia or strain. When they don't, the etiology should be explored under the care of a laryngologist. Factors preventing healthy phonation should be addressed directly before progressing with pitch goals.

For vocally healthy clients whose voice quality deteriorates with pitch modification in the absence of medical, surgical, or voice care issues outside of the session, immediately identifying the habits that may be contributing is crucial. The most common cause is excessive muscular tension in the larynx and associated structures. Again, utilizing resonance therapy and other techniques commonly used for dysphonia should be incorporated into the plan prior to continuing with pitch modification. In other words, back up and try it again before letting it go too long or too far.

Muscular Tension and Rigidity from Monotone Chant

Although a common way to start, using a chanting approach may be counterproductive in that its nature—sustaining one note and fixing the larynx in one position—can add tension for some clients. If this occurs, look for approaches that encourage variable pitch and more natural elevation and depression of the larynx such as pitch rolls or intonation work for potentially greater ease in vocal production.

Fear or Anxiety

Vocal imbalance or dysphonia that arise in the session may be a sign of emotional disturbance. For example, one client developed dysphonia during sessions and grew increasingly distressed. She was initially unaware of the change in her voice or the related emotions just below the surface until the providers were able to ask her directly at the time of the voice change. Upon reflection, she realized the performance anxiety she was having about the voice work was triggering similar pressures experienced in childhood. These deep-rooted conflicts were manifesting in voice. Once she was able to share this, the providers coordinated care with her psychotherapist.

Asking clients what they are thinking or feeling during unexpected or unexplainable voice change gives them an opportunity to become aware of and express emotions that may be arising in the moment. Changes in voice quality may simply be related to the challenges of the modification process itself (see Box 7–2 for example).

Issues related to repetitive daily stress or deeper unresolved concerns may arise. Support the client in the moment, and work with the client's psychotherapist for further support. More ideas related to attending to the mental health and wellness of the client are included in Chapter 8.

Box 7–2. Case Example: Emotional Block

A client who is trans AMAB developed progressive dysphonia in the session. After trying laryngeal massage and breath and oral resonance work with minimal change, we asked her if she was aware of what she was feeling. She started to cry and blurted out, "fear!"

When we probed further, she realized she thought she was incapable of being successful simply because she could not always hear her pitch and resonance changes during training sessions. This completely surprised us given her consistent growth, appropriate self-involvement in the process, and what we felt were good self-monitoring abilities. The new awareness of our client's anxieties allowed us to adjust our approach. We shared our experiences with her, and we also created tools such as audio files to practice identifying pitch and resonance changes in herself and others independently, but more importantly so that she could check her ratings against the providers' and develop a greater sense of self-efficacy.

She journaled after each practice to reflect on her small and large daily successes, as well as practice self-compassion and helpful self-talk. With time, she became a more confident learner.

Falsetto Phonation

Optimal breath support coupled with oral resonance is highly effective for achieving modal register phonation. A volume glide can be instrumental in helping a client shift from falsetto to modal phonation patterns at the pitch where falsetto is identified.

Starting with a supportive breath, have the client sustain a vowel at the target pitch with an easy voice, guiding them to very gradually add more volume. There will come a point where the quality of voice will shift from the thin quality of falsetto to the fuller quality of the modal register. This is the balance point we seek. There is no need to add much more volume past this point—we are not looking for loudness; we are looking for balance. Once the client is ready to replenish the breath, have them initiate the target voice and sustain it three to five times to stabilize. Ask the client to describe the difference in their voice. Progress from sounds to words and phrases. This exercise is depicted in Figure 7–2.

Maladaptive Postural Adjustments

Pitch modification can be challenging. To rise to this challenge, some clients compensate for the laryngeal adjustments that influence pitch by bringing the head back, protruding the chin, and elevating the shoulders. It is important early in the program to encourage clients to alter pitch supported by the breath and larynx rather than contorting the body and disrupting the postural alignment achieved earlier. The voice is influenced by shifts in head positioning, so be wary of drifting spinal misalignment. Additionally, when the client finds what they feel is target phonation, they may be tempted to stiffen so as not to lose it. Gentle cues for a "soft body" may be necessary until they are more confident in their ability to

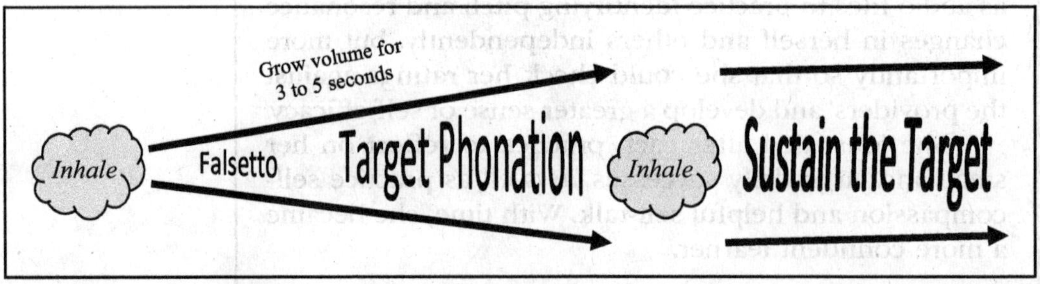

Figure 7–2. Volume glide.

return independently to the desired sound and feel. Reminding them that it is not one pitch we are looking for but rather a range of acceptability may help to relax this belief.

Two Approach Options

After warming up with basic resonance and pitch variation, begin to focus on pitch or resonance. Some clients will initially do well focusing on pitch as the primary goal and then address resonance secondarily. Candidates for this approach generally develop oral resonance organically as their pitch changes. Other clients will be more productive when working with resonance directly and can then let pitch follow. One of the advantages of focusing on resonance is that the client's anxiety in anticipation of pitch change is removed from the picture. We find this happens regularly with clients working toward a more feminine sound, elevating their pitch level. With time, clients become more comfortable and skilled in working with pitch more directly.

In either approach, it often happens that while focusing on a primary goal of either pitch or resonance, it stimulates more optimal production in the other. Having access to more than one approach will be helpful in getting the most out of voice modification with the least amount of effort. Before we begin, refer to a brief list of tips for working on pitch and resonance in Box 7–3.

Option 1: Focus on Pitch

We often set the target frequency during the assessment. The initial target set is highly dependent upon the initial potential. Many clients set one or two formal targets throughout an entire training program, but this can vary depending on your experience and your client's needs.

Setting target change of about 5 to 7 ST initially will be appropriate for many clients, however this can be quite variable client to client, and from transfeminine to transmasculine. It is motivating and practical to jump right into gender neutral; however, if there is too large of a jump, it can be stressful on the larynx and very discouraging for the client. The intention should be to find the level that presents with laryngeal ease and allows for upward intonation to occur with similar ease.

Box 7–3. Tips for Pitch and Resonance

- Be a good model; your client will be influenced by you.
- An aligned and relaxed body is essential yet is a common oversight when achieving optimal oral resonance. Good head position and relaxed abdomen are especially critical.
- Work slowly, giving the client time to hear and feel the shifts. Find language and experiences that work specifically for them.
- Make resonance an exploration of sound and feeling. Teach the client to enjoy the sensations in all parts of the vocal tract versus developing an aversion to what they have used all their life prior to transitioning. This may help reduce anxiety for upcoming direct voice work.
- If clients have poor body and sensation awareness, they will have a difficult time with oral resonance. Emotional trauma can lead to conditions for which counseling may be the best step before the client can move forward with direct voice work.
- Set flat and broad lip positions (as in a subtle smile) versus rounded lip positions to effectively shorten the vocal tract and enhance higher formant frequencies. Cuing for /i/-like postures early on can set the tone for the rest of the sessions. Contrasting flattened lips with rounded lips on /i/ and other vowels can anchor this learning.
- Using volume above an average conversational level or pitch level too far from target will make it difficult to achieve oral resonance.
- When intonation effectively stimulates oral resonance more than direct oral resonance modification does, by all means start with intonation goals at the target frequency. Further shaping can take place with greater ease once intonation skills begin to generalize.

When we identify a target, we are actually identifying a range where the quality, ease, and resonance is of similar consistency. A new pitch level is appropriate if it will be easily achievable and have a good quality. The client will report laryngeal ease within that range and room for intonation expansion as needed. The provider will note a sense of sustainability without compensatory tension, strain, roughness, or hoarseness.

In addition, the target pitch addressed from session to session will need to accommodate daily human needs such as sleepless nights, stressful days, newly arising reflux, allergies, new medications, dehydration, and situational voice strain. Being aware and flexible during these times reduces distress by normalizing variability.

Pitch Cueing Options

Voice modification is a new experience for clients, and learning to hear and manipulate the voice on command can be daunting. Pitch matching and the use of monitoring devices do not always help clients learn to control their voice when initially setting the target.

Visual Feedback Devices. Pitch monitoring devices are tools. They help to guide us in the proper direction. They do not take the place of what the provider sees and hears and what the client feels. This is important for the client to understand. Devices to monitor the productions are effective throughout the session. It is important that clients have a healthy relationship to these devices and are not so dependent upon them that they sacrifice developing their own "internal pitch monitor" and detach from the connection to their own bodies during this process. The external monitor—whether an app on a personal device or software on a computer—is a temporary guide and will be used less and less often both in and out of the session. More seasoned clients will be able to find their targets subjectively, and providers simply monitor that accuracy and provide feedback as appropriate.

Play with a few apps to find the one that is compatible with your devices, and get comfortable using them. They are fun and simple, and can be very helpful. Assist your client to select the apps that are most beneficial for them. They will need to monitor their own voice objectively at times both in and out of the session.

Once the target has been established, use an app with a piano keyboard (e.g., Pitch Perfect) to select and play the target level for the client to match to begin modification work. To identify a frequency of a speech sample, you can use any app that measures and displays frequency. Document and repeat your trials as needed for consistency. Some apps will record the voice and show the hertz and musical note and store the production for future reference. Clients can use headphones with the microphone to input a clear signal when there is background noise; an external microphone may not be needed in a quiet space.

Coordinate Language with Visual Cues. Referential language accompanied by visual cues such as drawings, a keyboard, or gestures may lead trans women more easily and effectively through the pitch shifting process. Indicate the broad space between their current voice level and the highest note (or the lowest note if they are masculinizing their sound) that they can reach. From there, guide them to come up (or down) a small portion of that, step by step, from where they are now until the first target level is identified. It is important that clients realize that this is not going to be the final product. It will feel artificial and it is! This is just our starting place.

Auditory Feedback. Auditory feedback is very important to help clients objectively assess their productions in the session and for documenting change over time. One of our seasoned clients was fine-tuning her resonance but was discouraged in one session, feeling there was no difference in her own voice from 3 months prior. When we compared her productions to the recordings from 12 weeks ago, her expression changed to surprise and she stated, "Oh my gosh! There is no reason to be embarrassed about my voice anymore! It *is* better!"

Listening to audio recordings teaches clients how to listen to themselves more objectively. In the session, auditory perception of distinction between the habitual and desired targets is necessary. Leave the recorder running to capture ideal productions or to play back and contrast two productions.

Also, because it is easy for clients to forget the target productions set for the home program, clients often report struggling to find the target sound on their own during home practice. In these cases, it is extremely important to record productions during the session, particularly with the provider instructions guiding them in the background. When the instructions are all so new, many clients simply do not recall with accuracy how they can be the most productive in their home practice. Listening to the recordings of themselves doing it during the session is constructive as well as encouraging.

It is important to note that for some clients listening to their own voice—for pitch, resonance, or for general consideration—on a recording can trigger gender dysphoria. Finding ways to approach this so that the anxiety does not outweigh the benefit is important. For example, listening to several speech samples that vary by how gender or other attributes are communicated may help increase the client's objectivity and reduce reactivity to their own voice.

Techniques for Pitch Modification

Slowly change the pitch until you both agree that the first target has been reached. It is helpful to begin by heightening the client's awareness of the sound and the feel of the baseline voice before shifting pitch level. This provides the client with a frame of reference for their upcoming productions and contributes to the decision-making process as they approach an effective target.

Adjusting the Frequency in Small Steps

- Using connected speech: The client either counts to five or says a short phrase aloud such as "my new level" in their comfortable voice, then moves up (to feminize the sound) or down (to masculinize the sound) in small steps on the scale. The benefit to this approach is that you get a feel for the client's quality and ease in connected speech that can then be shaped.
- Using sustained phonation: The client sustains a pitch on prolonged syllables such as "meee" to help with forward focus at their comfortable baseline pitch level. Then adjust frequency in steps (i.e., 2 to 3 semitones). This is particularly helpful for clients who need many experiences of mastery to build self-efficacy.
- Go up the steps of a scale: The client steadily moves along the scale using "do, re, mi." Move slowly, note by note to identify a target level.

Jump Right to It. Estimate a reasonable pitch target and have your client reach all the way to that level. Based on your assessment of their vocal quality and resonance, adjust from there by moving just a bit above, then below, until you find a good target. Target estimation depends upon baseline level. We tend to ask clients AMAB to jump into the gender-neutral frequency range (i.e., 145 to 165 Hz) and clients AFAB on testosterone to jump into the upper range of cisgender male norms (i.e., 120 to 140 Hz) if they are able.

Pitch Glides. Ask the client to do a pitch glide from their comfortable level toward their goal very slowly, on a prolonged syllable (for example: "meee"). If this is an effective approach, at one point in the glide you will perceive the vocal "sweet spot" where there is a distinct change in quality, resonance and ease (see Figure 7–3 for trans women). Identify the sweet spot frequency and have the client take a breath and sustain that level. Guide the client to describe the difference in the sensation compared to their baseline voice. Repeat until production is consistent and expand from there.

You will have to guide the client to the target pitch and resonance by applying judgment, cueing the client to "Go up/down a little more" and asking, "Do you feel the buzzing sensation more there?" Gradually go to the level where there is ease and clarity. For trans women, resonance often just falls more forward when the pitch is appropriate. It can be quite dramatic. Once it appears that the first target has been identified, we check the pitch against our experience and judgment (not too high or low), normative data (toward the goal area), and that there is room for ease in upward intonation (Gelfer, 1999).

What Is the Final Frequency?

The final frequency target is set when your client is using the previously set level functionally with oral resonance and intonation in all communication contexts with good consistency, ease, and endurance. You will observe that your client walks in the clinic door using it functionally and there will be minimal tension in the larynx or associated structures. Do not

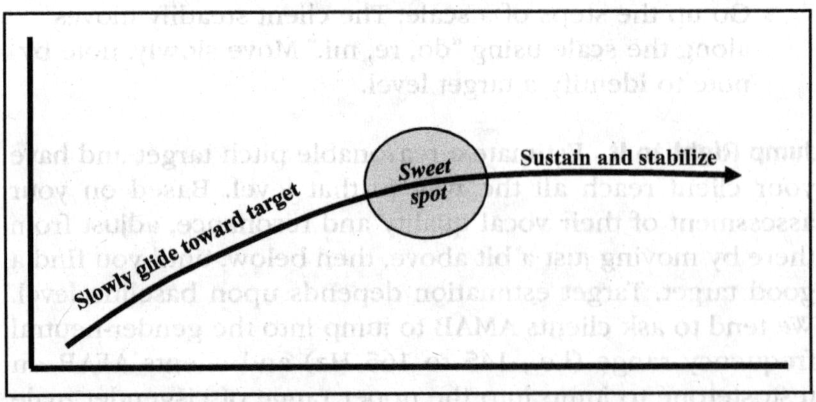

Figure 7–3. Pitch glide to sweet spot.

make a major adjustment in pitch from the initial target until oral resonance and intonation have been well established.

The time to stabilize the final F0 is determined by considering:

- normative data of cisgender males and females and research regarding levels of pitch and resonance influential to gender attribution (see Chapter 5),
- ease of intonation production with range for emotional expression (i.e., they aren't stuck in monotone F0),
- ease of healthy resonance at this level, and
- the client's comfort with this final level physically, mentally, and emotionally.

Option 2: Start with Oral Resonance

Some new clients have initial difficulty pitch matching or manipulating pitch skillfully, even with maximum cuing. To ease clients into these early sessions, it is helpful to establish the first target pitch level by focusing on oral resonance as the primary goal and pitch as the secondary goal. At this point, simply monitor pitch and focus on the resonance sensation. Most clients become more confident and skilled in directly monitoring their own pitch later in their program.

Shifting the shape of the vocal tract manipulates formant frequencies and changes the feel and sound of the voice. Perceptually, there is a distinction between the lower, heavier, darker sound of the male voice with the higher, smoother, lighter one more consistent with the perception of a female voice. In our experience, trans women will indirectly and spontaneously elevate their pitch to achieve forward focus.

As you guide them to explore sound in a variety of ways, aim for effortless, forward, clear, and pleasant productions. Direct the client to notice how and where they feel the sound, and how it sounds to them. Repeat each activity a few times until they are stable.

Resonance Cueing Options

The development of oral resonance can be challenging for clients. It can feel like they are grasping for an invisible target at first. In general, you will guide the client to feel a buzzing or vibration sensation in the mask of the face that may be perceived on the lips, palate, cheekbones, or eyes, or behind the nose, rather than in the throat. Several cueing options for this are described below. Using light contact on nasal consonants may help introduce oral resonance because of the strong sensation between the lips and front of the mouth during those sounds. Front vowels also facilitate forward placement. For clients who are not attuned to their body or physical sensations, using audio clips and demonstrating contrasting models can develop their skill and confidence with auditory discrimination.

Imagery

- "Place the sound in front of you/your mouth/your face."
- "Make the sound penetrate that wall in front of you."
- "Imagine your voice is on the outside of the body in front of you."
- "Put your voice up on the shelf in front of you."

Overshoot the Target

- "Feel the sound up here" (point between the eye brows, or the top of the head).
- "Feel it in your nose. Sound nasal. Now drop it to the roof of your mouth. Now your lips."

Client Flexibility. "Speak the tone":

- "Behind you and then in front of you."
- "Low in the body, and then high in the body"
- "With low energy and then high energy"
- "With a light voice and a heavy voice"
- "With tense lips and relaxed lips"
- "Louder and softer"
- "Stronger and weaker"

Descriptive Vocabulary. Ask clients how it feels to them. Use their vocabulary for effective productions. For example, one client felt like there was "a buzzing bee stuck in her head." Another client referred to the "pitch roll sensation" when trying to achieve oral resonance. A particularly creative client referred to the target resonance during volume glides as sounding like the close-up of the spaceship rushing by the screen in the *Star Wars* movie. She was able to use that as a cue for generalization to connected speech later in the session.

Avoid vocabulary that can be associated with effort, such as "Push it out here!"

Visual Representation. A visual representation of where to focus the resonance such as the one in Figure 7–4 has been very helpful to new clients. They often respond to an image like this with an understanding nod. The wave represents where to direct the sound within the boundaries of the front of the oral cavity.

Elicit Discovery of Resonance

Each of the following begins with a supportive and comfortable breath. Choose the technique that stimulates the best productions with the greatest ease. Explore several to find the best technique and starting level for your client.

Sustained Phonation. Guide the client to take a breath and sustain the word "mean" approximately 5 to 7 ST closer to the pitch target. Adjust up or down to get the best oral resonance. Pitch and volume remain the same throughout the 4- to 5-second production. The client is guided to feel the sensation

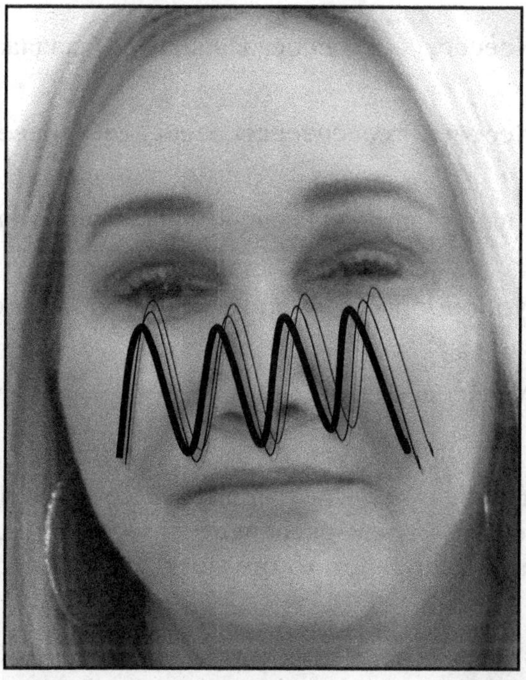

Figure 7–4. Oral resonance placement.

or oral resonance from the beginning to the middle to the end. The provider cues where appropriate for a forward production that has ease and clarity throughout. It should feel pleasant to the client. Try it first on the word "mean":

MMMMMMeeeeeeeeeeeeeeeeeeeeeeeeeaaaaaaaannnnnn
(mean)

Now have your client continue with the rest of the productions, slowly and consciously generalizing the forward placement for all of the following vowels and consonants in the word:

MMMMMMeeeeeeeeeeeeeeeeeeeeeeeeeeeeennnnnnnnn
(men)

MMMMMMaaaaaaaaaaaaaaaaaaaaaaaaaaaaaannnnnnnnn
(man)

MMMMMMoooooooooooooooooooaaaaaaaaaaaaaaaannnn
(moan)

MMMooooooooooooooooooooooooooooooooooooooonnnn
(moon)

and

NNNNNNeeeeeeeeeeeeeeeeeeaaaaaaaaaaaaaaaaaaaaaaaaarr
(near)

NNNNNNeeeeeeeeeeeeeeeeeeeeeeeeeeeeeeeeeeeeeeelll
(Nell)

NNNNNNaaaaaaaaaaaaaaaaaaaaaaaaaaaaaaaaaaaaannnn
(Nan)

NNNNNNoooooooooooooooooooooooooooooooooooooo
(no)

NNNNNNeeeeeeeeeeeeeeeeeeeeeeeeeeeeeeeeeewwwww
(new)

Experiment with other words loaded with nasal, liquid, and glide phonemes. Repeat each word several times, gradually reducing the prolongation to the standard production.

1. Mere
2. Meal
3. Kneel

4. Known
5. Real
6. Rear
7. Wren
8. Ran
9. Rut
10. Lean
11. Lear
12. Limb
13. Lamb
14. Loan
15. Loom

While sustained phonemes are often enough to stimulate the ideal target, some clients use unnecessary tension. Altering the pitch or volume in the production may boost the system just enough to place it and feel it more forward. The following two techniques can stimulate easy oral resonance in place of tension.

Volume Pulses. Repetitively and in a controlled manner, gently alter volume only. Pitch is static. The sound effect is similar to a buzzing bee. Gradually raising and lowering volume in a controlled and subtle manner will trigger the desired resonant quality. Increase volume only to the point of stimulating target oral resonance. Do not go louder. This exercise is depicted in Figure 7–5.

1. Begin softly on a sound, syllable, or one-syllable word such as /mi/ or /mu/.
2. Subtly increase and decrease volume in even pulses.
3. Maintain oral resonance throughout the production.
4. Pulse several times (usually 3 to 4 times) in one breath cycle.

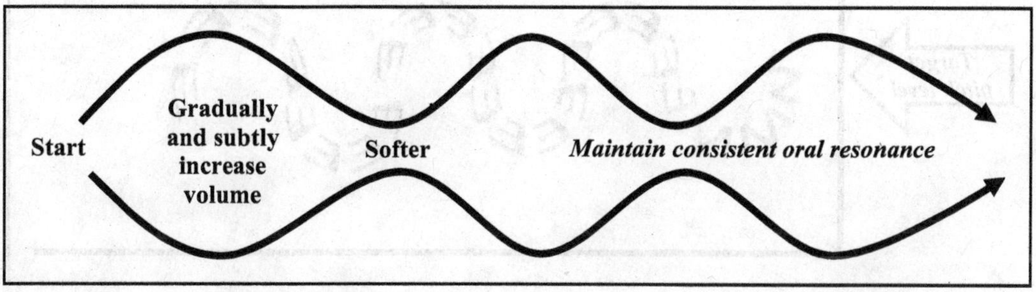

Figure 7–5. Volume pulses.

Pitch Rolls. For many clients, altering pitch by rolling it up and down with gradual shifts in pitch triggers oral resonance. Start at the target pitch and in a controlled manner repetitively alter pitch upward and downward in rolling "hills," maintaining a steady volume. Increase pitch to the point of stimulating target oral resonance, usually within 6 to 8 ST. The sound effect is similar to a police siren. Use vowels, syllables, or simple one-syllable words that stimulate the best resonance for your client. Encourage consistency throughout the entire production. This exercise is depicted in Figure 7–6.

1. Begin with sustained phonation to identify the starting pitch.
2. Gradually roll the pitch up and down in even hills.
3. Maintain oral resonance throughout the production.
4. Repeat a few times (usually 3 to 4 times) in one breath cycle.

Straw Phonation. Phonate into a drinking straw or other small tube to enhance and stabilize oral resonance (Titze, 2006). This increases air pressure above the vibrating vocal folds, maximizing the interaction between the vocal tract and vocal folds. Simply place a small straw between the lips and hold out a hum as you would with a kazoo. Use straw phonation with sustained phonation, volume glides, and pitch roles three to five times each, then remove the straw, guiding the client to duplicate the feeling of the resonance in the productions above.

Resonance will be used in connected speech, but for now you are looking for forward focus, vocal clarity, and ease while

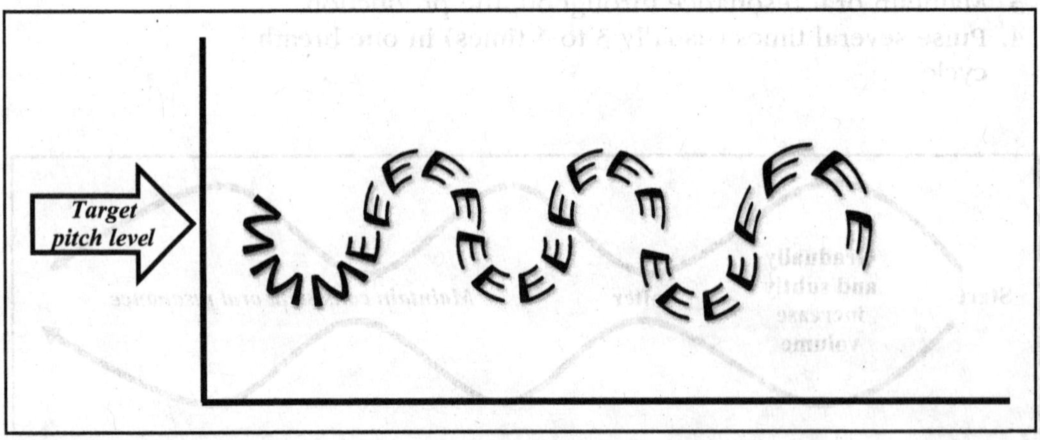

Figure 7–6. Pitch rolls.

monitoring and stabilizing the target pitch. In this new acquisition phase of voice modification, clients gradually increase reliance upon an inner model, reducing the need for your feedback and support. Their awareness and self-monitoring will increase with time and practice.

Integrate and Generalize

Whether you approach pitch or resonance first, stabilize the new level to help clients focus on function versus content as you integrate their pitch and resonance skills. Generalize by gradually increasing length and complexity of utterances.

If working toward feminine-sounding speech, instruct clients to apply a light contact to their consonants by transferring the lighter contact of voiceless stops and fricatives in the samples below to all consonants while maintaining forward placement of the vowels (Hirsch & Gelfer, 2012). This is especially helpful for trans females who have larger vocal tracts or whose consonant productions feel darker or heavier than desired.

1. Peach. Peach tea. Peach tea steeps.
2. Teeny. Teeny tiny. Teeny tiny feet.
3. Seek. Seek free. Seek free sweets.
4. Feed. Feed teens. Feed teens peaches.

Once stabilized, transfer the oral resonance and this lighter contact to longer utterances. Gradually broaden phonemic contexts. Proceed slowly and encourage feeling each production making sure the transitions from one word into the next is smooth. Try these examples:

1. Nearly. Nearly won. We nearly won. We nearly won more!
2. We know. We all know. We all know you. We all know your name.
3. Leave me. Leave me now. Leave me alone. Leave me alone now.
4. Will you? When will you? When will you know? When will you all know?
5. Mary won. Mary won nine. Mary won nine more. Mary won nine million more.
6. You were. You were married. Knew you were married. We knew you were married.
7. Morgan will. Morgan will need. Morgan will need more. Morgan will need more money.

8. Merrill wants. Merrill wants lean. Merrill wants lean meat. Merrill wants lean red meat.
9. Nancy wears. Nancy wears many. Nancy wears many hats. Nancy wears many more hats.
10. Where is he? Where is William? Where is William now? Where is William Moore now?

Then, apply new skill to these sentences:

1. Live a little!
2. Use your imagination.
3. Can you prove it to me?
4. Go ahead if you want to.
5. They finally got married.
6. You can't take it with you.
7. I feel like dancing tonight!
8. Use the power of persuasion.
9. Where would you like to go?
10. We all need some fun at times!

Beyond Pitch and Resonance

Once the target pitch and resonance has been successfully set, balanced, and briefly stabilized as an isolated skill in connected speech, we practice it with other communication skills, such as intonation modification.

The order in which you choose to address each goal is completely dependent on client potential and your clinical judgment. We want to foster as much of a positive experience as we can so that we can maintain newly developing skills with maximum success and minimal frustration. Blending both clinical and functional goals are extremely effective and provide some practical foundation for clients outside of the session.

PROSODY

Intonation

Intonation is very important in communication. As one component of prosody, it is more powerful than the words we use because it allows our emotions to be translated into vocal expression. The same words spoken in different situations with different attitudes or feelings may be used with a completely different intonation pattern. In the absence of body language and facial expression, shifts in pitch, rate, and other components contribute tremendously to the meaning of words.

To demonstrate how the rising point in intonation can change meaning, read the sentences below aloud elevating pitch for the emphasized word.

1. *I* am really happy!
2. I *am* really happy!
3. I am *really* happy!
4. I am really *happy*!

Aim and Purpose

As described in Chapter 5, clients with voice difficulties can benefit from intonation work to help reduce laryngeal tension, and improve laryngeal motion and vocal function. A natural and effective use of intonation is valuable in many contexts, though, so you may find that the client wants to work on intonation in their new pitch range for a variety of reasons that may not have to do with gender expression.

The benefit of intonation for our clients may be multidimensional. Intonation modification:

- assists to maintain or generate a more relaxed larynx, thereby enhancing functional ease and balance throughout the vocal change;
- creates a more affiliative and expressive communication style; and
- may contribute to how a person's gender is perceived.

It can be disconcerting for trans women to produce more variable intonation because it may sound and feel mechanical and fake. Discussing this ahead of time and being playful with it can be extremely helpful. With practice, the pattern will become more automatic and real. Remind clients that they have always expressed meaning and emotion through their voice, and that they will be using what feels right to them, as a foundation for building a new repertoire of melody patterns.

Equipment/Materials

- Audio recording device
- Illustrations
- Pitch monitoring tool

Use a monitoring method, whether it is objective or subjective. Encourage self-monitoring as early into the modification process as possible. We want clients to develop the ability to accurately self-monitor with regards to pitch (e.g., "I'm too low/on target/too high"), and intonation range (e.g., "I'm on target," "I'm not using enough range") both in and out of the session. Greater vocal awareness and confidence without assistance from a device or the provider will develop over time. The provider is always monitoring.

Measuring Intonation

Intonation Pattern. Patterns of pitch contours are often described and taught in accent modification training, a practice that has been suggested for working with trans people (Gelfer & Mordaunt, 2012). For example, a common pattern in standard American English is walk-jump-step-fall, as shown in Figure 7–7 (Edwards & Strattman, 1996).

In Figure 7–7, a sentence starts "walking" at approximately the speaking fundamental frequency (SFF) as a precursor to emphasis, "jumps" upward to the emphasized word, "steps" downward gradually in smaller increments, and then "falls" to below the SFF at the end of the utterance as a syntactic marker. The steps downward are important in that if they are too large, the speaker will run out of range. This requires awareness and control.

Appropriate pattern and range for each sentence will depend upon what the message is and how it is being communicated. For example, when a speaker has to emphasize a point with a higher frequency, such as in high animation, they

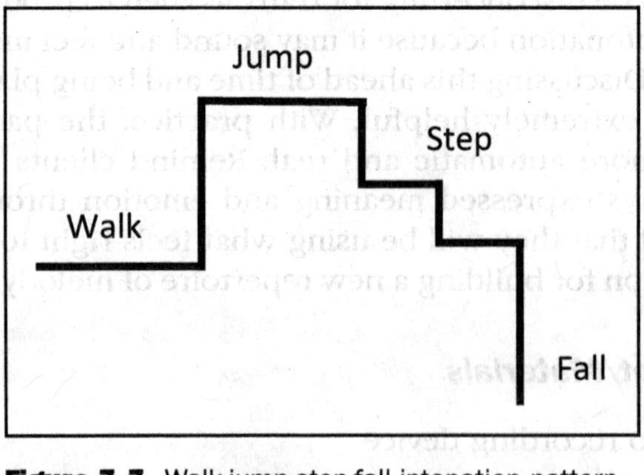

Figure 7–7. Walk-jump-step-fall intonation pattern.

may use broader intonation range and the SFF will elevate, which is why we have to be flexible with the original target frequency. The reverse is also true. If a speaker is relating information associated with a lower emphasis, such as feelings of concern, it can stimulate a lower pitch and narrower conversational range (Gelfer & Mordant, 2012). Another way to see it is that this would determine the approximate starting pitch prior to jumping, the height of the jump necessary to relate the message, and range and number of steps downward to complete the thought. There will necessarily be various cycles and ranges of consecutive patterns, but the core pattern will remain the same.

For most native speakers of standard American English, the rules are already in place. Native speakers already know what to stress and when to stress it depending upon the message intended. Our clients will adapt what they already know intrinsically while shaping it for authenticity. Trans people with foreign accents may target different patterns according to what is natural, and perhaps perceived as more feminine or masculine, in their language and culture.

Intonation Range. We can combine the above foundational intonation pattern with the target frequency range previously set to create a framework for setting an intonation range. This range must be flexible enough to accommodate a variety of communicative needs and true emotional expression. The intonation range can be trained and monitored objectively and subjectively.

The number of semitones above and below the speaking pitch is variable and dependent upon the message being relayed and the emotions involved—much more so than on the gender of the speaker. ST range appears to get smaller with more natural or higher level cognitive-linguistic contexts, so if we encourage trans women to use the wide ranges in conversation that are actually more common for reading contexts, we are probably contributing to the stereotype of women having "swoopy" intonation, as discussed in Chapter 4. Providers should set target SFF range according to speech context, and also consider emotional saliency. Here are some ranges reported by studies including trans speakers:

- Reading sentences: 12 ST (Gelfer & Schofield, 2000)
- Reading sentences: 6 to 12 ST (Fitzsimons, Sheahan, & Staunton, 2001)

- Picture description: 4 to 6 ST (Hancock, Colton, & Douglas, 2014)
- Conversation: 2 to 3 ST (Wolfe et al., 1990)

We typically set the range symmetrically around the SFF. For example, if the target frequency is 175 Hz for picture description, then we may aim for at least 2 ST above and below 175 Hz. Using an online semitone calculator (e.g., http://users.utu.fi/jyrtuoma/speech/semitone.html), it is easy to determine that the SFF should vary between 155 and 196 Hz. We can set the cursors on our recording software to these values and direct the client to play with their pitch variation so that their F0 trace reaches the top and bottom cursors.

Some clients will benefit from using a pitch app for objective feedback about their range. This monitoring is useful when applied strategically. Understandably, many trans people—and their providers!—can be overloaded with the visual tracking necessary with this method and lose connection to themselves during the process. This is particularly true when combining skills. Be flexible in how you approach monitoring pitch and intonation.

A simple subjective approach is the use of a rating scale, as introduced by Gelfer and Mordaunt (2012). Trans people can effectively use a scale, while the provider casually tracks the targets objectively, guiding the client as needed. Using a 1 to 5 scale like the one in Figure 7–8 allows the trans person and the provider to have the same frame of reference. If level 1 is monotone and inappropriate for communication (it may sound boring, lacking energy) and level 5 is excessive and also inappropriate (sounding dramatic, cartoonlike, or as if talking to an infant or puppy), then a level three is a good target. Provider models for each of the three levels are necessary. Use a sentence such as "I am really happy to see you" and contrast the levels by saying it at a level 1, 5, and then a 3.

Attaining Appropriate Intonation

Set the intonation range collaboratively once it is understood how the pattern they are learning relates to culturally appro-

1	2	3	4	5
(monotone)		(average)		(excessive)

Figure 7–8. Intonation rating scale.

priate standard intonation patterns and their previously set target pitch. Use illustrations, demonstrations, and models to help to make the target pitch and intonation pattern have meaning with regards to everyday voice use.

Intonation Cueing Options

Exaggerate. If intonation is consistently too restricted, overshooting it to a level 4 versus a level 3 can be helpful. The target can be dramatized further by using the level 5, then back off slowly for the desirable level.

Overlay Contrasting Emotions. Use emotion to stimulate more dynamic vocalizations for those who need greater inspiration. For contrast, try asking, "How would you say it if you just had a great day?" "How would you say it if you felt angry?" Surprised? Sad? Delighted? Scared? Note the difference. Select the target emotion where it is effective.

Use Personal Labels. Using client's descriptive language is more effective because it has more meaning and they remember the reference more consistently. A. X., who just began intonation modification, said that "The 1 (on the rating scale) sounds insincere, the 5 sounds ridiculous, but the level three sounds more real." We wrote her labels down for her future reference.

Technique for Intonation Modification. When the target pitch is achieved fairly independently, the exploration of more natural intonation can develop. See Box 7–4 for tips on addressing intonation.

With aligned posture, the client takes a moderate and comfortable breath. Starting at the target pitch, sustain a sound or syllable such as "mee" or "moo" while keeping the tone focus forward. Sustain for 3 to 4 seconds with oral resonance. Repeat approximately three times or until there is stability. Then begin to rock the voice upward and then downward, maintaining oral resonance. Move to single words and short phrases by starting with the word "up" while gliding upward and "down" while gliding downward. This exercise is depicted in Figure 7–9.

Based on the target speaking pitch and the intonation range you set objectively, using oral resonance, explore the edges of the intonation range. Always maintaining quality of voice, feel pitch movement during simple glides upward and downward. You are targeting clarity and ease throughout the intonation range. Gradually increase the range as appropriate toward the outer targets.

Box 7–4. Tips for Intonation

- Be a good model.
- A restricted total pitch range may impact initial success if not set precisely to client potential. If this is an issue:
  - □ start with a lower target frequency that allows the appropriate upward intonation range, or a higher frequency to allow for downward intonations, and
  - □ work to expand the usable frequency at the upper and lower ends of the client pitch range (such as using forward placement with pitch glides).
- Heighten client awareness early on if:
  - □ Lower intonation drops into glottal fry register.
  - □ Intonation is measured and artificially falling and lifting to the same level each time.
  - □ Melody pattern is too high above target. It will sound artificial. Some trans women may develop this pattern to hold their pitch up. If this habit goes on too long it can be difficult to break as clients may have adapted to the higher level and may perceive a more appropriate intonation range as "sounds male." Teach clients to surround their target frequency level, intending that their intonation will travel both above and below the target as is appropriate to the message.
- It is extremely important that clients feminizing their sound raise the pitch for intonation with the breath and the laryngeal elevators versus using compensatory facial tension, head lifting, and body tension. Investigate whether the target frequency originally set was too high making upcoming upward shifts difficult to reach. The frequency may need to be adjusted to allow for proper intonation patterns to occur.
- Discourage excessive volume during intonation modification. Because of the tensions and pressures needed for higher volumes, clients will not be able to maintain the vocal flexibility needed to produce needed intonational range.

In Figure 7–10, the dotted horizontal line represents the target SFF and the other lines represent a variety of intonation patterns. This visual may be helpful to show that frequency

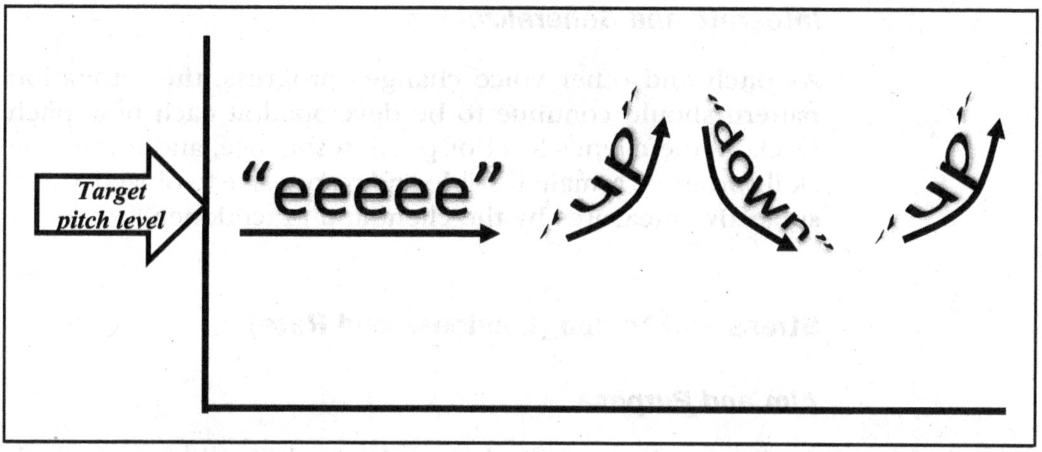

Figure 7–9. Rocking the pitch around the target.

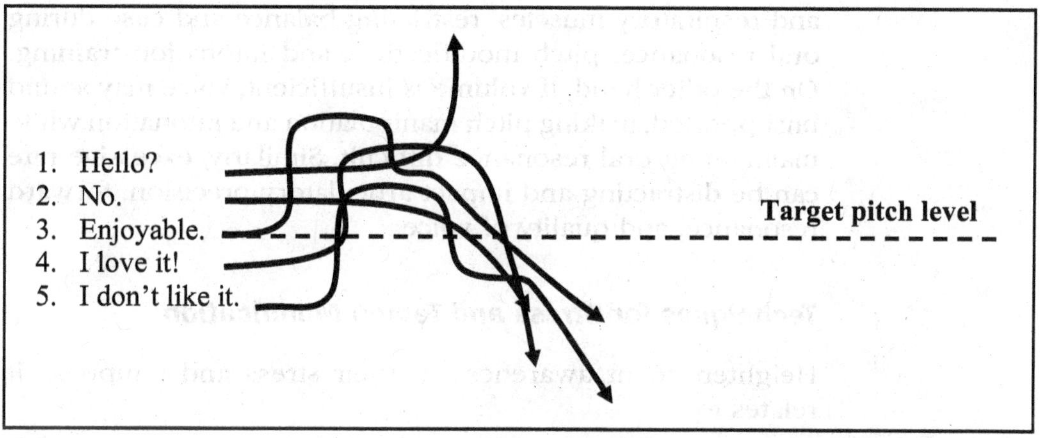

Figure 7–10. Variety of intonation patterns around the target.

may go above and below SFF depending upon the message. Some clients are resistant to go far from their target SFF, especially in the direction opposite of their ultimate goal. As with the other areas, progress up the cognitive-linguistic hierarchy as appropriate.

Whether intonation is going upward or downward, the goal is for all of it to be produced with oral resonance. There is a tendency for women to let a downward intonation bring a bright oral resonance down into a dark chest resonance. It is critical for them to maintain oral resonance across the entire sentence—it may be most challenging at the end of sentences when there is less breath to support the voice.

Integrate and Generalize

As pitch and other voice changes progress, the intonation pattern should continue to be developed at each new pitch level. As the client's level of pitch, resonance, and intonation skills progress remain flexible and responsive to objective and subjective measures by the client and practitioner.

Stress and Tempo (Loudness and Rate)

Aim and Purpose

As discussed in Chapter 5, there is not clear evidence that volume or rate plays a considerable role in gender attribution, but it could affect other speech characteristics that do. Excessive volume creates more pressure and tension in the laryngeal and respiratory muscles, restricting balance and ease during oral resonance, pitch modification, and intonation training. On the other hand, if volume is insufficient, voice may sound unsupported, making pitch manipulation and intonation while maintaining oral resonance difficult. Similarly, excessive rate can be distracting and impact articulatory precision, forward resonance, and quality of voice.

Techniques for Stress and Tempo Modification

Heighten client awareness of their stress and tempo as it relates to:

- gender presentation goals,
- vocal balance, and
- function in a variety of professional and social situations (e.g., intelligibility).

Engage in a discussion about loud talking or fast talking. Has it come up in their life in the past? Many clients are aware of being told in their past that they "are too loud" or "mumble." On occasion we have used a Sound Pressure Level meter or a recording as a feedback tool to help monitor increasing and decreasing levels. We set what subjectively feels like a good target range for that person and practice speaking there (see stimuli in Appendix 6–C).

Try a few exercises to improve the client's awareness of these behaviors, and how they change:

- Match the level of the provider's volume/rate to check in on themselves.
- Use a rating scale from 1 to 5. Model the three main levels: 1 (too soft), 3 (average), 5 (too loud). Discuss the difference and have the client demonstrate their production of each level in a short sentence such as "this is a level 1 (3/5) loudness level." Follow with progressive stimuli. You could do the same for excessive rate.
- Intonation training: Since intonation training has the effect of prolonging vowels for the rise and falls, it assists with slowing down articulation.
- Increasing articulation precision: Precise articulatory placement takes more time, and speech rate is automatically reduced.
- Learning phrasing, pausing between thoughts.

ARTICULATION

Articulation of a cisgender female is more precise and has a lighter contact than that of a cisgender male (see Chapter 5; Leung, Oates, & Chan, 2018). Lighter contact of consonants is also effective in creating a speech pattern associated with femininity in Western culture. Guiding clients to use a light touch may be helpful. As noted, targeting articulation may be a vehicle for change in areas known to contribute to gender attributions (see Box 7–5 for a case example of this).

If habitual final consonant distortions or deletions have been identified, articulatory precision may be enhanced by focusing on word closure. Word closure increases the consistency of the production of the final consonant in a word that would have otherwise been omitted. Focusing on the pattern of omission or distortion related to word (or syllable) endings can be highly effective. This also has the additional benefit of reducing speech rate to complete each word. Clients simply focus on finishing the word.

VOCAL QUALITY

Vocal Instability

Early in the process, it is natural for clients to feel as if they are walking a razor's edge when exploring different sounds while

Box 7–5. Case Example: Addressing Articulation

Robin, a 52-year-old architect, came for vocal feminization after she came out to her family. She had not transitioned at work and wanted to begin the process of vocal transition before she presented full time.

Evaluation revealed a low frequency when compared to cisgender male normative data and a heavy chest resonance. There was a significant under bite and difficulty approximating her lips without effort due to upper and lower misalignment of anterior teeth.

Diagnostic probes for oral resonance revealed difficulty achieving oral resonance in single words and short phrases. Articulation assessment revealed a general under articulation of consonants and groping for placement of some consonants on command. The client recalled she had speech therapy for l, r, w, and s sounds as a child and has been told in adulthood that she mumbles at times. She generally appeared to have low muscle tone.

Training of oral resonance was only possible with light articulatory precision of lingual and bilabial sounds. The slower speech and articulatory placement enhanced oral resonance and she began to sound more feminine. While this was a long training process for this client, it was necessary and rewarding in the end for both the client and the provider.

they are developing laryngeal and respiratory coordination and control. This is especially true for people taking testosterone who experience vocal fold changes that contribute to dysphonia and vocal instability. It is important to improve vocal quality and balance and to eliminate the chance of progressive vocal strain. Before direct vocal masculinization training with pitch and resonance work, guide clients to reduce excessive bodily tension that can contribute to laryngeal tension, as well as effort and tension of the larynx.

Begin with postural alignment, general relaxation, shoulder, neck, laryngeal, and lingual release to open up the vocal tract and release any tension prior to voice work. Diaphragmatic breathing is essential to support phonation at this lower pitch level and to keep tension out of the larynx.

Address vocal quality issues with techniques to reduce tension, roughness, harshness, and laryngeal effort. This may include easy onset and air flow techniques, and approaches to enhance laryngeal balance. Some clients have restricted pitch range, requiring the expansion of usable range with pitch glides. Once balance and ease are achieved, clients can shift with greater stability and maintain more efficient vocal function.

Excessive Breathiness

Occasionally clients AMAB wanting to sound feminine arrive with excessively breathy vocal quality. Further probing indicates they were influenced by advice from the internet on feminization of the voice. When breathiness is overdone it can have the effect of decreasing feminizing vocal features such as oral resonance, intonation, and emotional expression, and can eliminate carrying power and vocal flexibility. It can actually draw more unwanted attention from listeners. To enhance vocal balance and reduce breathiness, use techniques to reduce muscle tension and increase oral resonance.

VEGETATIVE FUNCTIONS

Some clients who are stable using their desired voice often throat clear, cough, and laugh spontaneously in the new level. When they cough at their desired level without thinking about it, they are often surprised. With all the work to bring the authentic voice into reality, something that comes easily can be a gift for them. However, it does not come easily to all; clients AMAB tend to struggle and begin to fear these potential voice betrayals. Below are some approaches to coughing, laughing, throat clearing, and sneezing in a sound consistent with intentional speech.

Throat Clearing

It is easier to start with throat clearing and progress into the cough because throat clearing has more control and there is a greater sense of success right at the start of this process. With lips together, say "hmmm" at target pitch with oral resonance. Gently produce the throat clear to avoid vocal trauma, and follow with another "hmmm." Put it all together to sound like: "Hmmm (clear) mmmmm." Try three in a row very gently. When there is some sense of stability, have the client gently and lightly go right into the "clear-clear-clear" thinking of forward focus and maintaining the target levels.

Cough

Extend the throat clear technique into a cough thinking "light and high." Repeat "mmm" three times with the lips together, as if tapping the back of the throat with the larynx. Generalize to an open-mouthed cough that is approximates a forward, light sound at the target level. It is the same tapping sensation, but with a "eh-heh eh-heh eh-heh." It may help to mix the two: "mmm mmm eh-heh eh-heh." Aim for a "tap" or "pop," but avoid a growl or grumble.

Do not encourage daily practice of the throat clear or the cough because of the obvious risk of vocal trauma. Rather, encourage coughs and clears as if acting or playing with it and only occasionally—two or three times each week.

Sneeze

Trans women are vulnerable to unwanted exposure of a deep-sounding voice during a sneeze. It is difficult to control, and at times they may not be able to; however, when they practice it, there is more of a sense of control and comfort within most clients. They must learn to be okay with the fact that while this is not always within their control, we do have some techniques to help them in the moment.

Consider the sneeze as three syllables: "me-yeah-choo." Start with the prolonged "mmmeee" to set the tone forward and as close as possible to the target pitch. Stretch out the second syllable, "yeah." in an upward pitch glide and let the last "choo" out in a falsetto range. The final "oo" may drift further up or back down in pitch—experiment to determine what sounds and feels more natural for the client.

Laugh

The laugh can be a lot of fun to work with for both the client and provider. How does your client usually laugh? Using their typical phonemic structure, build your practice around that. For example, one client's laugh is mainly a "hahaha" (versus "hehehe"). Since this requires an open vocal tract, we have to shape it to bring it more forward—similar to our resonance therapy approach.

- While faking a laugh, say "hmmhmmhmmhmm" at the target pitch or slightly above with closed lips and oral resonance.
- For the "hehehe" laugh:
  - ☐ Expand the "hmm" into "hmmmeeheeheehee," reminding them to feel that forward placement to enhance the higher formants.
  - ☐ Then shape into "hehehehe," feeling it forward in the vocal tract. Take a new breath and repeat.
- For the "hahaha" laugh:
  - ☐ Expand the "hmm" into "hmmmaahaahaahaa" with the flatter lips so it is really forward.
  - ☐ Finally, shape into the "hahahaha" again with forward focus at the target pitch. Breathe in and repeat "hahahaha"

This approach can be applied to any phonemic combination that is consistent with the original laugh, as long as the focus that approximates their target pitch with forward focus. Practice making any laugh as "real" as possible by prompting it with a joke, silly quote, or story.

BODY LANGUAGE, FACIAL EXPRESSION, LANGUAGE, AND CONVERSATIONAL STYLE

Some trans women are very aware of the tendency to control their environment with the use of their voice and the communicative style. Clients AMAB have reported imitating styles of male role models that did not come naturally to them to fit into society, and they are aware of the need to return to the patterns that they were innately more comfortable with earlier in their life. This does not appear to be the case for all clients, however. Other clients report being comfortable with their current verbal and nonverbal communication style. It is up to the trans person and provider to decide the needs of the speaker.

We begin by discussing and modeling a variety of communication styles considered masculine and feminine. We also discuss the additional factors of communication purpose, communication partner, and local culture that may influence the stereotypes. Several examples are presented to expose clients to a variety of verbal and nonverbal presentations.

Clients share their personal needs and desires based on this information. Those who are interested in pursuing more information and/or training work will watch a video of themselves during the conversational portion for more objective self-analysis. They are then asked to collect videos online of speakers whose communication style represents their inner self with greater alignment than their current communicative pattern. Sometimes this process leads to a client no longer being interested in habituating a particular pattern, other times the client becomes more confident about what and how to change.

CONCLUSION

Ultimately the direct voice approach, order of presentation, and specific techniques used are selected based on the talents, skills, experience, and intuition of the clinician as well as the ease, effectiveness, and individual needs and desires of the client. Therefore, each case will be approached differently. One of our graduate students was observing a session and turned in surprise to us and said, "It is amazing how different each one of our sessions look even though many clients have similar needs and goals!"

REFERENCES

Behrman, A. (2007). *Speech and voice science*. San Diego, CA: Plural Publishing.

Carew, L., Dacakis, G., & Oates, J. (2007). The effectiveness of oral resonance therapy on the perception of femininity of voice in male-to-female transsexuals. *Journal of Voice*, *21*(5), 591–603.

Edwards, H. T., & Strattman, K. H. (1996). *Accent modification manual*. San Diego, CA: Singular Publishing.

Fitzsimons, M., Sheahan, N., & Staunton, H. (2001). Gender and the integration of acoustic dimensions of prosody: Implications for clinical studies. *Brain and Language*, *78*(1), 94–108.

Gelfer, M. P. (1999). Voice treatment for the male-to-female transgendered client. *American Journal of Speech-Language Pathology*, *8*, 201–208.

Gelfer, M., & Schofield, K. J. (2000). Comparison of acoustic and perceptual measures of voice in male-to-female transsexuals perceived as female versus those perceived as male. *Journal of Voice*, *14*(1), 22–33.

Gelfer, M. P., & Mordaunt, M. (2012). Pitch and intonation. In R. Alder, S. Hirsch, & M. Mordaunt (Eds.), *Voice and communication therapy for the transgender/transsexual client: A comprehensive clinical guide* (pp. 187–224). San Diego, CA: Plural Publishing.

Hancock, A. B., Colton, L., & Douglas, F. (2014). Intonation and gender perception: Applications for transgender speakers. *Journal of Voice, 28*(2), 203–209.

Hirsh, S., & Gelfer, M. P. (2012). Resonance. In R. Alder, S. Hirsch, & M. Mordaunt (Eds.) *Voice and communication therapy for the transgender/transsexual client: A comprehensive clinical guide* (pp. 225–248). San Diego, CA: Plural Publishing.

Leung, Y., Oates, J., & Chan, S. P. (2018). Voice, articulation, and prosody contribute to listener perceptions of speaker gender: A systematic review and meta-analysis. *Journal of Speech, Language, and Hearing Research, 61*(2), 266–297.

Titze, I. R. (2006). Voice training and therapy with a semi-occluded vocal tract: Rationale and scientific underpinnings. *Journal of Speech, Language, and Hearing Research, 49*, 448–459.

Van Leer, E., Hapner, E. R., & Connor, N. P. (2008). Transtheoretical model of health behavior change applied to voice therapy. *Journal of Voice, 22*(6), 688–698.

Verdolini, K. (2000). Resonant voice therapy. In J. C. Stemple (Ed.), *Voice therapy: Clinical studies* (pp. 46–61). San Diego, CA: Singular Publishing.

Wolfe, V. I., Ratusink, D. L., Smith, F. H., & Northrop, G. E. (1990). Intonation and fundamental frequency in male-to-female transsexuals. *Journal of Speech, Language and Hearing Disorders, 55*, 43–50.

PART III

Finish Strong

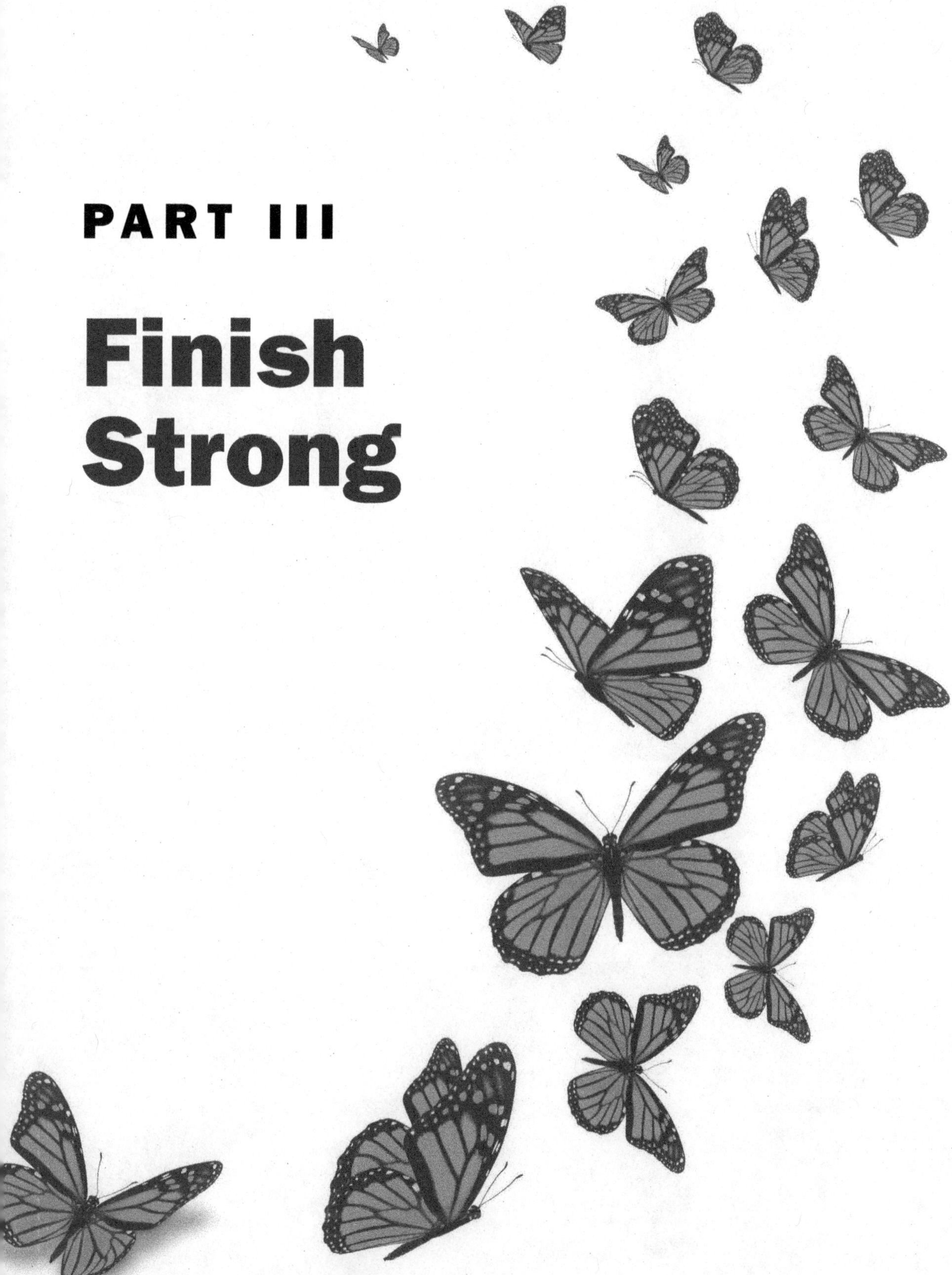

CHAPTER 8

Facilitating Progress

"So many things in my life have come easily to me, yet almost nothing about this process has!"
—Trans woman reflecting on her voice transformation process

Even in the best of circumstances, there will be times when clients plateau in their progress. Often these clients still appear motivated, attend all appointments, and deeply appreciate their provider's guidance. We may do everything "right," such as provide appropriate support, education, and direct training with creative and innovative home programs that fit the client's needs, and still progress seems slowed or even halts completely. Some clients may appear to be doing well in sessions but are not transferring skills functionally in daily life. Others may not seem to be responding as expected in the clinical situation beyond the occasional ups and downs that all clients experience. Still others appear to have limitations within a particular training area that could not be anticipated.

This can be confusing for the provider and possibly even the client. At times, clients are quite surprised when they realize through the tactful feedback of their provider that there has been a lack of growth.

The purpose of this chapter is to provide a framework for understanding and addressing these troubling instances. While the situations that arise are always unique and nuanced, understanding how humans approach change and how providers can facilitate the client's change will guide competent and compassionate care. Some of the more common obstacles experienced with gender-diverse clients are described with the authors' response. These responses are by no means prescriptive; on the contrary, a client-centered approach will include a highly individualized response based on your ethical expert intuition. We offer these cases as much for illustrative purposes as to prompt you to prepare for the times that finishing strong is in doubt.

TRANSTHEORETICAL MODEL OF HEALTH BEHAVIOR CHANGE

What contributes to successful behavior change? Why do some people practice regularly and persevere while others do not? This has been studied extensively, particularly in the area of health behaviors such as exercise, smoking cessation, and prevention of HIV and cancers (Bridle et al., 2005; Hutchison, Breckon, & Johnston, 2009). The Transtheoretical Model (TTM) of health behavior change provides a framework for understanding change and how it can be fostered. There are a variety of strategies that people use, and can be taught to use, that increase the likelihood they will progress toward their goal of change.

The TTM recognizes that change happens in stages (Procheska & Norcross, 2001; Zimmerman, Olsen, & Bosworth, 2000). The first is the *precontemplation phase*, in which the client has no intention of taking action. The second phase is the *contemplation phase*, in which clients become aware of the possibility of the need to change. They may weigh the potential costs and benefits of modifying their voice but are still generally ambivalent about it. When they begin taking baby steps toward change (e.g., doing research and gathering information to narrow down options) and commit to change, they are in the *preparation phase*. Not only is the client intending to make a change, they may also have tried some self-training over the Internet and inquired with friends and other providers about voice and communication services.

In the *action phase*, clients participate in regular sessions for voice training, follow through with their home program, and continually demonstrate regular growth. In this stage, change is still fragile, as the client is still reliant on the practitioner for feedback and encouragement so as to avoid returning to a previous stage.

The last phase is the *maintenance phase*, in which clients take responsibility for keeping up their new skills outside of the session. They are aware of the need to maintain their target pitch and oral resonance, release laryngeal tension if needed, and reset alignment and breathing as necessary.

The TTM tasks the practitioner to assess the client's readiness for change (i.e., identify which stage they are in). The client's readiness for change will escalate with the increase of two parameters: perceived importance of the change and their self-efficacy (Van Leer, Hapner, & Connor, 2008). Self-efficacy is the belief that they can make the change.

The practitioner then selects from a variety of psychologically based approaches to facilitate the behavior change required to achieve the goals. A strategy-stage mismatch will foster the client's ambivalence and likely lead to failure and dropping out. If the client is in the preaction stage, the practitioner should prioritize raising their awareness of the importance of change for them before starting direct voice techniques. On the other hand, when the client is ready and in an action stage, the provider can focus on practical strategies to adopt and habituate behavior change.

In an article applying the TTM to voice disorders, Van Leer, Hapner, and Connor (2008) provide 10 strategies to facilitate change or advance to the action and maintenance stages. These are listed in Table 8–1, alongside examples for application in the area of gender-expression instead. Notice they all are strategies the practitioner may introduce or explain, but ultimately the client is the one to do it.

MOTIVATIONAL INTERVIEWING

Motivational interviewing (MI) is a client-centered approach for increasing a client's motivation toward change. We as the

Table 8–1. Change Processes and Facilitating Strategies

Processes for Change	Facilitating Strategy	Example
	Preaction Stages	
Consciousness Raising	Education and awareness of unhealthy behavior	Learning about the limitations of speaking only in falsetto register
Social Liberation	Social norms support this change	Companies are increasingly including these services in health plan coverage.
Emotional Arousal	Experiencing negative emotions from the old behavior	Voice can trigger gender dysphoria.
Self Re-evaluation	Assess change in relationship to values and identity	Realizing that one does not want to continue to sound a certain way
Commitment	Set a firm goal	Email a practitioner for information.
	Action and Maintenance Stages	
Counterconditioning	Find substitute behavior	Hard swallow instead of throat clearing
Stimulus Control	Remove reminders of old behavior	Practice voice when visual presentation is consistent (i.e., hair, clothing).
Contingency Management	Reward positive behavior	Get dessert if resonance was maintained during the entire meal!
Helping Relationships	Seeking and using social support	Joining a local support group or online chat
Environmental Re-evaluation	Realize negative effect of behavior on social environment	Notice whether responses from others are influenced, and whether that is troubling

providers do not specifically encourage the client to change behaviorally but instead take an active role in helping them formulate their own reasons for change, creating movement toward behavioral change. During the motivational interviewing process, patients verbalize their own arguments for change and identify a plan of action. Clients who do this may have greater adherence to behavioral change than those who do not make such statements.

In her article, *Facilitating Behavioral Change in Voice Therapy: The Relevance of Motivational Interviewing*, Behrman (2006) discusses four assumptions that are foundational MI. First, motivation reflects readiness of the client to move forward. Readiness, however, is a dynamic state that changes with time. Second, client readiness for change is vulnerable to provider influence and is dependent on interaction style. Third, readiness to change is related to a state of ambivalence, an internal struggle about behavioral change. Finally, because every patient has the potential for behavioral change, it is the provider's task to release their potential and facilitate the process for change that is inherent in each client. All are directly applicable for working with transgender and gender diverse people through vocal transformation.

To help ambivalent clients make changes in their behavior, there are four general principles:

1. Express empathy: By relating an understanding of the client's communication using reflective listening we are demonstrating empathy. This may take the form of a statement such as, "I sense that you want to feel better in your alignment with your voice" or "It is clear that you work really hard in your awareness of your voice in the world."
2. Develop discrepancy: We help by also making the client aware of the discrepancy between the client's stated principles, values, and goals and the demonstrated vocal behavior, carryover habits, and practice. Once awareness of the inconsistency is illuminated, there is evidence that it engages the client toward greater commitment and implementation of necessary actions.
3. Support self-efficacy: Self-efficacy refers to the client's belief that change is possible, and they can have the confidence in themselves that they can do it. The provider guides the client to recall the positive changes they had made in the past to realize the power of their responsibility for all current and future acts toward change.

4. Roll with resistance: Resistance is a normal part of change, and by accepting it as a part of change, providers can guide clients to view it with introspection and insight rather than with negative emotions such as anger and fear. This opens up the possibility for the client to become the source of the solution.

Guiding the client throughout this process to construct their own case for change, we can address these principles with communicative strategies that support a client-directed focus. Most of what follows is utilized throughout training as appropriate and as an organic result of developing rapport and trust throughout the process. It is a way to maintain client engagement in their heightening identification of indecision and uncertainty within the process and taking ownership to move forward.

Specific techniques used in MI include:

1. Ask open ended questions (e.g., "Tell me about . . . ," "What do you think about . . . ?," "I wonder what . . . ") to encourage increased deliberation, enable an open dialog, and facilitate clinical rapport building. The new knowledge that is uncovered about the client may serve as an opening for discussion to gain a better understanding of their thoughts, feelings, and beliefs.
2. Affirm intentions and efforts expressed to make change. This act communicates appreciation and understanding to the client (e.g., "You really show determination in your thinking out this," "I hear that you're working hard," and "It's clear that you want to feel better").
3. Reflect the client's message in a statement echoing the client's meaning to show an understanding of the client experience. It builds the connection and helps to reduce ambivalence (e.g., "You feel that your voice is too low but doesn't affect your life," "I can see why you may be conflicted at home with your new voice," "But that makes you feel uncomfortable").
4. Summarize client statements that support a desire to make change and continue the momentum in the dialog toward growth while transitioning the discussion to a new focus. Summaries can help move toward change by exposing the discrepancies of the client. There are three forms of summaries. *Collecting* summaries are multiple statements elicited from the client supporting

their desire for change. *Linking* summaries connect past discussions with current ones summarizing a theme, supporting a discrepancy or line of reasoning assisting in the resolution of ambivalence. *Transitional* summaries are applied to shift focus and are often used to transition or close a session integrating all that has taken place throughout the session.

If the previous components of the session are working well, the client will use "change talk." Change talk involves creating a plan of action that will occur. Again, the act is completed by the client rather than the provider. When clients verbalize and create their own action steps, they are more likely to adhere to the plan than when they do not. The client will make clear statements about change and the benefits of these changes.

Change talk is divided into two categories. The first is *preparatory*, including desire for change, acknowledgment of their ability to change, reason for the change, and the need for the change. Preparatory change talk is an encouraging sign that real change is on the horizon. Even more encouraging is the second type of change talk: *implementing*. This includes statements of commitment to change, activation of preparedness and willingness, and taking steps to create the change.

The following conversation will illustrate how a provider can use MI with a client reluctant to practice with people outside of the session. T. H., a 39-year-old trans woman has been in training for 13 weeks developing her feminine voice. She is a physician and is presenting full time as a woman. She emphatically reports that she is motivated and wants this voice transition to take place, but she cannot make herself practice in safe communication contexts she has identified or in structured practice where she can focus.

T. H. knows she needs to, wants to, and fully intends to practice her home program as agreed upon at the end of each session. But once she is alone during the week, her resolve weakens, and she returns to the sessions hoping that maybe "pressure practicing" (what she calls practicing on the way to the session) in the car would be enough and that we would find that her status improved. Of course, it has not. She hasn't been able to explain her inability to practice the vocal skill that she wants so badly wants to adopt in daily life as her own. The source of such behavioral issues can run deep for some clients and may take a great deal of time to work through completely. This is not the case for all clients, however. Below is a conversation between T. H. and her provider, and examples of how to respond:

Provider: Do you have any insights as to what may be going on for you with this?

T. H.: [thoughtfully hesitating] Well . . . I am really good at what I do. I have always been successful at everything I have set out to do. Everything. I know that sounds obnoxious, but it is true.

Provider: You really sound confident as you talk about your successes . . . tell me more about this. **(Express empathy, ask open-ended questions)**

T. H.: Since I was a child, anything I thought would be challenging for me I simply would not even try to do. Therefore, everything I did do, I was very, very good at. I'm very good at my work, I am excellent at golf, and I am a championship chess player. I am very, very good at everything that I do. Even as a medical student, I rarely had to study, ever! And I always got "A"s.

That is why this [voice training] is so difficult. I have to face that I am challenged to do it! I am challenged to hear the differences in oral resonance. I am challenged to confront the fact that I have to spend more time than I ever have in learning to do something new. I can't avoid doing this. I have to be successful, yet this is so very difficult for me to do.

Provider: I wonder how you learned to only pursue things that you knew you would be successful with, that came easily. **(Roll with resistance)**

T. H.: I think it's because I grew up being trans. Everyday life was so difficult. For me it was survival. It took one element of challenge out of my life by avoiding things that I knew would require a great deal of strain on my part. I could not deal with the possibility that I may not do well with it.

Provider: I hear that that must have been really difficult, yet . . . am I sensing some real determination here to work through this? **(Develop discrepancy)**

T. H.: I know that I have no choice here, this is something that I have to do. I have to figure this out.

Provider: You and I have spoken a few times about what you called a "higher point of view." If there was a higher reason that you are confronted with this, what do you think that would be? **(Reflect, ask open-ended questions)**

T. H.: It is making me do something that I would never voluntarily face. It is making me have to confront the pain that this may not be easy for me, and I may not be perfect at it, and can I live with that? But the pain of not developing this new voice is stronger than the pain to accept another challenge in my life beyond the day-to-day living.

[Long pause] But I do see that I can't spend the rest of my life avoiding pain. But that is another thing that I'm very, very good at . . . putting things off for as long as possible.

Provider: It sounds like you are saying that it has felt helpful to avoid scary situations in the past, yet at the same time you are realizing that it may be holding you back in areas where you want to grow in the present. **(Develop discrepancy)**

T. H.: I guess . . . yeah . . . probably in a lot of areas.... but it is very hard for me to want to change this point of view. This is how I thought my whole life. It is very safe.

Provider: Yes, I can see how that would make you feel safer, and how you may feel that it is challenging to change. Is there anything you have in mind as a starting point? **(Express empathy, transitional summary, ask open-ended questions)**

T. H.: I guess I am starting to see that the jig is up. It is time to face the demons. I think I can do it, it is just that I don't really want to face it.

Provider: You seem really determined. You use the words 'I think I can do it' and I wonder—are there any . . . I'm not sure of the right word, shall we call them *small triumphs* that you can recall from the session that comes to mind at this point? Something that reminds you that 'you *can* do it' like you said. **(Support self-efficacy)**

T. H.: So I try to remind myself that if I can make my body do what it needs to do one time to use oral resonance, then I have the skill to do it, right? When I play golf and

I hit the ball just right, I know the path that the ball will take. All of my skills need to be basically in sync to trust the path that it will take. I keep telling myself that there is no difference with my voice. I have to learn it the same way. I tell myself, 'The only thing that stands between you and consistency is just creating the memory and the muscle memory to do it over and over and over again.' I've got enough glimpses here in the session with you to be confident that my physical being is capable of making the sounds. But I lose confidence when I'm at home practicing. I'm saying to myself, "Is that good? Is that the one I need to repeat again? It doesn't feel right . . . I don't think . . . does it? Is it really that different from the one that came before?" This is what makes it hard for me.

Provider: You seem to have a healthy inner voice telling you that if you can create the target voice one time, that means that you have the skill to do it all the time, is that correct? **(Reflect)**

T. H.: Yes, I know it is there but the truth is that I am terrified . . . I can't face not being able to do it . . . even though I just said that I know that I can. I need to change something . . . I need help.

Provider: You're sharing a new awareness: that fear can prevent you from moving forward and that you need to make a change to get help. **(Collecting summary)**

T. H.: I need to change something. I need help.

Provider: Yes, I hear that you need help to make a change. Do you mean additional external support to help you explore this new awareness? **(Affirm intentions and efforts)**

T. H.: Maybe through Katie? [Her therapist] I don't usually talk to her about this stuff, but maybe I should.

Provider: Oh, well that sounds like a really good start. How does it make you feel when you think about asking Katie about this? **(Affirm intentions and efforts, ask open-ended questions)**

T. H.: I'm just starting to see that this may be possible. I never thought about it this way before. It'll probably take me less time in the long run if I can figure out how to approach this without being so terrified.

Provider: It sounds like you are really thinking this through . . . first realizing that you have an old pattern that has been an old friend to you and made you feel safe as you went through your life. Then sharing that you are starting to see that it is preventing you from moving on with your voice work . . . and finally you are preparing to get yourself the support that you need to move forward. **(Linking summary)**

It is also clear that you see that you can develop this new voice . . . that you can learn it the same way you learned golf . . . and that you are confident that your physical being is capable of creating your new voice. What feels like a good first step to you? **(Support self-efficacy)**

T. H.: I want to give Katie a call and see if she can see me next week. I would feel more confident with her on my team. If she can help me work this through, it will be a big thing off my mind. Can I give you a call once I talk to her to discuss how we should move forward from there?

Provider: Of course!

T. H. left the session with a sense of resolve. After talking to her therapist, she arranged a leave from voice work to explore issues interfering with her progress. After 11 weeks she returned to resume voice training with greater ease and success. Taking her lead in the process, the provider slowly approached home program success by having T. H. journal appreciation of the small successes in vocal modification week to week and documenting experiences of self-compassion and unconditional acceptance, all of which was with coordinated support of her therapist.

T. H. is a good example of how a lack of self-efficacy, or belief that they are capable of this success, can prevent change. With the provider's motivational interviewing, T. H. came to see change as possible, and even committed a small step toward an action plan. Van Leer, Hapner, and Conner (2008) summarize four sources of self-efficacy that we can cultivate for our clients:

1. Mastery: Success early and often will build confidence, so set achievable goals. Break goals into smaller steps if the client continues to fail.
2. Vicarious experience: It would seem that no amount of theory or data is as convincing as seeing someone

do it, especially if you can relate to that someone. Connecting advanced clients to new ones, in group sessions or for a phone call or even a video recording (with permission!), boosts clients' self-efficacy like a cisgender person just can't.

3. Verbal persuasion: The good news is that encouragement builds self-efficacy. The bad news is that discouragement can crush it. Choose your words carefully.
4. Physiological and psychological state: Feeling uncomfortable, as T. H. did when she tried to practice at home, can decrease self-efficacy.

T. H. eventually accepted that her fear and anxiety was a normal part of being human and that as she denied herself this aspect of humanness it simply intensified. *Permission to be human* is the active acceptance of negative emotions. With professional help and some time, she learned that she was going to have painful emotions, but she had a choice as to how to experience them. She could stuff them down as if there was something wrong with them or she could choose to them flow out of her and dissipate, thereby allowing her, in time, to have room to experience more positive emotions. T. H. learned to have courage. Courage is not about not having fear. Courage is about feeling the fear and proceeding anyway.

Permission to be human is a principle introduced by the field of positive psychology and integrated into this client's vocal feminization program to ease her approach with herself. The following section considers what positive psychology can offer for facilitating transformation progress.

POSITIVE PSYCHOLOGY

Since World War II, psychology primarily has focused on disorder and disease, which is about what was lacking and what was wrong. What about studying those who were functioning well in life? Goodness and excellence are also states of being that can be studied and taught to others who need and desire it. What can psychology learn from them and perhaps integrate with traditional approaches to support well-being?

In 1998, Martin Seligman, president of the American Psychological Association, initiated a new emphasis in the field of psychology, referred to as positive psychology. The goal of positive psychology is to increase the process of positive growth or what he calls flourishing. Ben-Shahar (2009, 2017) defines it as the overall experience of pleasure and meaning. It is not just about a single moment but an overall state in which a person can endure emotional pain at times and still be happy overall. It is linked to having strong social connections and contributing to something bigger than yourself: the greater good.

Positive psychology focuses on what can create well-being by studying topics such as optimism, life satisfaction, gratitude, compassion, self-esteem, self-confidence, and hope.

Below are a few principles that may prove helpful with our transgender clients. They have to do with mind sets, emotions, and the decision to choose joy.

Perfectionist Versus Optimalist Mindset

How clients approach voice goals can be as important as the voice skills themselves. They can approach the development of their new voice from the point of view of the perfectionist or the optimalist. Perfectionists are often seen as people who set unrealistically high goals and expectations for themselves and then measure their self-worth against their perception of achievement, productivity, and accomplishment. They have difficulty coping when the goals set have not been accomplished (Parker & Adkins, 1995). Perfectionists are failure oriented. The focus is on what they are doing wrong, without recognition of what is going well. At all costs, tasks are approached by rejecting the possibility of making a mistake and facing inadequacies. Because it is impossible to achieve, there is a negative effect on self-esteem. Perfectionists approach tasks with tension and anxiety as they hold themselves to unreasonably high standards and may be discouraged from being engaged in future activities where there is risk of failure. They are therefore more rigid, defensive, and self-critical in their approach. The journey for them has only one direction, straight up to the destination; deviations in the learning process are not an option, from their point of view. This is of course a very difficult way to approach life (Ben-Shahar, 2009, 2017).

The optimalist is more adaptive. They don't like to fail either, but instead of rejecting the possibility of failing they include it as a part of life. They can accept failure as a learning experience rather than a cause to give up on the prospect of future successes. Optimalists tend to be more successful than perfectionists because they are more willing to take risks and less likely to shrink back from failure. Optimalists focus not only on the destination, but also on the process. Their journey will therefore be perceived not as a straight line as with the perfectionist, but something resembling more of an irregular upward spiral toward their desired destination. Their approach is not all or nothing, it is more nuanced. They can therefore be more flexible, self-forgiving, and open to external feedback. The root of optimalist is derived from the Latin *optimus*, which means *best*, versus perfect. What is the best for one may not the best for another (Ben-Shahar, 2009, 2017).

We can help clients at the start of training by explaining that vocal transition is a process, and as such, there will be many twists and turns, ups and downs, and variability from session to session. Ability to embrace a realistic approach to any voice goal is not only healthy, but also enhances the chance for greater success. As practice opportunities increase, both the good and not-so-good days contribute to learning and success. While becoming an optimalist is a lifelong journey, we can support our clients to appreciate the process, accept mistakes, and learn as they go. Progress is little by little, moment by moment.

While no one is purely optimalist or perfectionist, they can be viewed as being on a continuum (Ben-Shahar, 2009). Certain situations will bring out more of the perfectionist and others will stimulate the optimalist in all of us. We have found it helpful to discuss the perspective of the perfectionist and compare it to the perspective of the optimalist at the beginning of each client's training program. This often needs to be reinforced if we notice clients becoming more self-critical (Ben-Shahar, 2009). Being open to the fact that there is more than one way to approach the vocal transformation—and any aspect of life—can expose clients to the greater ease of the optimalist and may lead them to more of what they want with greater satisfaction and self-empowerment. A beginning client commented that exposure to the optimalist perspective helped her change her view during training: "When I stopped worrying about [oral resonance] being a certain way, sounding like my clinician's or other clients', it was easier for me to just let it happen and let my own voice come out."

Emotions

When we allow ourselves to be more connected with the body, as with the mindfulness work, it makes us aware of emotions that we may not have been aware of before. This brings us back to the mind-body connection. Our bodies store unresolved emotion from the past. Many of us for many years have spent a great deal of energy avoiding feeling the discomfort and pain of negative emotion.

Many gender-diverse people carry with them a lifetime of trauma, the most common expression of which is fear. As our clients practice mindfulness, postural alignment, respiratory control, feeling the body, and manipulating the voice as part of the transformation process, emotions tend to arise. This is normal and healthy. We do not have to fix them or make anything out of what we witness. Clients are responsible for their own emotions; however, we can give them safe space—physically and emotionally—to experience emotions.

A trans woman, C. D., shared the impact of being guided through her own process:

> Something that was really important to me and I have never forgotten was when I was struggling to understand where my feelings were coming from. One of the things you told me was that the feelings were always there, even before I was aware of them. The fact that I could not access them did not mean they did not exist inside me. The exact words you used, and I remember them so clearly, were "the body never forgets." Those were your precise words. That was kind of a thunderbolt that is hard to explain. It was a connection or an insight that I never formed for myself. I had never connected those three things: my breath, my body, and my feelings. Everything got easier after that. I began to understand and have my own personal emotional life that no longer over took me.

Reframe It

What happens to unexpressed emotions that sit dormant for 20 years? Do they go away? Unfortunately, they don't. They are stored in the body and can arise at the most inopportune times reminding us that we are unsettled, or that there is something amiss. They color our thinking and influence our decisions and direction in all aspects of our life. While the reality of this may at first be disconcerting, it can be viewed in a different way. Being able to see something from a new perspective can be life altering.

One of Linda's clients had been training much longer than the trans women she knew in her social group. It bothered the client deeply and brought up significant doubt about her potential voice development and therefore future life satisfaction and safety. During a discussion about this, Linda shared an insight with her.

> Linda asked, "Is it possible that you are meant to go a bit deeper in your transition than the people around you? It feels that your awareness of your personal growth is more pronounced than I see in many clients."
>
> There was a long pause as her face slowly lit up with recognition, and she said, "You know, I do feel that I am reconnecting more to a deeper part of me, beyond gender. It is almost as if I will not let myself go farther with my voice until I learn to be more aware of my body. And the more aware I am of my body, the more aware I am of me, but I don't mean my personality exactly. Like if there is such a thing as a soul, I feel that I know what this is now, I know myself in a bigger way."
>
> "What a beautiful thing to be able to say." Linda said as she hesitated and then asked the client, "Are you saying that you are learning to connect to your soul through your voice work?"
>
> She said, "Yes, I guess that IS what I am saying, but I did not realize that until just now!"

The experience was reframed to a new perspective. Just the possibility of greater potential for the client's personal journey not only helped her emotionally, but it freed her to explore her voice with less fear and resistance to the process.

Feel It to Free It

Emotions have a corresponding sensation in the body. For example, when Linda feels fear, she gets a tightness in her abdomen. It is disconcerting. Her first reaction is to avoid it by keeping busy or eating something sweet. Eventually she realizes what is happening. Then she tells herself, "Oh, I feel afraid right now. Okay." Then she finds a quiet spot on campus if she is at work and she sits with it. She lets it arise as she feels it. Sometimes there are tears, and sometimes not. They are allowed to come without judgment. After years of working with her emotions, it is easier to accept and move through. Slowly the tightness changes to lighter and lighter sensation.

Then it is gone. She feels freer. The space she is in appears brighter to her. Then she moves on in the day.

If you or your client is new to this process, it may be helpful to know that it is easier to keep ourselves calm and focused if we talk ourselves through this process step by step. Think of it as if you are helping your best friend through a difficult time. Self-talk such as, "It's ok. Let's go and find a quiet spot," can be very helpful versus the voice of panic that can sometimes arise when we feel out of control.

Within the clinical process itself, sometimes clients are not comfortable dealing with arising emotion in the session and sometimes they are. It depends on the client, the situation, and their relationship with the provider. For clients who are more aware of their emotions, this has become a natural part of sessions; it is more automatic for clients to release emotions freely and then move into whatever is next.

The role of the provider in this situation is to:

- provide a safe space,
- be a nonjudgmental witness,
- permit the process to occur in an organic way,
- allow clients to be responsible for their own experience, and
- provide a mirror for clients who need to see themselves as honored for their journey.

For others, emotions simply do not arise, and this is of course perfect for them. As providers, we work with what is in front of us.

It is helpful for both clients and providers to understand that it will not always be convenient in day-to-day life to just stop what we are doing to integrate unpleasant emotions. We do not always have the time or the privacy to deal with them in the moment. A very effective alternative is to take a couple of notes to remind us of the trigger (e.g., "I was criticized") and our reaction (e.g., anger: 'How could she say that!" and fear: "How can I face those people again?") and wait until we get to our car or get home to some privacy in order to make the most of each experience.

Letting Go of the Layers

Once we experience a particular emotion such as fear, and release it, we feel greater freedom and peace. However, like layers of an onion, there may be more that will rise again, perhaps with a different kind of intensity to it or a different angle to a similar triggering experience. Often when we go through this process, we are made aware of the connection this experience has with an old childhood trauma, and that the recent negative emotion has arisen in order for us to clear it out of our field of experience. The more we let go of the layers, the more we realize that life gets easier, and we feel lighter and freer.

Eventually, even a lifetime of chronic anxiety can level out to occasional stress and tension. It is important that we recognize these ups and downs as a part of life, look back to see the growth we have made because of them, and share our experience to help others.

Permission to be Human

Emotions will be a part of voice work. When we discuss this with our clients early in their care, we teach them that it is okay—even desirable—to give themselves permission to experience their fear, anxiety, and sadness so that they may experience joy, happiness, and well-being (Fredrickson, 2011). They may be working with their therapist to deal with the reasons certain emotions exist in their experience, but meanwhile we should be aware of whether the emotions are interfering with voice and communication goals.

One of our seasoned clients was especially mindful of emotions arising during her vocal transformation. She understood through the work with her psychotherapist that she may experience emotions as she goes through various phases of her process, and that it is natural and fine. So, when she found herself going through it, she was more able to just experience the emotions rather than judging herself or trying not to feel them and stuffing them out of her perception again. She was giving herself permission to be human. The paradox is when one tries to suppress, repress, or avoid painful emotions they only intensify. But when we let ourselves experience emotions, they are manageable rather than debilitating.

It may help some clients to understand that there is nothing wrong or immoral about emotions or about feeling anger or fear toward people in our lives. Emotions are not immoral, they are amoral (Ben-Shahar, 2007). They are above the moral domain. Negative emotion is not good or bad, it is like the law of gravity: It just is, and we can learn to accept it as such. When we view emotions as part of human nature, it becomes easier to accept them as we do the laws of physical nature.

Giving ourselves permission to be human should not lead to resignation and immobility (e.g., "Okay, I'll sit in front of the television and zone out because there is nothing that I can do"). Accepting the emotion and acknowledging its presence is followed by choosing the most appropriate action. We must be very clear about the distinction between emotions and behaviors.

There are certain things we cannot change, such as having anger or frustration occasionally. What we can change is our behavior, whether we choose to cry for another day, a week or 30 days or go out and look for positivity boosters in our lives. Our response to emotions is where we have the choice.

Positivity Boosters

If we lived in perfect circumstances, perhaps we could be involved in meaningful and satisfying activities all the time, but for most of us this is not possible. We may have jobs, home lives, or personal circumstances that may be draining or undesirable to us. Even in the best of circumstances, most of us go through periods of high stress, leading to a happiness deficiency. Fortunately, engaging in activities that are personally meaningful positively affects our lived experience, even in areas not directly related to these activities (Sheldon, Houser-Marko, & Diener, 2001). Even brief activities that are personally satisfying and meaningful can give us confidence and fulfillment that can trickle into other areas of our lives. These activities can function like a candle in a dark room—and just as it takes a small flame to light up an entire physical space, one or two happy experiences during an otherwise uninspiring period can transform our general state (Ben-Shahar, 2007).

An example of a positivity booster that may easily be discussed with clients is to ask them to notice one thing that makes them happy each day, and write it down or tell someone. Another is to list things they have enjoyed doing in the past or have thought about trying, and to try one of them within the upcoming week or month. For example: drawing, reading, crossword puzzles, baking cookies, being alone, being with others, grilling, gardening, cooking, listening to music, exercising, meditating, or watching or participating in sports.

Expressing gratitude can be a powerful positivity booster. Emmons and McCullough (2003) conducted a series of studies and found an overall effect of gratitude on psychological and physical well-being. Undergraduate students were randomly assigned to one of three groups, distinguished by what they had to write down (i.e., notice and document). In the first study, each week participants in one group wrote five things for which they were grateful, the second group wrote five hassles and the third group, the control group, wrote five things that affected them in the past week. Each week the participants also reported their mood, physical symptoms, reactions to support, exercise time, and general appraisals of their life.

After 10 weeks, the gratitude group felt happier and more optimistic. They had also exercised more and experienced fewer symptoms of physical illness. The second study was similar but instead of writing each week, participants wrote each day for two weeks, and the control group was instructed to write about ways they were better off than others. Again, the gratitude practice resulted in significantly more positive effects. They were also more generous and more likely to offer support to others. Overall, the studies in Emmons and McCullough (2003) suggest that a conscious focus on things they are grateful for may have emotional and interpersonal benefits for our clients.

Why does gratitude have such an impact? Because when you mindfully consider "What do I appreciate? What am I grateful for?" you are focusing on the good. "When we are thankful for the good in life, the good grows" (Ben-Shahar, 2014, p. 144).

As part of almost every home program, we ask the clients to write one gratitude at the end of each day after their voice journaling. It can be something as simple as, "I enjoyed a good cup of coffee this morning," "A stranger smiled at me today," or "My car started!" to as big as "I got a promotion."

The reason we do it is because most of our clients are very focused on what is wrong and are missing all of the tiny experiences that can be seen as positive or good or note-worthy and have the power to lift them. The focus on what is wrong or broken can weigh us down and mislead us into believing that there is something wrong with us or our lives. The power of appreciation of the good that happens in a day can be transformative.

The following is from one client, R. T.'s, evening journal:

> "I'm grateful that I focused on my quiet breathing for a full minute before I went into the meeting room. I was able to pause before telling Jack why we were going to try something

different than his idea, and I think it helped my tone of voice be less 'I'm irritated' and more 'thanks for trying.' I didn't hear my voice get tight and choppy. I'm grateful for the colleagues at work who support me."

CASE EXAMPLES

The following case examples illustrate how providers can help clients identify obstacles and sometimes overcome them to continue with transformation of voice and communication. Note that many of the instances involve emotions, often to the extent that professionals skilled in counseling and psychology are needed.

Struggling to Find the Way

L. B. was a 57-year-old retired government worker self-referred for voice assessment and intervention. She was generally in good health but reported a history of vocal fatigue when she used to work at her vocally demanding job. L. B. was AMAB but presented herself as a woman and desired others to see her as a woman. She felt she was perceived as a woman by others about 40% of the time, but never on the phone. Medications included estrogen and spironolactone. She reported a 2-year history of desire to change her voice to sound "more naturally feminine." The client had no prior history of formal speech and language training or therapy. She reported watching internet videos of vocal techniques for those in transition prior to coming for formal training.

L. B. exhibited shallow inspiration prior to phonation, and abdominal contraction and reduced airflow during phonation. Her posture was mildly rolled forward with significant bilateral shoulder tension and elevation, and hypertonicity of the suprahyoid and lingual musculature. L. B.'s voice quality was perceived moderately impacted (45/100), characterized by roughness (35/100) and strain (20/100), with low pitch (50/100) and excessive volume (35/100). Intonation was reduced (4 ST) and glottal fry was present. Mean fundamental frequency was 118 Hz for sustained vowel and 105 Hz for conversation. Her maximum phonation frequency range was 86 to 360 Hz (24 ST). The client scored 52/120 on the Transsexual Voice Questionnaire for male-to-female people (TVQ-MTF). Statements that rated as "strongly agree" included that her voice often makes her feel less feminine than she would like, and that her laugh in particular sounds like a man's.

The graduate provider completed posture and relaxation goals and began diaphragmatic breathing modification. Direct voice work was initially approached fairly traditionally. Pitch elevation work started at 145 Hz with oral resonance during sessions one and two. While she was fairly consistent with provider guidance, she seemed to work too hard to achieve the desired result. By the third session, she had not developed greater ease. While it was clear that she had access up to 360 Hz, she had difficulty raising her frequency high enough to reach the initial target on command without high efforts and strain.

With Linda's guidance, the graduate student provider shifted to oral resonance approaches to stimulate improved quality and ease; however, nothing attempted was fully forward and comfortable for her. They used recordings, demonstrations, models, sensory feedback, and negative practice using a variety of techniques including using a semi-occluded vocal tract for stimulating oral resonance. They transitioned to utilizing intonation modification to increase ease and flexibility with hopes of relaxing the larynx and creating improved resonance and quality without significant change. Finally, they took a step back and restructured the transformation approach in the following way:

1. Increased Breath: Focusing on increasing the depth of inhalation specifically assisted in lifting her pitch slightly without her conscious effort.
2. Decreased Volume: Reducing her volume by asking her to speak using "confidential voice." This made the greatest difference. Her frequency immediately floated up to 180 Hz without any direct pitch work. Her resonance improved. Her previous phonation pattern appeared to be produced with so much tension that reducing the volume reduced the vocal load, thereby increasing airflows and allowing for elevation of the pitch more naturally.
3. Intonation Modification: The client imagined aiming intonation into the space between her eyes and mouth, so that the highs were closer to the eyes, and the lows no lower than the oral cavity. These locations were purely used as internal markers. While the common cue for clients is to feel intonation in the mouth, lips, palate, etc., it can be effective to give a broader space

with which to draw their intonation. In her case, this improved laryngeal balance with greater oral resonance. It also had the effect of stabilizing her frequency to approximately 180 Hz effortlessly with greater oral resonance. She was able to move forward more traditionally from there.

Mental Health Conditions

Familiarity with psychological or mood disorders that affect voice work is advised so that clients can be directed toward professional care in a timely and caring fashion. Mental health concerns may be related or unrelated to the client's history of gender dysphoria or minority stress; however, there is evidence that the prevalence of such disorders is higher in trans populations (see Chapter 2). For example, the 2015 U.S. Transgender Survey reported that 39% of respondents experienced "serious psychological distress," compared with only 5% of the U.S. population (James, Herman, Rankin, Keisling, Mottett, & Anafi, 2016). A peer support hotline is easily posted in your waiting room, for example (the Trans Life peer support hotline is 877-565-8860 in the U.S. and 877-330-6366 in Canada; QLife in Australia is 1800-184-527 or online chat at qlife.org.au). See Appendix 2–A for additional resources.

Though empirical evidence is lacking in some areas, the World Professional Association for Transgender Health (WPATH) current standards of care identify the conditions of disproportionate prevalence in trans populations as anxiety, depression, self-harm, a history of abuse and neglect, compulsivity, substance abuse, sexual concerns, personality disorders, eating disorders, psychotic disorders, and autism spectrum disorders. These conditions left undetected or untreated can "complicate the process of gender identity exploration and resolution of gender dysphoria" (WPATH SOC7, 2011, p. 24). It is of note that abrupt discontinuation of gender-affirming hormones can worsen mood symptoms (Carmel & Erickson-Schroth, 2016).

To illustrate the impact of mental health conditions on voice and communication transformation, we will describe a client with a dissociation disorder. One study identified significant dissociative disorder in 10% of 64 "highly functional transsexuals" who completed the Dissociative Experiences Scale (Walling, Goodwin, & Cole, 2015). Whether officially diagnosed or not, some clients will find it difficult to feel because not feeling has become a protective mechanism from becoming aware of unpleasant sensations, memories, images, and emotions they may have suppressed for many years. Clients and providers can be surprised when emotional reactions come forward from simple tasks such as training breathing for voice productions.

When there is resistance to body awareness and its associated psychological blocks, it may be difficult for clients to soften their body, impacting the vocal process itself. Therefore, gently allowing the client to relax and follow a clinician's gentle voice in preparation for voice training can be helpful in and of itself with an open clinician and a willing client. This is illustrated in the following case description.

G. H. was a 42-year-old trans woman who was seen for 8 weeks for vocal feminization. She was presenting full time as female and worked as a background investigator. The beginning of her vocal transition was fairly typical. Her goals were to develop postural alignment and diaphragmatic breath support, and elevate frequency, intonation, and oral resonance. At approximately 6 weeks Linda and her graduate providers began to notice a pattern. Whenever they would work with oral resonance, G. H. would develop hypernasality. Once this was addressed with her by describing the issue, providing modeling, discrimination work, and negative practice, she would reset it appropriately and move forward in her program with ease. Oral resonance was consistent within the sessions themselves, but rarely generalized from session to session.

Finally, when Linda was called in to the session by the student providers for assistance, and sat with the client, G. H. blurted out, "I can't feel my body!"

Linda: Tell me more about that.

G. H.: I can't feel the vibration. I can't feel anything.

Linda: It's okay. Do you know when all of this started?

G. H.: I didn't notice it until we had to feel for resonance.

Linda: Can I hold your hand for a moment?

[*G. H. nods.*]

Linda: If you look at your index finger, can you feel it?

[*G. H. shakes her head, no.*]

Linda: Okay, now may I try something? [*G. H. nods*] I just want to touch the same finger, is that ok? [*She nods*] Can

> you feel that now? [*She nods yes*] Okay, fine. Now may I take this a step further? [*She nods*] I am going to let go of the finger, and I want you to tell me if you can feel it more easily than you could the first time we tried to feel it. Ready? [*She nods*] Can you still feel your index finger? [*G. H. nods yes and appears relieved*]

It was Linda's intention to bring G. H. back to her body enough to eliminate her panic, and to direct her to her psychotherapist for evaluation for body dissociative disorder. Her inability to feel her throat and facial muscles were affecting her ability to progress and creating a great deal of stress for her. The more clinicians would bring her into her body for her training, the more anxiety she would feel. People dissociate from their bodies as a safety mechanism to reduce the amount and severity of trauma memories and emotions that can arise from their past experiences. In her case, there were other fears that arose in the session such as making sure that she could see each person that was in the room with her (e.g., no one behind her), not being able to tolerate someone's hands on her neck for the laryngeal massage, and other patterns that triggered anxiety. It finally all came together into a more cohesive clinical picture. In consultation with her psychotherapist, all agreed that due to past trauma she was not going to be able to move forward with her voice work without some psychotherapy. To date, she is still receiving care and is planning to return to voice training when she feels ready.

Preconceived Ideas of Outcomes

Chapter 5 describes the importance and process for collaborative goal setting, in which the provider and client acknowledge certain limitation to individual agency—or the ability to control the outcome. As the ASSEMBLE model (Chapter 5, Hancock & Azul, 2018) prescribes, we:

> **A**cknowledge ongoing and dynamic agency of:
>
> **S**peaker's practices (e.g., self-presentation, lifestyle choices, self-attribution, responses to attributions from others)
>
> **S**ociocultural mediation of meaning-making practices (e.g., linguistic rules and standards, normative forces, socialization practices)

External **M**aterial forces (e.g., physical, chemical, biological, technical)

Biophysiological processes (e.g., genetic, hormonal)

Listening practices (e.g., perceptions, interpretations, attributions)

Elected professional interventions (e.g., behavioral, surgical, medicinal)

Nonetheless, some clients cling to what they subconsciously or consciously have been wanting for years. Many clients have shared that they have been planning what they will sound like for years prior to their transition. That image may change by the time they actually experience their own vocal transition, and it is just as influential in how they approach their vocal transition. Issues may not show themselves until they have gone almost all of the way through their vocal transition when they begin to see that there is no view in sight of the voice they have been waiting for.

An example of this is A. C., a 60-year-old who works in the computer technology field and positions herself as a woman (though AMAB) and requests she/her pronouns. When she got close to discharge after 8 months of sessions with Linda, she shared dissatisfaction with her voice. She felt it could be better. When her progress and recordings were reviewed objectively, A. C. could not be specific as to what caused her dissatisfaction. When she was asked how she related to her new voice, she appeared anxious and just repeated, "It doesn't match me" and "It doesn't sound female." Yet, she conversed at a resonant 180 Hz with 8 ST range and she had not been misgendered for approximately one month on the phone and related ease in all discussed communication situations. She consistently focused on what else she could work on rather than appreciating and accepting how far she had come.

When it was realized that she was unable to accept the exceptional vocal quality that she had achieved, discussions became more intense and probing became more purposeful around the issue of this ideal voice. It was not until the discussion about how aging changes the voice including and beyond gender that she was able to remember that she had a very specific idea of what she would sound like. It was not that she didn't sound female, it was that she didn't sound like a young female. She had subconsciously imagined that at the end of this process she would have the voice of her

25-year-old daughter. She overcame other signs of aging with hair replacement, reconstructive facial surgery, and breast and buttocks implants. Consciously or subconsciously, she had expected her voice work to disguise her age as well. Even though we followed the introductory protocol for the first training session to help client develop realistic expectations, she had not been able to integrate this information with her private anticipation of sounding like her daughter.

We discussed how aging impacts the inner body: The mucosal lining of the vocal tract becomes drier, absorbing and reflecting sounds differently; the vocal fold dimensions change and vibrate differently; muscle tone atrophies, thins out, and responds differently; the laryngeal structures themselves become more brittle and less flexible; and so on. She was surprised to say the least. Later she shared that she was secretly angry about this. It took her time to absorb this new perspective but eventually she commented, "How could I expect to sound 25 without a 25-year-old body?"

A. C. reports that she has been happier about her vocal product now that she is able to be more realistic. Over the next couple of weeks, she let go of the entire image that she had created and she finally was in awe of all that she had accomplished. She was also able to relax and allow an even more authentic voice to come through. Her voice was more expressive, flexible, and effortless, and reflected more of how she was feeling and who she was. She reports that now her thoughts are freed up from thinking so much about her voice, and she began to expand her life into areas of great joy such as taking the piano lessons that she always wanted. Life was more fulfilling to her once she was able to identify and let go of unrealistic expectations.

Attachment

G. R. was a 48-year-old trans woman AMAB who worked as a publisher and was seeing Linda for vocal feminization. She was highly motivated and determined to transform her voice. While she had made steady progress in all training areas and was consistent with her home program, after about 10 months there was a sense of resistance within the session. Her progress with incorporating oral resonance at each level of stimuli halted abruptly when she reached the conversational level. The more she was praised for her previous progress and encouraged to continue with her momentum and finish strong, the more she seemed to struggle. It did not fit what Linda was used to seeing in this highly competent client.

This continued until it became apparent that there was a disconnection between the client's current performance in sessions and her previous levels of understanding and vocal control. G. R. agreed that she also saw the inconsistencies, but did not understand them herself.

With some probing, the questions finally turned to the fact that she was close to reaching all of the goals that she had set for herself. When Linda asked her, "How do you feel about being close to finishing your program?" G. R. froze. She didn't know what to say. Finally, she said, "I know I want to get there . . . of course I want to get there . . . I don't know why I am hesitating."

G. R. was asked if she would share what some of the positives were for being able to reach her goals. She responded with the discussion of the freedom from fear of societal reactions, family dynamic improvements, and ease in the workplace. When she was asked for negatives about being able to reach all of her voice training goals she started to say, "How could there be any?" but then hesitated. Later she was able to share that she was concerned about being "cut off" and afraid of losing contact with her provider, someone with whom she could be with without worrying about being judged.

With some support from her psychotherapist and assurance that she is not cut off from needed voice support and follow-up care as needed, the pressure eased, and she was able to relax and move forward. It is extremely important for clients to have access to psychological support, and sometimes providers are a large part of that whether they are aware of that or not. As recommended in Chapter 3, have a list of trans-friendly counselors, psychologists, professional or peer-led support groups, conferences, and hotlines. Not all clients will be receptive to or ready for these activities, but knowing there are resources if and when they are ready is sometimes enough to ease their distress about seeing you less frequently.

Part-Time Presentation

For some clients, until they are able to present as themselves full time, they simply cannot be free to develop vocally. R. S. is a 32-year-old analyst who participated in the beginners' vocal feminization group. She attended sessions regularly and was motivated to develop a female voice. She demonstrated a great deal of anxiety during her beginning breathing, pitch, and resonance training. This was perceived by her providers as trying too hard, being highly self-critical, and having personal discomfort with the process. She was unable to express to us what she was feeling and was insistent that she was fine to continue.

Rebecca Pereira was her graduate provider at that time and shares her experience of what followed:

> It appears that full presentation can facilitate progress for many reasons beyond the fact that clients have more time to practice because they are living fully as themselves.
>
> As a third-semester graduate student, I was familiar with the concept [of vocal feminization] and was aware that one's voice could be misaligned with their gender identity; however, I didn't truly understand what the effects of misalignment and alignment would look or sound like, until I met my client, R. S.
>
> R. S. is a transgender woman seeking a natural, feminine-sounding voice who reported a significant misalignment between her masculine-sounding voice and her gender. When I first met her, she was presenting as male professionally and as herself socially. She presented with a low, monotone, strained voice with significant laryngeal tension. R. S. also presented with notable nervousness and frustration, which were consistent with her reports of misalignment between her voice and gender. Throughout the first several sessions, these emotions were hindering her progress in all goal areas: oral resonance, intonation, and diaphragmatic breathing.
>
> This continued until the day she transitioned at work and she arrived at vocal feminization group presenting as herself as well. The moment she walked in it seemed as if the fairy godmother in Cinderella transformed Cinderella's ragged dress into a beautiful ball gown. R. S. was beaming with a confidence that had previously never been observed. She looked relaxed and was able to recompose herself after challenging trials within the oral resonance portion of the session.
>
> She achieved more progress in that one session, in all goal areas, than in all previous sessions. Instinctively, I knew that. Emotionally, I felt it. Statistically, my data supported such observation. Above all, my client reported that she felt more

aware of her voice and the sensation of oral resonance for the first time. Though R. S. has more work to do in voice training and currently perceives her voice do somewhat misaligned with her identity, she is one step closer to her goal.

To be a part of this moment in someone's transition in becoming themselves was indefinable and an honor to be a part of. As a student clinician, this moment highlighted the importance of learning about all the variables that can influence a person's ability to communicate emotionally, psychologically, and physiologically. As a future professional, this moment affirmed that my duty as a speech-language pathologist is to serve all those with communication barriers and impairments, which certainly includes those in the transgender population who seek vocal feminization. In this case, if she did not present fully, she would not be so far along in voice training.

Sometimes it is difficult to present your gender acoustically if you are not presenting it visually. Ironically, it is a similar disconnect that intervention is addressing: looking feminine but sounding masculine can be dysphoric, lead to misgendering, and generally is a reason the client sought you in the first place. Yet it is common for clients AMAB to begin sessions before they present their gender 100% of the time (i.e., not out at work yet), so they may come to sessions in business suits and ties. In attempt to alleviate this source of blockage, we leave beautiful scarves in the clinic for clients who feel they would benefit and feel more in alignment while wearing them during the voice work. In addition, some clients leave their own scarves or tops here for use until they present full time. Explore with your clients some simple solutions to increase their comfort and facilitate congruence while they work with you.

Resistance and Readiness

Despite our best preparations and efforts, clients will still get stuck sometimes. Do the best you can, but then surrender and be patient. This sounds obvious, but it is worth stating: We can't always perceive, let alone modify, the client's behavior. C. E.'s case was a humbling reminder of this.

C. E. was a 52-year-old security specialist who had transitioned to presenting her gender at all times and had been in voice sessions with Linda for 10 months. She had progressed fairly steadily between periodic professional traveling for 5 to 10 days each time. She now was experiencing inconsistent follow through with her generalization practice between sessions.

She and Linda would agree on a home program at the end of each session and prepare attached audio files and written instructions for practice. Then she would come in the following week as if it never occurred. She would share what she would do between sessions, which did not resemble their discussion and did not appear to be effective, as there was little generalization and growth of skills that they could objectively document.

When Linda reviewed the home plan from that previous week and found that there was no follow through, she asked C. E. what her experience was with her home program. C. E. appeared confused. It was as if she recognized it, but was not really sure why she did not follow it.

This went on for weeks. They discussed it, used MI, which they thought was quite helpful, but she would revert back again and again. Linda thought it was related to personal stress in her life, which they discussed and decided to share with her therapist in the context of voice training progress.

One day, she walked into the session and she was completely different. Her voice was more consistent and she appeared completely comfortable using it. There was complete engagement as she began sharing her week.

> Linda: There is a freedom in you today that I have not seen before that appears to be related to your vocal presentation. I am wondering if you see this as well.
>
> *C. E.: I do . . . I do . . .*
>
> Linda: What was the shift that allowed you to present your voice in just this way today? I'm just wondering if you even know the answer to this question.
>
> *C. E.: I have an idea. Part of it I think, and this isn't unique to my voice, is that change happens when one part of me that I can't always consciously access, decides it's ready for it to happen and not a moment before.*
>
> *I wish I could explain . . . I don't mean explain it rationally, because it's something else, something that drives a lot of my behavior. Maybe it's the subconscious that determines this. I think it's also something we hadn't really talked about before . . . which you asked me about.*

After struggling to practice the skills I had worked so hard to develop, you asked me this question: "What was I afraid of?" You were basically asking me . . . what were the fears holding me back from finding and expressing the voice inside. I may be paraphrasing a bit, but that's what I heard. And we hadn't really discussed that before, you know? As often happens when something profound happens during our time together, it may not seem like it really sank in, but a few days later it burled its way under my skin if that makes sense because it's not just about voice, it's about all kinds of fears that I've kept to myself.

Some I've done better at conquering, some I struggle with a lot. My relationship with my children is something I struggle with a lot for example. But it feels like fear and resistance are connected *sometimes. So even if I wasn't being verbally resistant in the session consciously, I still think there are ways that it came out. And you pointed that out to me on more than one occasion, which were not necessarily comfortable conversations, but I've learned that they are necessary.*

So it feels like that's part of it somehow. I don't know that it's a coincidence that after we had that conversation I was willing to stand up in front of the group at work for the very first time and talk about myself. And now look at me, being videotaped for a work promo. And now feeling hopefully ready for the really big presentation coming up next week. I had to be willing to at least acknowledge the fear in order to move forward.

Now I am coming to understand and embrace the fact that I have a voice! That I can share it with others and believe it's worthy of being heard.

So that's part of it too.

Linda: So you've always known that you had the mechanics, but it was not until you felt you had a voice that represents who you are, until that connected for you, could you allow this voice to come fully forward.

C. E.: Yes, it's really about self-acceptance about my imperfections and that I can be afraid. From the beginning you have seen how I struggled with self-acceptance. I didn't like that my voice was not the voice that I wanted.

Now it's at the point where there is something I can see that has a feminine aspect to it that I was not willing to accept before. And I must say, and this is something you taught me, I can embrace the voice I do have and how different [improved] it is from the voice I began with! This is entirely about acceptance. And I got a lot of that from you. I think that is intimately connected with feeling safe enough and loved enough so that whatever my scared and naked self was at, I could share that here in the session and that I would be embraced. I think for me, this goes well beyond my voice. That has made every difference.

In retrospect, C. E. had been in a stage of contemplation about moving forward, still feeling two ways about this step. She was not ready for the action stage of change until she discovered and began dealing with her fears in counseling. While it seemed to the practioner that she had not grown for a long period of time, something outside of her provider's perception was growing and may have been blooming for a long time. Finally, the blossoming was evident in her vocal expression in a way that they could now talk about.

Through open discussions and sharing perspectives as the client approaches discharge, we gain important insight regarding remaining resistance or fears that may prevent a client from moving beyond the provider's services. S. J., a woman AMAB, began to realize her constant questioning was blocking progression and finally adjusted herself to be more trusting of the provider and the process. She reflects on her realization and the impact that "acting on faith" had in her transformation:

I have been looking at the work that you are asking me to do, and why I so resist this whole process. I am always asking myself the question, "why?" And after weeks of contemplation, I think the answer is that there is no real answer to that question! I just have to go forward on faith. Which I think will help both of us. It will make me a more compliant client, but more importantly it will also work to push all the inner junk away from blocking the process and sort of let me move forward in my vocal transition. 'Cause everything I have done in the last five years has been an act of faith.

Transition is an act of faith. You never know if any particular step is the right thing, because everyone around you tells you, "it is not right!" and "it's wrong." And so you do it and you see, "oh this is fantastic!" I think acting on faith is one of my superpowers. So as I'm doing the breathing, staying aware of what I am doing, trusting that this is the next step as you guide me, I'm letting go, in faith, and turning myself over to your guidance. I'm realizing, yeah, just do what the nice lady says instead of resisting it or controlling it and always asking why, why, why.

I'm not overly logical anymore. In fact, my heart and my brain are actually conversing together every once in a while. I lived a life where my heart and my brain were at odds with one another through my entire life. So my brain would keep me alive, the heart would be dangerous in that it would tell me to be something else. But I started listening to my heart, and—I'm surprised to say—the brain still works nicely! I'm happy with that. But I realized, they are not two separate things. They are two amazing interconnected, beautiful things and my brain is much better with my heart alongside of it.

It is very important to keep communicating with clients but understand that they may or may not be ready to express themselves through their voice. Resistance to change is not uncommon. Even when vocal skills are in place, a readiness of their inner being is required. In C. E.'s words, "This goes beyond gender and yet is a part of it."

CONCLUSION

Each client's transformation will be unique. Common to them all is your role as facilitator of voice and communication change. Never is that privilege more daunting than when the client's progress is stalled. Evaluating their level of readiness for behavioral change and any underlying obstacles requires time and skill but is vital to resuming progress. Whether that progress will occur sooner or later is not entirely up to us, but we hope the information in this chapter helps you navigate bumps in the process.

REFERENCES

Behrman, A. (2006). Facilitating behavioral change in voice therapy: The relevance of motivational interviewing. *American Journal of Speech-Language Pathology, 15*, 215–225.

Ben-Shahar, T. (2007). *Happier: Learn the secrets to daily joy and lasting fulfillment*. New York, NY: McGraw-Hill Education.

Ben-Shahar, T. (2009). *Pursuit of perfect: Stop chasing perfection and find your path to lasting happiness!* New York, NY: McGraw-Hill Education.

Ben-Shahar, T. (2014). *Choose the life you want: The mindful way to happiness.* Chapel Hill, NC: Algonquin Books.

Ben-Shahar, T. (2017). *The joy of leadership: How positive psychology can maximize your impact (and make you happier) in a challenging world.* Hoboken, NJ: Wiley.

Bridle, C., Riemsma, R., Pattenden, J., Sowden, A., Mather, L., Watt, I., & Walker, A. (2005). Systematic review of the effectiveness of health behavior interventions based on the transtheoretical model. *Psychology and Health, 20*(3), 283–301.

Carmel, T. C., & Erikson-Schroth, L. (2016). Mental health and the transgender population. *Journal of Psychosocial Nursing, 54*(12), 44–48.

Cole, C. M., O'Boyle, M., Emory, L. E., & Meyer, W. J. (1997). Comorbidity of gender dysphoria and other major psychiatric diagnoses. *Archives of Sexual Behavior, 26*(1), 13–26.

Emmons, R. A., & McCullough, M. E. (2000). Counting blessings versus burdens: An experimental investigation of gratitude and subjective well-being in daily life. *Journal of Personality and Social Psychology, 84*(2), 377–389.

Fredrickson, B. L. (2011). The role of positive emotions in positive psychology: The broaden-and-build theory of positive emotions. *American Psychology, 56*(3), 218–226.

Hancock, A. B., & Azul, D. (2018). *Theory-guided, person-centered voice and communication support for gender-diverse people.* Presented at the World Professional Association of Transgender Health Conference, Buenos Aires, Argentina.

Hutchison, A., Breckon, J., & Johnston, L. (2009). Physical activity behavior change interventions based on the transtheoretical model: A systematic review. *Health Education and Behavior, 36*(5), 829–845.

James, S. E., Herman, J. L., Rankin, S., Keisling, M., Mottet, L., & Anafi, M. (2016). *The report of the 2015 U.S. Transgender Survey.* Washington, DC: National Center for Transgender Equality.

Parker, W. D, & Adkins, K. K. (1995). Perfectionism and the gifted. *Roeper Review, 17*, 173–176.

Procheska, J. O., & Norcross, J. C. (2001). Stages of change. *Psychotherapy, 38*(4), 443–448.

Sheldon, K., Houser-Marko, L., & Diener, E. (2001). Self-concordance, goal attainment, and the pursuit of happiness: Can there be an upward spiral? *Journal of Personality and Social Psychology, 80*(1), 152–165.

Van Leer, E., Hapner, E. R., & Connor, N. P. (2008). Transtheoretical model of health behavior change applied to voice therapy. *Journal of Voice, 22*(6), 688–698.

Walling, D. P., Goodwin, J. M., & Cole, C. M. (2015). Dissociation in a transsexual population. *Journal of Sex Education and Therapy, 23*(2), 121–123.

WPATH. (2011). *Standards of care for the health of transsexual, transgender, and gender nonconforming people* (7th ed). Retrieved from http://www.wpath.org

Zimmerman, G. L., Olsen, C. G., & Bosworth, M. F. (2000). A stages of change approach to helping patients change behavior. *American Family Physician*, *61*(5), 1409–1416.

CHAPTER 9

Completion and Connection

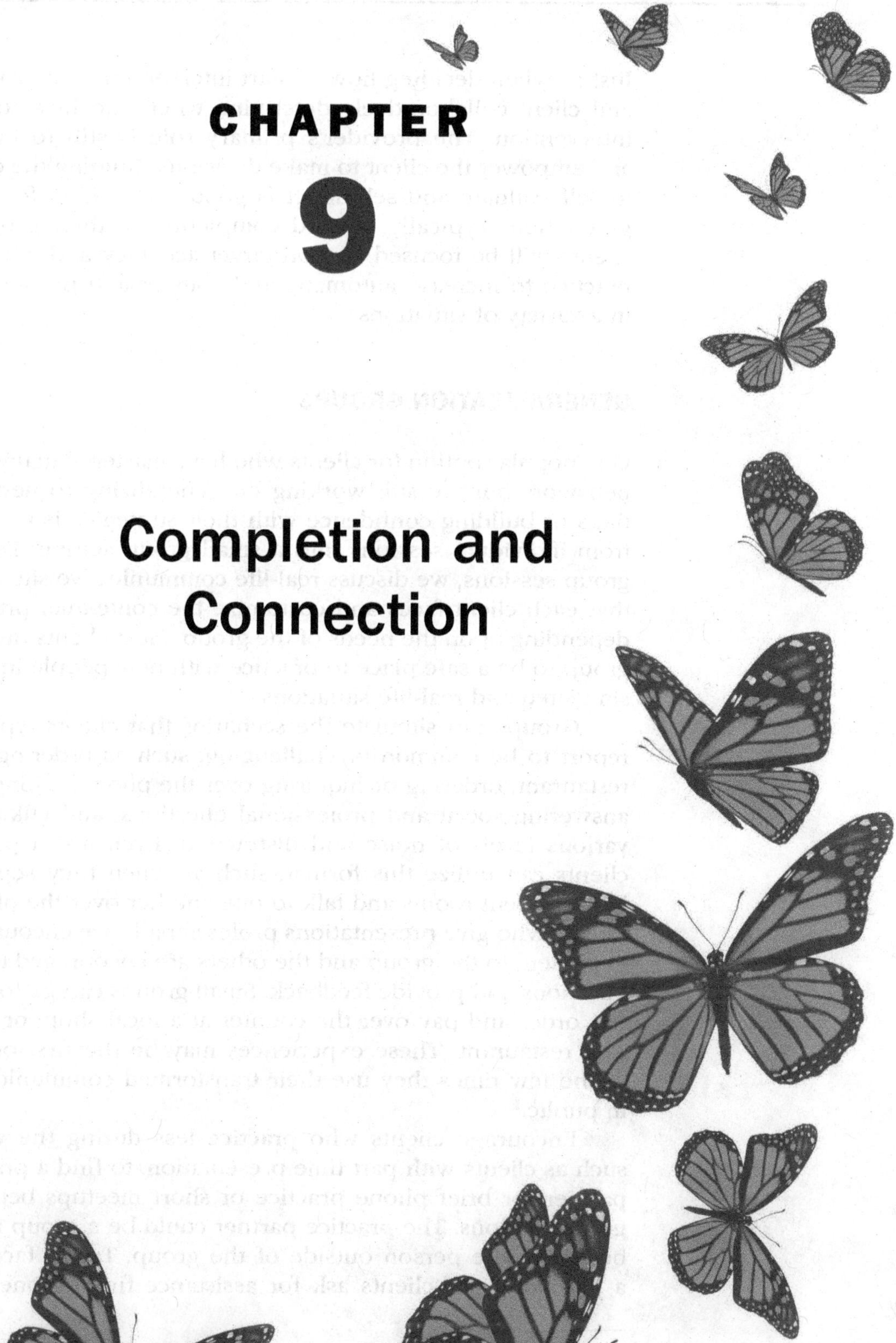

Just as when deciding how to start intervention, the provider and client collaboratively determine when and how to end intervention. The provider's primary role is still to inform and empower the client to make decisions. Guiding the client to self-evaluate and self-direct is good preparation for their graduation. Typically, toward completion of their program clients will be focused less on target accuracy and more on practice to increase automatic and comfortable productions in a variety of situations.

GENERALIZATION GROUPS

One popular option for clients who have mastered many new behaviors but are still working on generalizing to new settings or building confidence with their strategies is to move from individual sessions into a small group setting. During group sessions, we discuss real-life communicative situations that each client faces and customize the contextual practice depending upon the needs of the group. Most clients find the group to be a safe place to practice with new people in both simulated and real-life situations.

Groups can simulate the scenarios that clients typically report to be common or challenging, such as ordering in a restaurant, ordering or inquiring over the phone, asking and answering social and professional questions, and talking in various levels of noise and distraction. Even just a pair of clients can utilize this format, such as when they separate into different rooms and talk to one another over the phone. Clients who give presentations professionally are encouraged to present to the group and the others are encouraged to ask questions and provide feedback. Small groups can go for coffee, order and pay over the counter at a local shop, or meet at a restaurant. These experiences may be the first or one of the few times they use their transformed communication in public.[1]

Encourage clients who practice less during the week, such as clients with part time presentation, to find a practice partner for brief phone practice or short meetups between group sessions. The practice partner could be a group member, or a safe person outside of the group. Try to facilitate a partnership if clients ask for assistance finding one. The

[1]Some Toastmasters International chapters are specifically for LGBTQ people who want this sort of practice.

accountability and mutual support facilitate continued progress and the independence from the provider that they will need upon discharge.

In addition to a new practice context, the group setting provides opportunities for clients to give and receive support from one another as they share their communication challenges and successes. Vicarious experience is invaluable for building self-efficacy (Bandura, 1994; Van Leer, Hapner, & Connor, 2008). Ideally these groups would be co-led with professional counselors to help navigate the complex thoughts, attitudes, and emotions that often come with moving toward independence.

BUILDING INDEPENDENCE

If group options are not available or acceptable to the client, tapering frequency of sessions (i.e., from weekly sessions to monthly, then to bimonthly) is another way to ease into a maintenance phase. Whether the client needs to be independent for a short time during their program for some reason or indefinitely at the completion of a program, help them plan to be successful. The key word is "plan"—not hope, not assume. Specifying intentions and establishing habits are important. As they progress toward completion, they take more responsibility to maintain and build on their momentum.

A few practice attempts with independence can be enlightening. Because of the university calendar, the authors' clients have to be independent for the 6 to 8 weeks between semester sessions, knowing they will return to continue their program the following semester. The authors introduce the semester break as a valuable opportunity to practice being independent and learn what will work for clients. A short-term maintenance plan for the increasing intervals between sessions may include some of the following:

- Follow specific exercises and activities listed in a home program, including privately at home and more informally in public contexts.
- Log duration of vocal warm-ups at the start of the day and before practice.
- Continue to journal and document their intentions, vocal experiences, and gratitude.
- Intentional and regular meetings with their practice partners (i.e., weekly).

CONFIRMING PROGRESS, AFFIRMING CLIENTS

Set your sights on a strong finish. Preparations for finishing the intervention program should start well before the final session. Clearly defined goals and responsible data collection help us identify when we are nearing program completion. The pitch and intonation data often predict when clients can demonstrate ease and consistency in communicating in a variety of contexts. Charting assessment results over time for both objective and subjective data can show clients how far they have come. The most convincing evidence of transformation tends to be the audio or video recordings collected throughout (see this book's companion website for an example of these). When clients experience moments of acceptance—either of themselves or from others—with increasing frequency, they are nearing completion of their program.

With advanced clients, discuss the progress on general goals in addition to those specific to each client's unique needs and desires. One empowering way to do this is by asking the client to put their status and accomplishments into words and say them aloud in their transformed voice or communication style. Explore any resistance or exceptions they add to the statements, such as "except when I laugh," so that you can address those in your final sessions. Client-generated statements would be best, but statements from questionnaires (e.g., Voice Handicap Index, Transsexual Voice Questionnaire for Male-to-Female) or the statements below could be used as examples.

- I do not have to strain or use effort to communicate the way I want to.
- I am knowledgeable and confident about caring for my voice.
- I have reached my voice development potential.
- I am close to my potential. I am ready to continue progress independently.
- I am comfortable/satisfied with (or, I accept) my communication function and effectiveness.
- I understand what I can—and can't—do to influence how I attribute my gender.
- I understand what I can—and can't—do to influence how others attribute my gender.
- I have knowledge and strategies for communicating with people in a way that I am comfortable with.

Sometimes clients end services before clinical goals have been met in cases of unavoidable or external causes, such as relocation, a change in financial or health status, life stress, difficulty attending sessions, and a variety of other personal issues. There may be options for the client to continue care with a different provider or format. Refer to the considerations and ideas for facilitating access to care discussed in Chapter 3.

You may feel surprised when a client begins to hint or abruptly announces their readiness to end the sessions. Yet, it is very common for an individual's goals and criteria for success to morph as they go through voice transformation and transition in general. Other possibilities are that they are not ready for the extent or pace of change happening (see discussion of stages of change in Chapter 8) or that they are reconsidering alternative interventions for voice change (see discussion of hormone and surgical options in Chapter 5). Gently probe what led the client to consider discharge by using the motivational interviewing techniques described in Chapter 8. You may discover the need to educate or motivate, but most importantly you want to understand and attune to the client's needs and wants.

SEND-OFFS

Completing the intervention program may feel bittersweet for the provider and the client. Therapeutic empathy you developed early in the relationship likely continued to grow. Consider sharing your perspective of the experience together and what you appreciate about the client.

Offer practical tools or approaches for maintaining their level of success. It may be most effective for the client to develop what feels appropriate for them, but the following materials and ideas have been useful for clients and may spark more ideas.

- The client can follow warm-up, relaxation, and vocal exercises, either written or recorded on audio or video. This may include activities such as self-massage and neck stretches, realignment of the spine, general relaxation or meditation, pitch glides, and other activities specific to the needs of the client.
- The client can listen to audio recordings of their successful communication practice both in and out of

structured practice. The provider's reinforcement and feedback in the background may feel supportive to clients. Hearing themselves may be reinforcing, and also provide a cue if they begin to forget the target sound.

- Reflection journals are very helpful reminders for not only tracking progress day to day but also to set intentions at the start of every day for their anticipated communicative situations and to express gratitude at the end of each day for the small (and big!) things they appreciated that day.
- Find a circle of support. This could be gender support groups, psychotherapy, and family support—whether it is their family of origin or their newly created family of supportive friends and acquaintances.
- Continue with communication partners for knowledgeable reinforcement in a safe communication situation.

Clients are encouraged to follow up with clinicians if needs arise after they have successfully completed their program. It is advised, however, to clearly mark completion of their program for purposes of closure and celebration.

GIVING BACK

At the voice clinic at the Speech and Hearing Center of George Washington University, many seasoned clients have volunteered to share their experiences with future clients, providers, and graduate students. It is a way to bridge from a personal transformation to a shared one. Not only is it extremely helpful for their audience, but those who communicate their support and experiences are also excited to use what they have learned to help other people, essentially giving back with gratitude for what they have been given previously. It is empowering to be able to give in an area that was once so gratefully received. Another benefit, particularly for clients who are vocally ready for discharge but not quite psychologically ready for independence, is comfort in maintaining a connection to the provider. The following are examples of ways clients have been able to give back:

- Newly formed client introductory groups benefit greatly from past client personal visits and video-recorded messages. Having discharged or seasoned clients attend one session per semester, per group gives incoming clients the opportunity to ask questions that they may not otherwise ask.

- Student providers benefit from the perspective of a seasoned or past client who can share their experience of being a client retrospectively. One clinician asked a question that she felt that she could only ask a previous client, "What can we do to make our clients feel more comfortable in the training process?" The speaker simply responded, "First, be yourself; secondly, realize that you don't have to be transgender to share experience. Maybe you don't know what it's like to be transgender, but you know what it's like to have a bad day, you know what it's like to be challenged, and you can share those experiences with us."
- At an annual holiday party, past and current clients meet in the holiday spirit. Not only does it give new clients and past clients the opportunity to meet each other and share some of their experiences, but also practitioners can informally learn how clients continue to transform over time. It is a wonderful way to stay in touch with past clients on a casual basis.

One client shared that it wasn't until she could sit in front of a group of cisgender people and state that she was a transgender woman that she could she fully embody her newly aligned self. She felt completely renewed, "as if the chains had been taken off" of her body. Describing her experience impacted her audience and made a difference in her own life, too.

CONNECTIONS

Connection is central to the entire transformation process. Part I of this book addressed how we can connect with ourselves and others to meet important emotional, mental, physical, or logistical needs. Part II revolved around the client connecting to their voice. Part III demonstrates how connection is crucial for support during challenges of transformation.

A final important connection to mention is the connection among providers. In 2006 the authors connected to each other through a shared interest to serve marginalized people well. Since then, they have been fortunate to connect to many clinicians who also serve or are learning to serve gender-diverse populations professionally. A large motivation for this book was their desire to connect with more colleagues and support so many good intentions. In the authors' university setting, they are privileged to provide training and research experience for graduate clinicians in addition to collaborating on research and program development.

We implore you to connect with colleagues doing like work, as well as with students or mentees. As more providers become interested and learn to provide competent and compassionate care, there should be a natural expansion of the availability of services in a variety of places. With that will come opportunity for beautiful communities of clients and providers, connected by the powerful process of transformation.

REFERENCES

Bandura, A. (1994). Self-efficacy. In V. S. Ramachandran (Ed.), *Encyclopedia of human behavior* (pp. 71–81). New York, NY: Academic Press.

Van Leer, E., Hapner, E. R., & Connor, N. P. (2008). Transtheoretical model of health behavior change applied to voice therapy. *Journal of Voice, 22*(6), 688–698.

CHAPTER 10

Important Voices

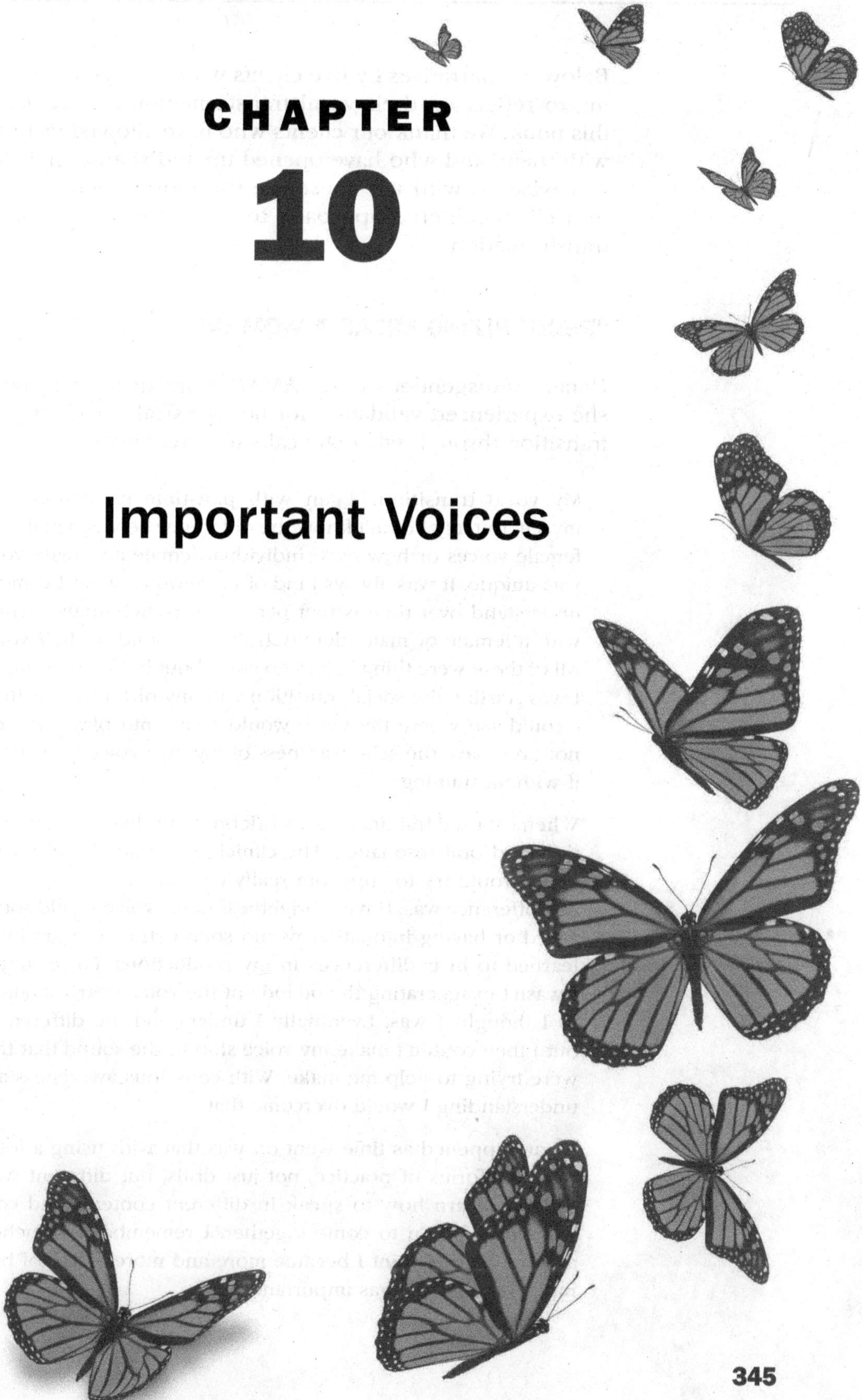

Below are narratives by five clients who were graciously willing to reflect on their vocal transformation for inclusion in this book. We thank our clients who have allowed us to work with them, and who have opened up and shared their needs and wisdom with us. These are the most important voices in a client-centered approach to voice and communication transformation.

"RECOGNIZING ME AS A WOMAN"

Dena, a transgender woman AMAB, helps us understand how she experienced validation for her physical, social and vocal transition through what she calls her "acid tests." She says:

> My vocal transition began with part-time presentation as myself. Initially I didn't know the difference between male and female voices or how each individual female and male voice was unique. It was always kind of mysterious. What I came to understand over time is that people overwhelmingly identify with a female or male identity from the sound of their voice. All of these were things I had no clue about before training. As I was starting the social transition with my physical transition, I could see where the voice would come into play but I did not even have the self-awareness of my own voice to work on it without training.
>
> When I started training, we'd work on things like pitch, intonation, and oral resonance. The clinicians would model for me and I would try to copy, but really couldn't understand what the difference was. Having brightness to my voice would sound weird or having intonation would sound strange. I gradually learned to hear differences in my productions. For example, I wasn't exaggerating the melody of the voice nearly as much as I thought I was. Eventually I understood the differences, but I then couldn't make my voice shift to the sound that they were trying to help me make. With conscious awareness and understanding I would overcome that.
>
> What happened as time went on was that with using a lot of different forms of practice, not just drills, but different ways to try to learn how to speak in different contexts and copy women, it began to come together. I remember somewhere around the midpoint I became more and more aware of how much psychology was important in this.

During that time, I started to have periods where I would hear myself speak and I would know that was me speaking. Then it started to happen in spontaneous conversation. What I found was that once I was able to start doing that, then I could see that the voice was one of the first things that people tune in to. I could just see that they were more readily recognizing me as a woman right away and the voice is part of that. If it was another woman standing next to me, we would start talking as women talk to each other and I knew it was happening. I had the experience of hearing myself for the first time and it was exciting and fulfilling. I was able to present easily and readily as myself. Over time it became more automatic and it's a wonderful thing, it truly is.

Once I reached that point where I started getting positive feedback, it helped me to keep maintaining my voice and finally got to the point where it would take me some effort to go back to the old way.

I had a couple of important experiences that were acid tests for me. They were experiences that were dominated by cisgender men.

One was with my auto mechanic. I went to these blue-collar guys to work on my car. I had used them for a number of years but I had not gone for a year or so. It's a situation where first I talked to the guys on the telephone and they recognized me as a woman on the phone. When I met them in person, they'd say, "Yes ma'am," or "Let me bring the car around for you," or manners and ways of speaking that indicate that they are recognizing me as a woman. And then there was one time when I wasn't sure if they remembered me as a male, and accepted me anyways or didn't. But I later found out for sure that at least one of them did remember me because of a telephone conversation we had and he was again saying, "Yes ma'am" and recognizing me as the woman on the phone. Then I realized as I talked further that he had known me from quite a while back. So this would have been before I started transitioning. I knew that he obviously had recognized me but treated me as who I was and clearly the voice is a big part of that. Obviously there were times on the phone where the voice was primarily what gave people the cue that I was a woman. That was a big deal.

The second experience took place in North Dakota, where I had to do work in a place where there were many new people around me for several hours a day. I kept wondering how this was going to go and whether they would recognize me as a woman. It became clear that they did when there were guys opening the door for me. One day, I stumbled getting into one of their pickup trucks with a really high step up. When we got to our destination, he got out first and walked around to help me get out. There again, I feel the voice was very important.

Both experiences happened around the time that I was completing my voice training program, and they helped me get comfortable with my voice. They gave me the sense that things are right in the world and that I'm in the place that I should have been in all along. I was finding my voice in the world and I wanted more and more of it. My new voice is empowering me to put my past behind me and it is giving me the reward and peace and rightness and that inner happiness that I now know is possible.

"I BECAME MORE EXPRESSIVE"

For some clients, realizing that they have to give up the idea of how they will sound for the evolution of their natural voice to occur takes time. Ali, a transgender woman AMAB, shares how it was only in giving up the ideal that she found her real voice.

Before my vocal training with you, my personal expression was sort of nonexistent. If I went into a room or a pub or a restaurant full of people, I might not say 15 words in a whole night. I was even afraid to talk with people I knew the best. I felt like the more I spoke, the greater my risk would be and the more unsafe I would feel. You never knew when somebody was listening. I don't want to sound paranoid but all transgender women know that's a possibility.

My experience at the start of vocal training was terrifying. I had put enormous pressure on myself to succeed. I mean I've been sort of planning my transition since I read about Christine Jorgensen when I was 8 years old. So that's a lot of fantasizing. I am certain that that ideal voice changed over the years, because someone else would come into prominence in the media.

I think the fear of speaking partially dissipated rather rapidly as I pursued vocal training. My psychotherapist, who has worked with me for 18 years prior to my transition, mentioned that he thought my personality and self-confidence was blooming after our first intensive vocal training weekend together. Until he had shared that with me, I wouldn't have thought of it that way, but he was correct. I was lighter.

An important aspect of training for me was to understand that nobody knows in advance how they're going to sound at the end of voice training. We discussed this the first day, but if I really had accepted that, then how could I be upset with the new voice that developed? But the truth is that it was challenging. I knew that without a congruent voice my life would never be as much as it could be. And of course, the congruent voice, which I had a mental image of, was Taylor Swift. Not much more could be dissimilar in our body types, vocal apparatus, and therefore the sound of our voices. Even as a physician, I initially thought I could reproduce the voice I wanted with more effort and more time. I didn't realize that no matter how hard I tried I could not get there.

After almost a year of training I was quite frustrated and probably didn't recognize the progress I had made. And then Linda [Siegfriedt] gave me The Talk. It was important for me to understand that I had to give up the delusion. I realized that our uniqueness requires us to accept the new voice that emerges instead of waiting for a voice that will never come. I left that session feeling heartbroken. Like there was no tomorrow. But of course there was a tomorrow and over the next week or two, I gradually accepted what we all inherently know to be true about ourselves. I can't sound like any other human in the world. Only me. I began to find a new stride and much more comfort in my speech and in casual conversation. That was for me a turning point. To know I don't have to sound like someone else . . . What a freedom!

I became more expressive. I lost my fear of trying to communicate with others that I did not know and that's a remarkable thing. Then, in having me speak to a group of student clinicians, you helped me scale another hurdle. It was the first time that I was able to be truly myself in front of a group. For that I will be forever grateful.

I feel like I have made real progress with my voice. I'm not where I thought I would be, but in reality, I had no idea where this road would go. Before vocal training I would sit in a room surrounded by talking, happy people, but never joining in the conversation. Now, I join. And that's the way vocal training changed my life going forward. A great deal of the fear I lived with is gone. It's a peaceful feeling as they say.

I have no regrets. There are things I either don't yet like or have not gotten used to, but I have had a different voice for 60-some years so it's going take some adjustment, and I'm much happier now!!

"HAVING A VOICE THAT 'FIT'"

Reana's journey included the daily anxiety that most clients AMAB like her face—with an additional challenge. Her work requires her to do public presentations in the media. She shares how she was able to present as herself on radio and podcasts after vocal training and hard work.

All I ever wanted to do was live as my true self. While that is a nearly universal sentiment, it's especially powerful for transgender people who grow up saddled with the pain from a fundamental disconnect between who they know themselves to be and how the rest of the world sees them. For me, that meant wanting to live and be seen as my true self, as a woman.

For many transgender people, the process of transitioning—of living life in the gender you identify with—involves making your external presentation to the world match your internal view of yourself. Just think about the ways you present to the rest of the world: your clothes, your hair, your face, the way you walk—these are all facets of yourself the rest of the world sees. And as you move through the world, other people make instant, subconscious assessments of who you are: young man, middle-aged woman, teenage girl, and so on.

For transgender people, simply moving through the world can be a highly self-conscious and anxious experience. Shortly after I transitioned, I battled a low-level, gnawing fear while at the grocery store, on the subway, walking down the street, working out at the gym, and during all the daily, mundane moments of my life: "Do they know I'm transgender? Do they think I'm a man? Am I at risk of embarrassment, humiliation, or even physical attack?"

Fortunately, it did not take long for that anxiety to dwindle and eventually disappear. After weeks and months of daily interactions with all kinds of people in all kinds of situations it was clear that my outward presentation to the world matched my inner self. I was seen, treated, and recognized as being a woman. There really are no words to adequately describe how freeing, empowering, liberating, and life-affirming that felt! And voice therapy was a vitally important part of the long, involved process to reach that point.

Unless you sing or speak for a living, most people don't really think about their voice very often. Sure, most of us suddenly become aware of our voice when we hear a recording of ourselves: "Oh my goodness! Is that what I really sound like?" But in your daily life, how often do you consider what you sound like, much less why you sound like a woman or whether you sound like a man?

And voice is a key way, in fact a very powerful way, you communicate to the world around you who you are. And the world can be a very difficult place indeed if people see a woman but hear a man. So for me, taking the time to work on my voice through voice training was extremely important. I spent a lot of time practicing, went to classes, and soon become quite focused on things I had never thought about: pitch, resonance, and intonation.

It is difficult to explain the embarrassment and pain from being misgendered—to be presenting to the world as a woman and be called a man. Of course, the flip side of that is the joy of validation: For example, being asked, "What would like to order today ma'am?" at a restaurant generated my own internal happy dance. That is easier to achieve when every aspect of your outward appearance is female.

But of course, on the phone, there is no other way to present than through your voice. Talking on the phone proved to be one of the earliest real-life tests of my voice training. An important part of gender transition involved changing my name, and then calling banks, utilities, insurance companies, magazines—all the thousand different places where your name is attached to an account—and telling them to change my name and my gender marker from male to female. My goal when starting those conversations was to hear, "Hello ma'am, how are you today?" when I began speaking to the customer service representative. Not only did that provide self-validation, it also smoothed the way when I had to explain to a complete stranger that I'm a transgender woman who needed to update her account information. The series of small successes I had with those phone calls, mostly made before I went to work as my true self, helped build my sense of confidence.

Having a voice that "fit" was especially important for me at work. My job involves a great deal of interaction with other people, sometimes in very formal settings. Most daunting of all, I sometimes speak publicly, including occasional media interviews. I was especially concerned about radio interviews and podcasts, where literally the only "face" to the listener is your voice. Without voice training, I never would have been able to present my real self in those circumstances. Not only would anxiety about my voice hamper the ability to do my job, it would distract the listener—instead of listening to what I was saying, they would instead listen to how I was saying it.

I remember the first time I had to give a major presentation as my true self in a public forum, in front of cameras and all the rest. That's of course a bit nerve-wracking to begin with: You need to be clear, concise, on point, respond well to questions, and portray a command of the material. At the same time, I needed to focus on the quality of my voice. For the first couple minutes the butterflies in my stomach nearly overwhelmed me, but I soon calmed down and did what I normally do when speaking publicly. I read the room and could tell: People were listening to the content of what I was saying, not the way I was saying it, which felt like a huge victory!

And that is one of the ironies of successful voice training. If you work with your provider, do your homework, and get over your initial frustration and discomfort ("This is never going to work!"), your ultimate reward is that most people won't notice how you're speaking. So in my case, during say, radio interviews or on the phone, people hear a woman talking to them, which is what they expect based on my name. Or if I'm meeting with some external clients for work, they see a woman and they hear a woman. The voice and external presentation match, which means they don't really notice my voice at all.

To put it another way, really the best way to tell whether my voice is working is the lack of response from people. And that has been my experience. My voice matches the way I look and the way I feel. I move through the world talking to people in person and on the phone; never once have I had someone say, "Your voice sounds very female." I could not ask for more than that.

It's now been three years since I began living my life as myself, as a woman. Over that period of time the voice that I worked so hard to achieve has become my voice, my way of speaking. Sometimes when I'm tired or distracted I have to make a conscious effort to think about how I am speaking. But most of the time I just speak.

It is literally impossible to describe the wonderful rush of liberation that comes from being able to finally live as yourself. Voice training was a big part of that. It is not easy. It does not happen overnight. You need to work and practice. You will become frustrated and will need to keep practicing and working through your frustration. But progress, dramatic progress, is possible and can be achieved. Like so many other valuable things in life, the rewards do not come easily, which makes them sweeter when you do attain them. The ability to speak, to literally have a voice that speaks as my true self to the outside world, is the most wonderful reward from voice training.

"FINDING MY OWN VOICE"

Morgan, who was AFAB but positions as transmasculine of center, genderqueer, or nonbinary, shared their vocal journey with testosterone while exploring the evolution of their voice in life, work, and as they participate in a choir as a newly developed upper baritone.

Prior to hormone replacement in my late forties, 4 years prior to this writing, my voice was merely a functional tool in my life. I had brief choral experience as a soprano in my twenties but no vocal training or appreciable skill. In hindsight, I felt rather disconnected from and dysphoric with the quality of my voice. This most manifested during singing.

Voice was one of the few physical changes I did not imagine much about prior to transition. Rationally, I knew my voice would deepen. Naively, some parts of me assumed I would be able to keep my upper range to some degree if I practiced or used it. This felt important due to my work with children of all ages. Voice change began rather soon after starting testosterone (T), within a few months.

Initially, my speaking voice began to sound "froggy" or hoarse. At work (the last place I came out about being trans), I was blatantly asked what was wrong with my voice. Not ready to risk my employment, I responded with feigned ignorance and blamed allergies, perhaps. Privately singing along to songs, I discovered missing pockets midrange, then rapidly lost all of my upper range. I needed to clear my throat multiple times daily (for years that increased with voice use); vocal fatigue was a problem I dealt with multiple times a week.

Despite the drawbacks of losing most of the range I usually sang in, the ability to yell, effectively project my voice, or make my realistic cat meows anymore, I discovered something precious! I could physically feel my voice in my body! It seemed to resonate all the way to my belly. I love how rich, strong, and full it feels both inside my body and out loud when I sing.

Despite hearing of options for vocal training in trans support groups I self-selected out. My insurance would not cover costs and the resource seemed more useful for transfeminine people in a clear survival sense. I had also discovered at a conference for transgender health that there are smartphone apps one can purchase that provide a bit of vocal therapy direction. They have evolved with pitch meters and exercises to help one achieve desired gender presentation. This helped me get started.

My origin story includes childhood trauma background. Trauma therapy in part involved learning to pay attention and be aware of what I feel in my body. I am grateful and lucky to have survived long enough to find the psychological and physical security I needed to embrace my identity and transition. Transition is an embodiment of my self-acceptance and self-love.

In more ways than one, transition is still working its magic slowly empowering me. A couple years after starting T, I was reminded how inspiring live music is and how choral productions have a way of creating a powerful gestalt. I still am not a singing talent, but I can contribute! Boldly (translate that as: anxiously and not impressively), I auditioned for and joined a large Gay and Lesbian Association (GALA) chorus. The safety and acceptance I receive here are crucial to my continuing and overall success.

The journey has been challenging. In this TTBB chorus (a four-part chorus: Tenor 1, Tenor 2, Bass 1 [Baritone], and Bass 2), I am an upper baritone (though I likely should have started as a lower baritone). The beginning was hardest. Finding the right octave to sing, especially standing near tenors or upper registers, was not easy. Holding low notes—while they feel and sound fabulous, I ran out of air immediately! Binding was impossible. Breath control seemed hopeless. Nobody seemed to know anything helpful about issues unique to transmasculine voices, especially late starters.

I found it difficult (and still do at times) to know what to strive for without a voice of reference. In *passaggio*, a given note sounds and feels different approaching from above or below. While, at first, my voice was mostly like a new toy, now it is more like this challenging enticing complicated instrument I am slowly learning how to play. I had accepted my range would be less than two octaves. I thought I was becoming a bass—and was truly ok with it.

Out of the blue relatively recently (after over 3 years on T) my range started opening up again. It is not all useful for singing, consistently reliable or available, but I have more range than ever with improving control. My upper registers sound better and stronger than they used to. Currently, I am also challenged by air somehow slipping into my stomach when I am singing in my upper range (worse if nervous) and randomly delayed onset of sound as I strive to start in higher notes.

Each step of the way I am feeling and associating within my body how to generate desired sound. Transitioning has opened my eyes anew to white male privilege, sexism, and even racism all around me. As my life improves, I have a responsibility to help others, especially my trans siblings and the many in life who face unfair inequalities. My life, both metaphorically and literally, has become about finding my own voice and learning to better use it.

The ways I could have benefited over the past 4 years from working with a speech-language pathologist varied based on where my voice and transitioning process were at any given time. Only your clients can tell you what they need most or struggle with or carry fear/anxiety about. The setting needs to feel safe and welcoming enough for them to share. Sometimes it just helps to know what is possible or likely. My sincerest thanks for the available info and supportive providers I found along the way.

RESONANCE

Grace is a transgender woman AMAB. She shares how her experience started as a physical vocal journey as she learned to manipulate the sound of her voice, but ultimately became an emotional journey that lead her into a deeper part of herself.

I first began to see Linda [Siegfriedt] early in my transition process, more than a year before I transitioned to live as Grace full time. I knew from the beginning that feminizing my voice would be important so that I could express myself in words the way I also wanted to in my appearance and my feelings.

At first, I was motivated at least in part by the fact that I was extraordinarily tall for a woman and I would already be standing out far more than I would wish to. I thought that having an unconvincing feminine voice would increase the risk of being misgendered, which in turn could increase the risk of many other things that trans women often rightly fear.

I was certainly naïve about what voice feminization would entail. Like many, I suppose, I imagined that changing my voice was fundamentally a matter of pitch.

Unlike any other aspect of training my voice, pitch had the undeniable virtue of objectivity. Ascertaining the quality of my voice was an art, but measuring the frequency was an app. There was a gold standard of idealized femininity I could aspire to: 220 Hz, the A below middle C on a piano. I started with a voice perhaps half that, an entire octave down. Get to work, Grace.

I had always believed that exertion equaled excellence in life, but now everything was upside down. The more I clenched my vocal cords together to raise my pitch, the less feminine I sounded. More was not better. This was the first of many paradoxes I would encounter. The more I relaxed my muscles, by contrast, the higher my voice could naturally go. Pitch was not an objective; it was an outcome of doing everything else well.

I learned that there are a great many other signs we use subconsciously to distinguish the qualities of voices we perceive as male or female. In many cases, the fundamental pitch was not even the most important cue. Often the variety of pitches we use in the context of a phrase or a sentence for emphasis is even more important, a characteristic known as intonation. This is one quality I have come to appreciate a great deal—finally hearing a voice that expresses melody and not monotony.

It has also been an opportunity to reflect not only on what I sounded like in my prior life as a male, but also what that meant. As men often do, if I wanted to emphasize a point, I would rely more on varying loudness than pitch. Of course, this is the privilege men sometimes assume subconsciously; to be the voice that speaks the loudest and often the longest is a way to assert one's self in the hierarchy of men above of other men, and very often above women.

I think to live in privilege is a little like being a fish unaware that it lives in water. It's an invisible substance that surrounds and sustains it, and as the fish moves privilege causes ripples that push other things barely noticed out of the way. My cisgender female friends nod knowingly when I describe the new sensation of being a female in a meeting, of being talked over and down to. Welcome to the sisterhood.

It has taken me time to learn that sometimes softness is louder than loudness. It has taken me even longer to learn that saying my words carefully does not have to be a sign of tentativeness. It can be recognized as a measure of thoughtfulness and of genuine interest in another, something few of us ever experience enough of in this life. I would never have imagined these to be among the presents that my efforts to change my voice would bestow.

As Linda has pointed out to me in kindness on a great many occasions, each of us will find that we have skills in our transition that come easier to us, and some that are far more difficult. The best analogy I can think of to learning to speak as a woman is learning to swim. First I learned to float, but that was not enough. Then I learned to kick my legs in ways unfamiliar to them, and then, even harder, to keep kicking when I wasn't thinking about kicking. Progress. Now to master the skill of simultaneously moving my arms as though digging horizontally in sand.

Better, but not there. Then, I had to learn how to breathe sideways in the brief moment when my mouth was above water. Now combine all of these learned abilities so that they are seamlessly and effortlessly coordinated, even graceful. Welcome to voice feminization therapy.

For me, the most formidable challenge by far has been resonance.

Why do a piano, a trumpet and a violin all sound so recognizably different when they are all playing middle C? Why do the voices of men and women share this quality in a way in which we subconsciously gender voices the same way we identify musical instruments? Resonance.

One characteristic of a resonant voice can be expressed at least partly as the harmonics or overtones it produces. Bells, for example, are highly resonant. Bob Dylan, maybe less so. Resonance sounds simple as a theory to recognize, but I have found achieving it far harder to do. I was beginning from a difficult place. One reason a bassoon and flute sound different is the size of the chamber used to produce the sound. I learned that the size and shape of the vocal cavity within the mouth greatly contributed to the resonant quality of a voice. The smaller the cavity, the more feminine a voice was likely to sound. My vocal cavity was sufficiently large for explorers to go spelunking in.

Resonance, feminine or not, is the product of vibration, and especially how and where it is produced. The further upward and forward the origination of vibration, the more feminine the overtones of my voice would be. At first the resonance in my voice originated in my chest and throat, which made me sound less like an opera singer and a lot more like an aging R&B singer. My voice only started to sound truly feminine when the resonance was focused at the front of my mouth. In some ways, it's an act of trickery, of positioning the tongue and teeth and lips to make the vocal cavity seem much smaller to the breath passing through it.

Learning to achieve effective resonance is in certain respects an exquisitely sensitive exercise in biofeedback. What felt like minute differences in how relaxed my throat was, where my tongue was positioned, and the shape of my lips made an enormous difference in the resonance of my voice. Did the back of my teeth vibrate when pronouncing a vowel? Did my upper palate quiver when articulating a D? Were my lips humming when I pronounced words that began with M and N? The exercises to teach me this discriminatory skill seemed endless.

Nine. Nearly nine. Nearly nine million. Nearly nine million men. Nearly nine million men now. I'm certain I could be unattractively tattooed with these phrases by now, but they served an important purpose. Repetition and analysis are one way we progress from conscious effort to unconscious mastery. I first imagined that I would progress the most from using my voice in public, but the opposite was true; I was far too entangled in what I was saying to attend to how I was saying it. Only when resonance became second nature from sitting in front of Linda would it carry over to interactions everywhere else.

I often found that practicing voice feminization was much harder for me than other skills I had already mastered, to my bewilderment and often frustration. I wanted the process of changing my voice to be a straight, smooth upward line toward whatever ideal I was capable of achieving. [The line] looked a lot more like spaghetti. There were times when I would record myself repeatedly reciting the same passage and despairing that I could never sound as I might wish to. At those moments Linda's encouragement made every difference. Even if I did not have faith my voice would ever become more feminine, Linda had faith, and I could have faith in her.

Yet my voice did get better. To my surprise, I found that achieving a feminine pitch came more easily to me than it did to some, although consistency can be harder. I relished practicing intonation, because I could finally learn to sing in prose. Some weeks I would take pride in the smallest accomplishment—I was articulating my Ts and Ds a little better, for example.

Resonance, however, proved obstinate. My throat and tongue and teeth and lips would all be properly positioned like actors in a dress rehearsal. The voice that emerged, however, was calling from a limbo between male and female. The male undertones had largely vanished. At the same time, I would listen to it and feel that a believably feminine voice was a planet or more away from me.

I had always imagined myself to be a diligent student, and perhaps outwardly I was. Linda could see, however, there was a place far deeper inside of me that resisted cultivation and kindness. My breath.

Perhaps this should have been evident to me sooner. I would wince to hear a recording of my voice when I lived as a male. It sounded strangled and nasal to me, more the voice of a cartoon character than a person. It was scarcely surprising in hindsight, for it was the weakly vibrating air that emerged from a constricted self I was hardly even conscious of.

To express my whole self meant that I would need to speak from my whole body. The wellspring of my authentic voice existed far inside of me, below my tightened chest and inside of my frightened skin.

In a strict sense this could be called breathing from my abdomen, learning to properly employ my diaphragm as the engine of my inhalations and exhalations. But this is too clinical of a description to explain my experience. By now I was used to being mindful of my mouth. My throat. Now I was being asked to be mindful of my breath. Inhale fully and then count to three and then slowly exhale and let the belly relax naturally and—I don't know where the tears came from. They were welling up unbidden from inside some buried chamber of my spirit, first as a trickle and then erupting like lava. Hormones and gender therapy had given me permission to cry, but this felt different. A moment ago, I was studious and analytical, and now my battered heart heaved inside its frame. Linda would look at me with gentle eyes and softly ask me if I could name where these feelings were coming from. I could not.

The sadness felt overwhelming and endless, like a tide that just kept coming in. Linda would sometimes lead me outside to the sunlit garden she lovingly tended, where my bare feet could sink into the grass and belong again to the earth.

The simplest touch could trigger sorrow. An innocuous phrase in practicing my vowels: no one really knows my name. A kind silence that reminded me anew that I had at last found refuge. The key was never really what was most important. It was the hidden box it unlocked.

People often say their goal in life is to be happy, but I don't think that is the choice life gives to us. We have a choice to feel—happy, sad, infatuated, scared, and every other emotion sought and unsought—or not to feel. I don't even remember the day when I made my choice as a boy who really wasn't, but I made it.

After a while, denying one's feelings is no longer an act of will, it is as natural as being right handed. The conceit I maintained that a feeling denied was a feeling deflected, however, was profoundly untrue. All the fear, all of the loneliness, and yes, all of the joy didn't evaporate, it simply found a home in me I had chosen not to reside in, the very place from which my true voice emanated. The body never forgets.

Now my body was a chrysalis, a shell in which the woman I was always meant to be was being birthed. My genuine voice began to emerge into the air as I learned how to breathe, becoming a butterfly in Linda's garden. The fear that had been the original impetus for voice feminization therapy had been transmuted into desire.

Linda had given me a book she had written called *Buds, Petals and Blooms*. It was filled with close-up pictures of flowers in her garden, pinks and purples pinker and purpler than could be imagined. The book was hardly over a hundred words, written in a language that children understand, and adults feel. "Every bud dreams of itself in bloom," it began. I tried many times to use it as a practice aid for my voice, but I could never make it to the end without collapsing into sobs. I still can't.

When I began this journey, I had been entirely incorrect about what I might sound like when my spirit at last began to bloom. It was never about changing my voice. It was about finding it.

INDEX

Note: Page numbers in **bold** reference non-text material.

B

C

M

N

O

P